The Alzheimer's SOLUTION

The
Alzheimer's
SOLUTION

A Breakthrough Program to Prevent
and Reverse the Symptoms
of Cognitive Decline at Every Age

Dean Sherzai, M.D., and
Ayesha Sherzai, M.D.

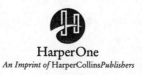

HarperOne
An Imprint of HarperCollins*Publishers*

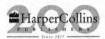

Permission to use art on page 150 granted by The Royal Melbourne Hospital Radiology.

HarperCollins books may be purchased for educational, business, or sales promotional use. For information, please e-mail the Special Markets Department at SPsales@harpercollins.com.

FIRST EDITION

Designed by SBI Book Arts, LLC

Library of Congress Cataloging-in-Publication Data is available upon request.

ISBN 978–0–06–266647–5

17 18 19 20 21   LSC   10 9 8 7 6 5 4 3 2 1

We dedicate this book to two of the
greatest men we've ever known:

our grandfathers,
Dr. Zahir and F. M. Zikria,

who planted the seeds of knowledge and
discovery, and ultimately lost their lives to the
very disease we set out to cure.

All profits from sales of *The Alzheimer's Solution*
will go toward the Healthy Minds Initiative, a nonprofit
working to empower communities, families, and
individuals to achieve optimal brain health.

Contents

The
Alzheimer's
SOLUTION

Introduction
The Alzheimer's Epidemic

If you would have told us fifteen years ago that we'd be writing the first book about the only scientifically proven solution to the international epidemic of Alzheimer's disease, we never would have believed you. Fifteen years ago we were young neurologists practicing medicine the way we'd been taught. We were hopeful that the billions of dollars donated to fund Alzheimer's research would soon result in a cure, some kind of pill that could affect the pathology we'd learned so much about. We pursued the most prestigious fellowships in our field—at the National Institutes of Health and University of California–San Diego—and worked with leading researchers at the forefront of the fight against Alzheimer's. We wanted to find a solution. And we did, eventually—just not the solution we expected.

It was during those fifteen years that we uncovered promising scientific research about the factors that significantly influence Alzheimer's disease, research we will reveal to you in Chapter 2 of this book and that revolutionized the way we practice medicine. It was during those fifteen years that we conducted one of the most comprehensive studies on the incidence of dementia and designed a groundbreaking protocol for Alzheimer's treatment and prevention, work that began at Loma Linda University and then took us to Cedars-Sinai in Los Angeles before we returned to Loma Linda to continue our research and serve communities throughout Southern California and beyond. And it was during those fifteen years that we treated thousands of patients suffering from mild cognitive impairment to Alzheimer's disease with our innovative NEURO Plan, helping them reverse symptoms, prevent further decline, add years to their lives, and change the trajectory of their health.

So many of these patients have shared their stories with us. They've told us that their parents or grandparents had Alzheimer's, and that developing the disease themselves was their single greatest fear. They've told us about the humiliation of having to rely on caregivers to meet their basic needs. They've assumed there was no treatment, that they would be ostracized if others found out about their condition. Some of these patients are in denial. Some of them are having trouble remembering names or have gotten lost in a familiar place. Some of them already have a formal Alzheimer's diagnosis when they arrive at our clinic, unable to express themselves or recognize their loved ones. If you've picked up this book, then there's a good chance you or someone you love has one of these stories. You may be feeling little hope for the future. We know you are looking for something, anything you can do. We know you are incredibly afraid.

There is reason to be afraid. While every chronic disease you can think of—cardiovascular disease, diabetes, cancer, stroke, HIV—is in decline, deaths due to Alzheimer's have increased by nearly 87 percent in the last decade. The next decade could be even worse: 10 percent of people over the age of sixty-five will develop some form of dementia, and people over the age of eighty-five have a 50 percent chance of developing the disease. Many of us can reasonably expect to live beyond eighty-five, especially as treatments for cancer and other major diseases continue to improve. This means that almost everyone, and certainly every family, will be affected by Alzheimer's.

In 2016, Alzheimer's disease was the sixth-leading cause of death in the United States. Some researchers believe that Alzheimer's is grossly underreported on death certificates. Oftentimes the official cause of death for a person with Alzheimer's is a dementia-related condition like aspiration pneumonia. This means that Alzheimer's may in fact be America's third-most deadly disease, behind only heart disease and cancer. The question is no longer *if* we will develop the disease, but *when*.

As if the emotional costs weren't high enough, there are also staggering financial costs. Alzheimer's is by far the most expensive disease to manage, with costs reaching $226 billion in the United States this year, and $604 billion worldwide. This annual cost will likely increase to several trillion dollars over the next few decades, overwhelming our already strained health-care system. In 2015, the World Health Organization estimated that the total number of people with Alzheimer's worldwide will rise to 135.5 million by 2050. By then, global costs will surpass twenty trillion dollars. This figure doesn't take into account the vast amount of unpaid caregiver hours. In 2015 alone, caregivers provided an estimated eighteen billion hours of unpaid care. The demands of this disease could crash not only our health-care system, but our entire financial system.

Fifteen years ago, we had no idea our field of study and research would play a crucial role in our health as a nation, and as a species. Back then we accepted the conventional approach to neurology, though we could see it came up painfully short for patients with cognitive decline. That approach went a lot like this: Patients were examined, put through comprehensive neuropsychological testing, and sometimes underwent brain MRIs. A diagnosis would be made based on the stage of cognitive decline, and in a follow-up appointment with family members, patients would be told that their disease was chronic and had no treatment. They were given pamphlets for nursing homes and encouraged to make major life decisions now, while their faculties were still intact. Many of these patients were then passed off to primary-care physicians, as it was believed there was little a neurologist could do beyond diagnosis and symptomatic treatment. Because of this conventional approach, patients assumed their symptoms were completely driven by unfortunate genes. They believed decline was inevitable, that nothing could be done. The whole process was devastating for our patients and it was devastating for us.

If this sounds familiar to you, we want you to know there is hope. There is a way to prevent cognitive decline, to slow its progression and improve quality of life for those who already have a diagnosis. What conventional medicine hasn't told you or your loved ones, or any of the nearly six million people living with Alzheimer's in the United States, or the forty-seven million people living with Alzheimer's worldwide, is that within the normal life span, 90 percent of Alzheimer's cases can be prevented. This figure bears repeating: 90 percent of grandparents, parents, husbands, and wives should have been spared. Ninety percent of people living with Alzheimer's or dementia didn't have the resources or knowledge they needed to prevent this devastating disease. Ninety percent of us can avoid ever getting Alzheimer's, and for the rest of us, the 10 percent with strong genetic risk for cognitive decline, the disease can potentially be delayed by ten to fifteen years.

This isn't just an estimate or wishful thinking: it's a figure based on rigorous science and the remarkable results we've seen in our clinic, which we will share with you in this book. As it turns out, the solution to Alzheimer's has been hiding in plain sight. We now know that Alzheimer's disease and overall cognitive health are deeply influenced by five main lifestyle factors represented by the acronym NEURO—Nutrition, Exercise, Unwind, Restore, and Optimize. Direct links exist between poor nutrition, lack of exercise, chronic stress, poor sleep, the extent to which we challenge and engage our brains and neurodegenerative disease. The truth is that the choices we make every day determine our cognitive fate—but there is almost no awareness of this crucial fact, despite the veritable crisis we're in when it comes to Alzheimer's.

Why aren't we more aware? Why aren't there public service announcements about the cognitive effects of a high-sugar diet and sedentary behavior? Why doesn't every physician tell their patients that they can control the process of cognitive decline and even increase the power and resiliency of their brains? How could so many of our patients have gone to doctor after doctor and still not encountered anyone in the health-care system who knew how to intervene and change the very behaviors that were accelerating the disease?

If you want answers to these questions, you've come to the right place:

- If you have a loved one with Alzheimer's disease and want to help slow the progression of symptoms, you're holding in your hands the only proven solution to do so.

- If you're experiencing mild cognitive impairment, our NEURO Plan will help you reverse symptoms and avoid a formal diagnosis.

- If you're concerned about the health of your brain because of chronic conditions like high blood pressure and high cholesterol, or even diabetes and heart disease, our comprehensive protocol will address the risk factors for every chronic disease, including Alzheimer's and all other types of dementia.

- Maybe you're the primary caretaker or spouse of someone struggling with Alzheimer's. Spouses of Alzheimer's patients are 600 percent more likely to develop the disease themselves. This book will help you change your lifestyle and dramatically reduce your risk of developing cognitive decline.

- If you have no signs of decline but want to significantly improve your cognitive function and keep your brain healthy as you age, this program will help you, too.

After fifteen years of research and practice, we are certain that lifestyle has a profound effect on the health of the brain, and we know that lifestyle medicine, a field of medicine devoted to addressing the factors that contribute to chronic disease, is the only way to both avoid and treat Alzheimer's. The brain is a living universe. It responds to how you care for it, what you feed it, how you challenge it, the ways in which you allow it to rest and restore. Modern life significantly increases the risk of cognitive decline. Processed foods high in sugar and saturated fats are toxic for the brain. Most of us spend all day sitting at a desk or in traffic, but we need regular movement in order to stay healthy. We experience tremendous stress without the proper tools to manage that stress. Almost none of us are consistently getting a good night's sleep, and our jobs often require repetitive activity, the exact opposite of what the brain needs to stay resilient as we age. But despite these very real challenges, it's well within our power to preserve and even improve the function of our brains.

The problem for so long was that no one believed it was possible. Nearly everyone in the medical establishment is convinced that lifestyle intervention is futile. Our own medical training taught us that lifestyle change is impossible, and the way we conduct Alzheimer's research is based on the assumption that people can't change. We had to make a decision fifteen years ago: keep believing what we'd been taught, succumb to a system that refused to consider the role of lifestyle in cognitive health—or find another way.

Together we vowed to help people however we could. Dean earned a Ph.D. in health-care leadership to learn about the intricacies of behavioral change and how to empower individuals and whole communities. Ayesha completed a combined vascular neurology and epidemiology fellowship at Columbia University, where she focused on public health and the complex vascular aspects of neurological disease. While she was at it, she also went to cooking school—she knew her patients would only change their diets if she could make healthy food delicious. We brought all our skills to bear at Loma Linda University, where we conducted retrospective lifestyle studies that showed healthy behaviors were associated with longevity and dramatically lower rates of dementia. We observed these same profound effects in our clinic. There we had the unique opportunity to care for two radically different populations: our patients from Loma Linda, California, which has a large population of Seventh-day Adventists who embrace plant-based eating, regular exercise, and community service, were some of the healthiest people in the world; those in nearby San Bernardino, California, an underserved area plagued by chronic disease and lack of access to basic health care, were some of the sickest. We consistently found that people living a healthy lifestyle had a much lower prevalence of dementia. By contrast, those who lived unhealthy lifestyles got dementia more often, and it usually emerged earlier in life. Seeing the striking effects of diet, exercise, stress management, sleep quality, and cognitive activity on a daily basis changed our whole perspective on Alzheimer's. The truth was undeniable: a brain-healthy lifestyle all but guarantees you will avoid Alzheimer's disease.

Now, as the codirectors of the Brain Health and Alzheimer's Prevention Program at Loma Linda University, we've guided thousands of people through the highly personalized process of lifestyle change. Every day we sit down with patients and look for the seed of potential change, one small aspect of healthy living that we can start with and build upon. We've helped people with a wide range of mental and physical limitations. We've become veritable masters at midlife behavioral change in patients who are less than enthusiastic about changing anything. Step by step we proved the establishment wrong: people can change their lives. And if you picked up this book today because you're worried you are at risk for cognitive decline, or you want to do something about the symptoms you're now experiencing, the NEURO Plan is the solution you've been waiting for.

Our plan is so much more than a simple three-, five-, or seven-day plan. It's far more comprehensive than a rushed doctor telling you to "find ways to mitigate stress," "get more sleep," or "watch your diet." Our NEURO Plan not only defines what a brain-healthy diet actually is, but also teaches you how to design your own. How do you systematically reduce your refined sugar intake, especially if you love sweets? How do you decrease your consumption of meat not just by cutting it out but by replacing it with healthy—and delicious—alternatives? The answers are in this book. How do you avoid sedentary behavior if you have a desk job and are forced to sit all day? How did we teach a middle-aged, overweight man with diabetes and balance issues to start biking, a practice that eventually transformed his life? The answers are in this book. Why is sleep so important to brain health, and what practical steps can you take to ensure you're getting the restorative sleep you need? Which commonly prescribed medications could dramatically increase your risk of dementia? The answers are in this book. Everything we offer here is grounded in science, and each chapter ("Nutrition," "Exercise," "Unwind," "Restore," and "Optimize") is accompanied by a personalized program that allows you to assess your unique strengths and resources. We've even changed our own lives with the NEURO Plan. Our whole family, including our children, lives a brain-healthy lifestyle, and we've included our personal stories along with numerous patient stories as examples of how to apply what you learn. These same methods are the foundation of our work at Loma Linda, where we're now conducting the most comprehensive research to date that explores lifestyle risk factors and the development of neurodegenerative disease. What we've discovered will change the way you think about Alzheimer's forever.

There is no cure for Alzheimer's disease once it has manifested, but you can be cognitively active, reverse debilitating symptoms, and add happy, healthy years to your life—even with an Alzheimer's diagnosis. Lifestyle matters. It's the best defense we have, and it's easier than you think. We felt it was our duty as doctors to share what we've learned. Our hope is that you use this book to transform your life and help turn the tide of Alzheimer's.

The Truth About Alzheimer's

In November of 1901, a young German physician named Alois Alzheimer was working at the Frankfurt Psychiatric Hospital when he was assigned a new patient. Her name was Auguste Deter, and her husband reported that she was suffering from paranoid behavior, emotional outbursts, and increasing confusion. Some nights she would scream for hours, he said. Other times she was unresponsive. When asked to write her name, Deter struggled with the letters, repeatedly saying, "I have lost myself." She seemed to have no understanding of time or place and little to no short-term memory. Though memory problems in old age had been documented for centuries—by the ancient Egyptians, Romans, and Greeks—Alzheimer had never seen or read about a patient with memory deterioration at such an early age: Deter was only fifty years old. He took a special interest in her case, checking on her even after he was transferred to another hospital in Munich. Unfortunately, Deter declined rapidly and died in 1906. When Alzheimer examined her brain, he found both amyloid plaques (abnormal protein fragments that aggregate outside brain cells) and tau tangles (twisted protein fibers that cut off the supply of nutrients within brain cells). These same plaques and tangles are considered the hallmark pathology of what we now call Alzheimer's disease.

Since this first case of Alzheimer's was discovered over a century ago, doctors, scientists, and researchers have hypothesized about the cause, the physical manifestations, and the solution to this terrible disease. Is it caused by a single gene? Can it be cured by a single drug? Does it progress suddenly or develop over a period of time? Is it modifiable or susceptible to changes in the environment? Are we stuck with the symptoms once the disease has taken hold?

In asking these questions, and never being able to answer them with the research available to us, scientists and doctors have perpetuated some troubling myths about Alzheimer's disease that create a great deal of confusion and anxiety. That's why we need to begin by dispelling these myths and revealing what the research tells us. As you'll soon learn, the prognosis is not as dire or inevitable as we may have thought. Alzheimer's has many causes that are intertwined in a complex disease picture. Rather than a simple game of tic-tac-toe, Alzheimer's is more like three-dimensional chess: what matters is the combination of your age, your overlaying genetic risk profile, and how your lifestyle choices either protect or damage your brain. You can't control your age. You can't control your genetic risk profile. But you can control your lifestyle. You can control the health and resiliency of your brain, and by doing so, significantly delay or completely avoid the anguish of Alzheimer's. If all of us—doctors, patients, and leading researchers—understand that our lifestyle choices have a profound impact on cognitive function, we can abandon a wasteful approach doomed for failure, and we can stop the needless suffering.

1.

Myths and Misunderstandings

When it comes to Alzheimer's, the most damaging myth of all is that lifestyle has nothing to do with the disease. Most of our patients are convinced that genes determine everything, that their daily choices have little to no impact on what happens to their brains. By the time they come to our clinic, they're already experiencing brain fog, short-term memory problems, and other symptoms of cognitive impairment. They think that the process of decline started when their symptoms first emerged. The disease and the symptoms, they assume, must share the same time line. But the truth is that Alzheimer's develops decades before a diagnosis. It's during those decades that the brain becomes increasingly vulnerable to what we eat, how much we exercise, our ability to manage chronic stress, the quality of our sleep, and the ways in which we challenge our cognitive abilities. Only later on, often when we reach our sixties or seventies, is the brain unable to compensate for our less than healthy choices, and that's when we first begin to notice changes in thinking and memory. The purpose of this book—and our life's work—is to make this connection clear, and to show you why lifestyle medicine, and specifically our NEURO Plan, is so effective at treating and preventing neurodegenerative disease.

COMMON TERMS ASSOCIATED WITH ALZHEIMER'S

Acetylcholine: A chemical messenger integral to learning and memory.

Activated Microglia: Small cells that help with the clearing of waste and damaged neurons.

APOE4: A gene responsible for production of the protein apolipoprotein E, one function of which is to help regulate cholesterol in the brain. There are three types of apolipoprotein genes (APOE2, APOE3, and APOE4). APOE4 appears to increase the risk of developing Alzheimer's, and APOE2 is protective against Alzheimer's.

APP: Amyloid precursor protein, which is found in many cell membranes, is a protein responsible for making amyloid, the abnormal protein associated with Alzheimer's disease.

Atherosclerosis: Hardening and narrowing of the arteries due to the buildup of cholesterol plaques, which compromises blood flow throughout the body.

Atrophy: The shrinking of an organ that results from cell degeneration.

Beta-Amyloid: Abnormal protein fragments that aggregate between brain cells and disrupt neuronal function.

Brain-Derived Neurotrophic Factor (BDNF): A protein responsible for the growth and proper function of neurons.

Cytokines and Chemokines: Signaling molecules that support the immune system by attacking foreign substances.

Dopamine: A chemical messenger involved in many behaviors like reward-motivation and motor control. The decreased production of dopamine is a prominent feature of Parkinson's disease.

Free Radicals: Molecules that are missing an electron and thus unstable and highly reactive. In the brain, free radicals can damage neurons and DNA.

Glia: The most common type of cells in the brain whose function is protecting and supporting neurons.

Glutamate: The most abundant neurotransmitter in the brain.

Inflammation: A naturally protective function of the immune system for fighting harmful bacteria and viruses. Acute inflammation helps us recover from injury. Chronic inflammation puts us at risk for diabetes, heart disease, and cognitive decline.

Microvasculature: The smallest blood vessels in the body.

Myelination: The process through which a neuron's connections are coated with myelin, a fatty membrane that facilitates communication between cells.

Neurons: Cells that make up the nervous system, which includes the nerves, spinal cord, and brain.

Neurotransmitter: A chemical messenger in the brain that facilitates communication between neurons.

Oxidation: A chemical process that involves the transfer of electrons, thereby creating free radicals.

Tau Tangles: Twisted protein fibers inside neurons that cause neuronal damage and contribute to Alzheimer's disease.

Vascular Health: The state of health of the vascular system, which includes arteries, veins, and smaller vessels. Lack of optimal blood flow to the brain due to atherosclerosis (hardening of the arteries) can starve the brain of oxygen and glucose, thereby accelerating the development of Alzheimer's disease.

REGIONS OF THE BRAIN

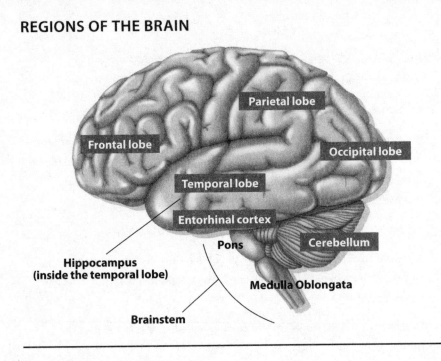

The Four Main Pathways to Alzheimer's

Four interconnected biological processes are responsible for most of the degeneration that contributes to Alzheimer's and other dementias. You'll see these terms throughout the book, so it's important to understand what they mean. The first is inflammation. Inflammation is a naturally protective function of the immune system for fighting harmful bacteria and viruses. Acute inflammation—the redness and swelling of a cut on your finger, for instance—increases blood flow to the injured area and facilitates healing. This type of inflammation is essential—without it we wouldn't heal. Chronic inflammation, on the other hand, occurs when the inflammatory response is activated long term, often because of constant irritants like high-sugar diets, unmitigated stress, and many other unhealthy lifestyle choices. When inflammation is chronic, it turns from protective to destructive. Tissues are damaged instead of healed. The body actually attacks itself when inflammation goes unchecked. If you were to look at the brains of people with Alzheimer's, even early on in the disease process, you'd see evidence of chronic inflammation in the form of cytokines and chemokines (proteins that support the immune system by attacking foreign substances) and activated microglia (small cells that help with the clearing of waste and damaged brain cells). Activated microglia become so hyper-responsive in clearing waste that they harm neurons (the cells of the nervous system) and their supporting structures, resulting in both cell death and structural damage. This is why chronic inflammation is widely considered a main factor in the development of Alzheimer's.

The second process is oxidation. Oxidation occurs naturally when oxygen reacts with other substances, and by doing so changes them. A banana turns brown when you leave it on the counter—this is oxidation, and this same chemical reaction happens in our bodies. Oxidation results in the formation of oxidative by-products called free radicals. Free radicals are molecules that are missing an electron and thus unstable and highly reactive. Their high reactivity compels them to steal electrons from other molecules. In the brain, free radicals steal electrons from neurons, glia (cells that support neurons), and organelles (small cellular structures located within cells), as well as proteins, lipids, fatty acids, and even DNA—all of which results in permanent damage. Because the brain works harder than any other organ in the body, consuming 25 percent of the body's oxygen, it's especially vulnerable to oxidative reactions. The brain is also a kind of vacuum-sealed system. The energy to clear oxidative by-products must come from within this system—there appears to be minimal outside help. Though the brain has special cells and molecules that help break down and neutralize free radicals, these cells and molecules are damaged over time by poor diet, lack of exercise, chronic stress, lack of quality sleep, and general aging. When the brain's natural clearance system is compromised, free radicals become especially harmful.

Glucose dysregulation is another biological process that contributes to Alzheimer's and is especially common in the early stages of the disease. The system responsible for maintaining glucose often begins to falter as we age, especially when we consume a diet high in sugar and refined carbohydrates (though in some cases there is also a genetic component to glucose dysregulation). Abnormal production and usage of glucose affects the pancreas, hormones, enzymes, and cells that make up this system, and because glucose is a major source of energy for the entire body, the consequences—like impaired immune function and inability to clear harmful waste products—are far reaching. These negative effects are compounded in the brain due to its considerable energy requirements.

One dangerous consequence of glucose dysregulation is insulin resistance, which is a change in our sensitivity to insulin (a hormone that allows our bodies to harness the energy of glucose, and glucose's most important regulatory mechanism). Glucose fuels our brain cells, but it can only be actively internalized—or brought into the cell—in the presence of insulin. When insulin binds to the cell, the cell's receptors are prompted to bring glucose inside. But when there's too much glucose in the bloodstream, two significant problems arise: 1) Insulin levels rise and cells become desensitized to its effects. It's as if there are fewer locks (receptors) for the key (insulin) to open. The result is that glucose levels rise outside of the cells, but because the receptors aren't working properly, glucose can't be internalized. The cells then end up starving from lack of glucose even as the bloodstream is flooded with it; and 2) High insulin levels in the blood initiate a cascade of other harmful processes including inflammation, oxidation, dysregulation of lipids (fats), and tau phosphorylation (which creates the aberrant form of tau protein strongly associated with Alzheimer's disease). You can find more information about insulin resistance and the brain in Chapter 3. Many people are unaware that they're insulin resistant, but this pathology alone can lead to cognitive decline and Alzheimer's. Once you've progressed from insulin resistance to a diagnosis of diabetes, the most dangerous consequence of glucose dysregulation, your risk of cognitive decline is even greater. Studies have shown that individuals with diabetes experience brain shrinkage in the hippocampus, an important memory center.

Lipid dysregulation is the fourth biological process responsible for the changes associated with Alzheimer's disease. Lipids are fat-like substances that form the building blocks of cell walls, hormones, and steroids, and are integral to cellular structure, energy storage, and signaling—all life-sustaining functions. Lipids are pervasive throughout the body and compose more than 50 percent of the brain's dry weight.

Lipid dysregulation occurs when the body is subjected to excess lipids, inflammation, oxidative damage, and other forms of stress. In response, lipid transport and metabolism are impaired, which leads to lipids being oxidized (creating even more harmful oxidative by-products). There are many disease-promoting effects of lipid dysregulation, but here we want to shed some light on two of the processes in this complex system that are relevant to Alzheimer's: 1) Cholesterol is a type of lipid whose processing and clearance is altered during times of stress. Aberrant cholesterol begins to accumulate in the blood vessels, eventually forming plaques that clog arteries and cut off the blood supply to small vessels. The end result is microvascular disease (damage to our smallest blood vessels). Over time, macrovascular disease (damage to larger blood vessels) can develop as well. Both micro- and macrovascular disease are downstream consequences of lipid dysregulation in the vascular system, and as you'll learn throughout this book, vascular disease is a major risk factor for dementia; and 2) This improper clearance and processing of cholesterol and other lipids can also lead to a cascade of damage that ultimately contributes to the formation of amyloid plaques (the brain pathology strongly associated with Alzheimer's disease). APOE4, the most researched gene connected to Alzheimer's, has been implicated in lipid dysregulation in the brain. This gene encodes a protein responsible for clearing both lipids and amyloid, but because this version of the protein is inefficient at clearing waste, lipids and amyloid accumulate outside brain cells and begin to damage neural tissue. Later in life, the cumulative trauma of lipid dysregulation, vascular disease, and improper clearance of amyloid, combined with years of inflammation and oxidative stress, can ultimately manifest as Alzheimer's disease.

All four biological processes are interconnected, though Alzheimer's disease can be primarily driven by one or more of them. That is, Alzheimer's has different pathways to the same end result. A person with a diet high in cholesterol and saturated fat may develop vascular disease first, which leads to inflammation and then oxidation, whereas a person with

RISK FACTORS

PROTECTIVE FACTORS

1. Aerobic exercise, resistance training, and balance strengthening. Learn more in Chapter 4.

2. Walking meditation, mindful breathing, yoga, and others. Learn more in Chapter 5.

3. Learn more about beneficial and harmful foods on page 126.

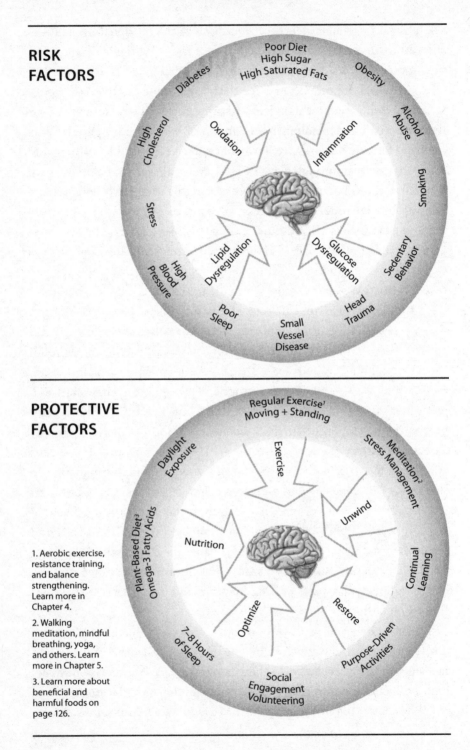

a diet high in sugar may start with insulin resistance, which then leads to vascular disease and inflammation.

The combined effect of these processes in the body results in the formation of amyloid and tau: the cascade of biological changes comes first, followed by the physical pathology of Alzheimer's (except in rare, early-onset cases where amyloid and tau appear to drive the disease process). In this way, Alzheimer's disease is really a constellation of several different disease pathways that ultimately manifest in the symptoms and pathology we call Alzheimer's. What's so incredible is that all four pathways are deeply influenced by lifestyle. Our daily choices are the driving force at the onset

KEY FACTS ABOUT ALZHEIMER'S

The past hundred or so years of research have yielded these key facts about Alzheimer's disease:

- Alzheimer's is a progressive disease of the brain that impairs memory, thinking, mood, and problem solving.
- Alzheimer's disease is one type of dementia that accounts for 60 to 80 percent of dementia cases.
- The majority of patients notice the first symptoms of Alzheimer's in their midsixties to early seventies.
- Alzheimer's is grossly underreported on death certificates, making it likely the third leading cause of death in the United States.
- The pathology associated with Alzheimer's disease includes:
  - Amyloid plaques and tau tangles in the brain;
  - Loss of connections between neurons;
  - Eventual atrophy, or shrinking, of the brain.
- Inflammation, oxidation, glucose dysregulation, and lipid dysregulation are the main biological processes that drive the development of Alzheimer's.

of Alzheimer's and throughout the entire progression of the disease. As we'll show you in Section Two, each one of these pathways can be controlled and even reversed by how you live your life.

With these biological processes mounting in the brain for decades, why don't cognitive symptoms appear earlier? How is the brain able to withstand daily assaults without showing signs of distress? The answer is that the brain is naturally—and profoundly—resilient. Redundancy is part of the brain's elegant design. With eighty to ninety billion neurons and close to a quadrillion connections, as well as overlapping arteries that supply multiple brain regions with nutrition and oxygen, the human brain can make pathways around damage. It can sidestep closed vessels and neurons destroyed by plaques, inflammation, and oxidation. If it takes a hit in the form of a stroke or injury, other parts of the brain can take over. Studies have shown that in strokes, for instance, parts of the brain near the damaged tissues compensate for lost function, as do mirror regions on the opposite side of the brain. The brain is also capable of regenerating some cells, though this capacity is limited. In Alzheimer's patients, cognitive symptoms emerge only after there is so much damage that the brain's innate resiliency can no longer compensate. This is what's so insidious about Alzheimer's: we only become aware of the disease once the damage is considerable.

Despite the brain's tremendous ability to withstand damage, it's extremely sensitive to stress at the cellular level, especially in regions like CA1 of the hippocampus and the entorhinal cortex, both of which are implicated in memory. As we explained earlier in this chapter, the brain has a very difficult job. It consumes more energy than any other organ in the body as it processes input and interprets the world around us. It also has the greatest output in terms of heat, energy, and waste products. These waste products—including oxidative by-products—are especially damaging if not properly cleared. But again, we can't see or feel the damage right away. It takes years for the trauma to accumulate, and during that time, we're usually focused on other bodily systems. In patients with diabetes, for instance, we monitor kidney damage, filtration, and the buildup of creatinine, all clear indications of glucose dysregulation. At the same time, elevated glucose in the blood is also destroying the brain's microvasculature (the smallest blood vessels), as well as billions of neurons and glia. In patients with cardiovascular disease, we address direct damage to the heart, vessels, arteries, and veins. Meanwhile, arteries harden in the brain, decreasing blood flow throughout. The brain really is the "end organ" of the body—stress experienced elsewhere accumulates in the brain over time and ends up causing exponentially greater damage.

Alzheimer's and Genes

Our bodies come preloaded with a set of key data points in the form of DNA. This genetic information is a product of our family's biological history—we inherit it from our ancestors. Most people have heard that Alzheimer's is an inherited disease, and because of this they assume it can't be prevented or influenced. Our genes do in fact play a role in the disease process, but they are far from the only determinant. To date, more than twenty different genes have been implicated in Alzheimer's, most of them affecting immune response, clearance of harmful by-products, and vascular health, but none of them guarantee that you will develop Alzheimer's disease.

APOE4, the most-researched Alzheimer's gene, is responsible for producing apolipoprotein E, a protein that helps regulate fats. Those who carry this gene are less resistant to Alzheimer's and may also experience an earlier onset (by fifteen to twenty years). Though having APOE4 means you have a greater chance of developing the disease, Alzheimer's is not a foregone conclusion. Risk doesn't necessarily mean disease. To understand how APOE4 affects our Alzheimer's risk, we first need to learn how genes work.

Genes are stretches of DNA that determine specific traits. Each parent provides you with a particular form of any given gene. These gene variants are called alleles, and they can be dominant or recessive (where only one set of alleles determines the trait), additive (where the allele's characteristics add up to determine the trait), or multiplicative, as in APOE4 (where the effect of multiple alleles is exponential). Let's look at a few examples. First, here's how dominant and recessive alleles determine eye color: Your father passes along a dominant allele for brown eyes (B), and your mother passes along a recessive allele for blue eyes (b). Because (B) is dominant to the recessive (b), you will have brown eyes. Skin color is determined in an additive manner. The main gene responsible for skin color produces the pigment melanin, the amount of which determines the precise shade of our skin. Having fewer alleles—and therefore a lower level of melanin—means lighter skin. Having more alleles—and therefore a higher level of melanin—means darker skin. APOE4 works in a multiplicative way, such that having more alleles exponentially increases your risk of Alzheimer's and also lowers the age of onset:

- If you have no APOE4 genes, you have the standard 50 percent chance of developing Alzheimer's at age eighty-five.

- If you have one copy of the APOE4 gene, you have a 50 percent chance of developing the disease at age seventy-five.

- If you have two copies of the APOE4 gene, you have a 50 percent chance of developing the disease at age sixty-five, twenty years earlier than those without the gene. Individuals with two genes have twelve to twenty times the risk of developing Alzheimer's as those with no APOE4 genes.

It's important to note that none of these scenarios—even having two copies of the APOE4 gene, which accounts for only 2 percent of the population—guarantees that you will develop Alzheimer's. If you don't implement healthy lifestyle practices, you'll have only a 50 percent chance of someday developing the disease. And for the great majority, roughly 90 percent of us, adopting a brain-healthy lifestyle can completely eliminate the risk.

For the other 10 percent, those with genes like presenilin 1, presenilin 2, or amyloid precursor protein (APP) that put them at an especially high risk, the effect of lifestyle is even more startling. Consider individuals with Down syndrome. Among those individuals between the ages of fifty and fifty-nine, one in three suffers from Alzheimer's disease. Fifty percent of those over the age of sixty develop the disease. This increased risk of Alzheimer's has to do with how Down syndrome arises. Individuals with Down syndrome have three chromosome 21s, and the genetic code in chromosome 21 produces APP, a transmembrane protein responsible for making amyloid, the abnormal protein associated with Alzheimer's disease. These individuals therefore have a greater than normal amount of APP, and the potential for higher levels of amyloid.

Whether APP functions normally or contributes to the pathology of Alzheimer's depends on the action of enzymes (proteins that initiate or propagate chemical reactions in the body). These enzymes cleave APP into smaller pieces as part of the body's natural process of clearing amyloid. When this process goes smoothly, amyloid is cut and cleared away by the brain's innate waste disposal system. When this process goes awry, beta-amyloid accumulates in small units outside of the neurons, where it then coalesces and starts to form plaques. These plaques cause inflammation that damages both cells and their supporting structures.

Given the role of APP in forming amyloid plaques, we would expect almost all Down syndrome individuals to develop Alzheimer's—but they don't. Studies have shown that individuals with a lower prevalence of diabetes and heart disease have a lower risk of developing Alzheimer's or a later disease onset. Again, this is despite a genetic abnormality that should guarantee Alzheimer's. As part of our work at Loma Linda, we're currently investigating which healthy behaviors confer the most protection against disease in Down syndrome individuals. By studying the risk factors common to all chronic diseases—obesity, inflammation, cholesterol metabolism—we hope to learn more about how to lower the risk of Alzheimer's no matter the genetic profile.

Even more powerful proof that genes do not guarantee disease comes from studying identical twins in their sixties and seventies. Researchers at King's College London followed 324 female twins over the course of ten years to investigate whether muscle fitness predicted changes in cognition. Despite the exact same genetic profile, the twin with greater leg muscle fitness experienced less cognitive decline than the twin who was not as physically fit. When researchers looked at the twins' brains using MRI (magnetic resonance imaging), they found that those with stronger legs had bigger brains. This study shows again that lifestyle changes—in this case, exercise and muscle strength—can supersede genetic risk and dramatically influence cognitive health.

WOMEN AND ALZHEIMER'S

Many of our patients are surprised to learn that two-thirds of people with Alzheimer's are women. One in six women develop Alzheimer's after age sixty-five, while for men the chances are only one in eleven. Women in their sixties are twice as likely to develop Alzheimer's as they are to develop breast cancer. We don't know for sure why this is. Longevity is at least part of the equation: women live longer than men and thus are more likely to develop the disease. But even when longevity is taken into account, women still seem to have a higher risk. Women who have the APOE4 gene are twice as likely to develop Alzheimer's as men who have the same gene. Some researchers have posited that women have traditionally had less access to intellectually challenging jobs and higher education, both of which are protective factors against Alzheimer's. Women who have multiple children are at a greater risk for stroke later in life (both ministrokes and regular strokes), and there is a clear relationship between vulnerability to stroke and vulnerability to cognitive decline. Hormonal changes during menopause also affect the brain at both the neuronal and vascular levels, which in turn could promote cognitive decline.

The remaining twenty or so genes that have been implicated in Alzheimer's affect the processes that initiate and propel the disease forward. Some of these genes govern the immune system and can either slow its response, resulting in the buildup of waste products that damage the brain, or cause an overactive immune response, which subjects the brain to chronic inflammation. Other genes impair our clearance system, again leading to the buildup of molecules that harm neurons and their connections. Additionally, genes associated with lipid metabolism and vascular health affect the vessels supplying oxygen and nutrients to the brain, and can promote vascular disease, vessel blockage, and neuronal damage.

While we don't get to choose the genes we inherit, we do have control over how those genes are expressed. This relatively new scientific concept is at the heart of epigenetics, the study of environmental factors that regulate gene expression by turning genes on and off. Epigenetics is concerned with all the life experiences that can affect how your genes are expressed, everything outside of genetics that influences your health. We know that genetics accounts for at least some of the risk of developing Alzheimer's, but epigenetics plays an even greater role in determining our cognitive fate. Research has shown that our genome actually changes over time when exposed to harmful environmental triggers like poor nutrition, sedentary lifestyles, pollution and chemicals, and chronic stress (both mental and physical). All these factors can influence the genes of developing embryos and the elderly alike. Whatever environment we're exposed to, be it the womb or an aging body that's been dealt some decades of unhealthy living, we are constantly subjected to epigenetic processes. New studies show that environmental stressors accumulate as we grow older, which makes epigenetics especially relevant for those in their sixties and seventies who want to age well and avoid chronic disease.

One of the main biological processes studied in epigenetics is methylation, a metabolic process in which a methyl group (a compound made up of one carbon atom and three hydrogen atoms) is passed from one molecule to another, ultimately altering gene expression. This process is a critical aspect of the modification and elimination of heavy metals (which can be toxic in the body and brain), regulation of gene expression, regulation of protein function, and RNA processing (transforming DNA's genetic information into proteins). Changes in the prevalence of methylation in certain regions of our DNA have been implicated in aging and seem to be especially associated with neurodegenerative diseases like Alzheimer's. For example, a deficiency in B vitamins (caused by poor nutrition) is a major contributing factor to impaired methylation pathways, resulting in aberrant DNA repair and subsequent dementia.

Epigenetics will have wide-reaching implications for complex chronic diseases like heart disease, diabetes, cancer, and dementia. We can combat all these diseases simply by reducing the environmental factors that put us most at risk: sugary and processed foods, pollutants and heavy metals, lack of exercise, and stress. Decreasing the amount of sugar in your diet, for instance, impedes glycosylation, another epigenetic process responsible for high inflammation, impaired adaptive responses at the cellular level, and oxidative stress—all of which damage the proteins and DNA of neurons. Physical exercise regulates many cellular processes, resulting

EPIGENETICS IN ACTION

Several important studies illustrate the role of epigenetics in the development of neurodegenerative disease. The Honolulu-Asian Aging Study found that Japanese people living in the United States have a higher prevalence of Alzheimer's than those living in Japan. There was little genetic variance among the men in this study, so the increased risk of Alzheimer's can be attributed almost solely to the epigenetic influence of poor diet, lack of exercise, and other unhealthy behaviors that are common in modern American life. Other studies have shown that in the United States, children of immigrants from China and Japan suffer more from chronic disease than those children who stayed in Asia. Here, too, the genetic similarity among subjects points to the epigenetic processes that promote disease.

In countries like China and India, we're seeing the epigenetic consequences as people move away from traditional lifestyles and adopt more modern ways of living. Diets high in vegetables and grains have been traded for animal products, refined sugar, and saturated fats. Instead of moving throughout the day, people are more likely to be sedentary. All these unhealthy behaviors change our gene expression and promote chronic disease. These dramatic—and unfortunate—lifestyle shifts give rise to the paradox of affluence: so-called

---

in methylation changes that improve the metabolism of amyloid and oxidative by-products in the brain. Exercise also boosts the genes that encode brain-derived neurotrophic factor (a protein responsible for neuronal growth) and promotes connections between brain cells. Every day we're learning more about how our lifestyle choices alter both the expression of our genes and our risk of someday developing a chronic disease.

Alzheimer's and Age

When Jeanne Calment turned ninety, she decided to sell her apartment in Arles, France, figuring she only had a few years to live. The winning bid came

progress leading to more disease. China now has the world's largest diabetes epidemic, with 11.6 percent of adults developing this chronic condition, and many millions more with prediabetes. China is also ranked second for obesity, behind only the United States. Both diabetes and obesity are major risk factors for dementia, which is also increasing exponentially. Alzheimer's Disease International estimates that China had more than 6.4 million Alzheimer's patients in 2009; another review in 2010 found that roughly 9.19 million Chinese were living with dementia. China has a rapidly aging population, a severe lack of nursing facilities and specialists, and little understanding of the challenges of Alzheimer's or how lifestyle affects the disease. India is experiencing a similar increase in Alzheimer's cases—more than four million people in India have some form of dementia, and that number is projected to increase dramatically as the population becomes more urban and influenced by Western lifestyles. In India, as in so many other developing countries, Alzheimer's is underdiagnosed and poorly understood. We fear these countries are not equipped to handle the explosion of lifestyle diseases that awaits them. This is why understanding the role of epigenetics in neurodegenerative disease is so critical to addressing the global epidemic of Alzheimer's.

from her forty-seven-year-old lawyer, who agreed to pay her a monthly rent until she passed away, allowing him to acquire the apartment for a bargain. Calment's lawyer died of cancer thirty years later, having paid more than double the apartment's value. To everyone's surprise, Calment was still alive. She even lived on her own until her 110th birthday. When Calment was 118, she underwent neuropsychological testing and a brain scan. Her cognitive scores were consistent with those of people in their eighties and nineties. Her brain showed no evidence of neurological disease.

Another enduring myth about Alzheimer's disease is that it's a natural consequence of aging. Research has definitively shown that Alzheimer's is a unique process of degeneration, and we have numerous examples of people living long—even extremely long—lives and never developing the beginning stages of cognitive decline. Age is a major risk factor for Alzheimer's only because the older we get, the more likely that we will have experienced the cumulative effects of inflammation, oxidation, glucose dysregulation, and lipid dysregulation over time.

Each decade of life has the potential to cause the brain significant stress and predispose us to developing Alzheimer's later on:

In early childhood, physical and emotional trauma can cause considerable stress. Atherosclerosis (hardening of the arteries that supply oxygen to the body) starts during childhood because of lifestyle factors like poor nutrition and lack of exercise. Perhaps not surprisingly, physical neglect and emotional abuse sustained at a young age have been associated with memory deficits in adulthood. Most of the brain's myelination (the process of coating the neuron's connections with a fatty membrane called myelin, which facilitates communication between cells) and cellular growth happens in our first five years (though myelination continues through our teens and early twenties). Both myelination and the number of cellular connections help the brain develop its resilience in the face of later traumas. Stress has been shown to significantly affect growth in developing brains. This means that if you have fewer connections and less cognitive resilience to start with, you'll have a much higher risk of developing dementia once you reach your sixties and seventies. Children who experience early trauma are also at a much higher risk for lifestyle intermediary diseases like high blood pressure, diabetes, and high cholesterol, which increase their risk later in life for both stroke and Alzheimer's disease. Sports-related head trauma is another risk factor that can predispose children to developing cognitive problems. A 2013 study in *Radiology* found that repetitive "heading" in soccer was associated with structural changes in white matter that could later contribute to cognitive decline.

In our twenties and thirties, we continue to accumulate the early traumas to our brains that push us into risk. During these decades many of us experience academic and professional stress, subsist on unhealthy foods, and often skip both exercise and sleep. All of these behaviors set the stage for declining health in midlife.

As we progress into our late thirties and forties, we may see the first signs of chronic disease—high blood pressure, high cholesterol, prediabetes— all of which adversely affect the brain. Later on, in our fifties and sixties, cumulative vascular disease emerges in the form of cholesterol plaque buildup, microvascular damage, and ministrokes so small we don't notice them on regular brain scans. The brain's waste disposal system also gets overwhelmed with inflammatory by-products and other toxins, which promotes the buildup of amyloid and tau.

By the time we reach our sixties and seventies, the hallmark signs of the disease begin to show up in MRIs and other laboratory tests. The first indication of Alzheimer's is the presence of beta-amyloid plaques (which usually emerge in our sixties); tau intracellular tangles form shortly thereafter (usually in our seventies). Both of these toxic proteins cause hypometabolism, where brain cells use glucose (their main fuel) less efficiently, especially in the temporal and parietal lobes, two areas of the brain that are uniquely susceptible to Alzheimer's. Changes in metabolism then cause changes in structure. The brain loses connections, neurons, and overall volume, and the hippocampus (which regulates emotions and short-term memory) and other key regions of the brain start to atrophy. This is when we finally begin to experience the debilitating psychological and cognitive effects of Alzheimer's—impaired memory (especially short-term memory), executive function (our ability to perform complex tasks), and visuospatial sense (our ability to quickly and accurately interpret what we see).

Though there are instances of early-onset Alzheimer's, when the disease emerges in the late forties and early fifties (and amyloid and tau begin accumulating in the thirties and forties), these cases are extremely rare. Generally, the disease appears after the sixth decade of life, once the brain has accumulated enough trauma to make its damage known. As we enter our eighties, we are even more likely to experience these cognitive changes. The longer we live, the greater our risk.

The Failures of Alzheimer's Research

A recent study published in *Alzheimer's Research & Therapy* examined all Alzheimer's clinical trials that took place between 2002 and 2012. Researchers found that 244 compounds were tested during this decade in a total of 413 clinical trials. Of these compounds, only *one* drug was approved: Namenda, a glutamate blocker that can temporarily lessen some of the symptoms of Alzheimer's but has no effect whatsoever on the underlying disease process. The overall research success rate for the whole decade was just 0.4 percent. This means that the rate of failure was a staggering 99.6 percent, one of the highest failure rates for any type of disease research in the world. When it comes to slowing or stopping Alzheimer's disease, the current success rate is 0 percent.

FDA-APPROVED MEDICATIONS FOR ALZHEIMER'S

To date, the FDA has approved five medications for the treatment of Alzheimer's symptoms. Cholinesterase inhibitors (Aricept, Exelon, and Razadyne) are used in early to moderate cases of Alzheimer's and are designed to target short-term memory loss, confusion, and impaired thinking and reasoning. This type of medication works by preventing the breakdown of acetylcholine, a chemical messenger integral to learning and memory. Cholinesterase inhibitors do not stop Alzheimer's from progressing, but they may lessen symptoms for a limited time (an average of six to twelve months for roughly half of patients, though there are rare cases of symptoms lessening for up to four years; the other half experience no effect). In more advanced Alzheimer's patients, memantine (Namenda) can help block a specific type of neuron receptor called NMDA, which binds to glutamate (the most abundant neurotransmitter in our brains). Some people experience a slowing of the symptoms of cognitive decline, but this effect is only temporary. Namzaric is a new combination drug (a mixture of Aricept and memantine), and is sometimes prescribed for people with moderate to severe Alzheimer's. All these drugs can have debilitating side effects (nausea, vomiting, dizziness, nightmares, headaches), and they have no effect whatsoever on the progression of Alzheimer's.

The newest drug in development, Aducanumab, has shown some promise in a group of 166 people: it effectively removed amyloid without the severe side effects of other medications. In a small subgroup of forty people, this drug was shown to significantly slow the progression of Alzheimer's, but several studies have demonstrated similar results that could not be replicated in a larger group. A phase 3 clinical trial is now in progress, with results expected by 2020.

Alzheimer's research is the greatest—and most costly—misunderstanding of all. It doesn't take a brilliant neuroscientist to see that there's something very wrong with the way we're conducting research. How could we invest so much scientific knowledge and so much money—the NIH (National Institutes of Health) has spent billions of dollars on Alzheimer's research and is projected to spend $991 million in 2017—only to fail over and over again? Why has this been happening for decades, and why do we stubbornly adhere to the same approach despite these glaring failures?

The answer is simpler than you might think—once you understand how the research works. Below are the major misunderstandings about Alzheimer's that have impeded research and significantly delayed our search for a cure.

Single Molecule Research

Modern medical research is fundamentally misguided when it comes to curing a chronic disease like Alzheimer's. Almost all our research is disease based, meaning that scientists focus on developing a cure in the form of a single drug. The NIH, the main funding agency that determines which types of research receive financial support, adheres to a simplistic model that has guided medical research since the eighteenth century: infection—bacteria—drug—outcome. This method has led to many spectacular breakthroughs. In the early twentieth century, for example, our biggest killers were infectious diseases. Cholera took tens of millions of lives worldwide before an antibiotic was found. Now we know that a single dose of doxycycline can be used to treat this once dreaded disease. Cholera still affects developing nations today, as do other infectious diseases like malaria and tuberculosis—and that's why this model has persisted. Though treatment for these diseases may sometimes require multiple steps, the underlying principle is almost always a single drug designed to eradicate a specific infectious agent.

When it comes to complex, chronic diseases of aging, especially diseases of the brain, this research method doesn't make sense. Acute, infectious diseases like cholera usually involve one element that emerges and immediately damages tissue, invoking a strong immune response from the body. Chronic diseases, by contrast, represent layers of cumulative damage that add up and become more complex over time. The problem is that scientists don't investigate this vast and multilayered damage. Instead they take a single, myopic snapshot of the disease—usually one element in a much more complicated, much larger disease picture.

In the case of Alzheimer's, this element is amyloid (and to a lesser extent tau). There is indeed evidence that amyloid has something to do with Alzheimer's. Amyloid plaques were identified decades ago as we discovered the early-onset genes implicated in Alzheimer's: presenilin 1, presenilin 2, and APP. It's clear that amyloid is propagated on some level as the disease progresses, but there are many other processes parallel to amyloid that contribute to Alzheimer's (like inflammation, oxidation, glucose dysregulation, and lipid dysregulation).

There is also ongoing confusion about amyloid versus tau in the progression of Alzheimer's. As far back as the 1990s, some researchers claimed that it was in fact tau intracellular tangles that were more closely associated with the symptoms of cognitive decline. New evidence suggests that tau tangles emerge later in the process and are better predictors of Alzheimer's and its progression than amyloid plaques. A 2017 study published by researchers at Mayo Clinic in the journal *Brain* concluded that tau may actually start the process of cognitive decline, meaning that drugs targeting amyloid may not be complex enough to treat or cure this disease.

Despite the evidence we now have, scientists still seem blindly focused on amyloid, ignoring all other findings that don't conform to this single molecule approach. They're unwilling—or unable—to look at Alzheimer's as it really is: a complex, multifactorial, temporal disease that requires a complex, multifactorial solution. This inability to understand the complexity of Alzheimer's has wasted billions of dollars and prolonged suffering for decades.

Inadequate Models

Alzheimer's drugs are developed and tested on animal models—mostly rats and genetically altered mice. In one sense these animals are appropriate models for human disease because we have many genes in common. To date, roughly four thousand genes in humans and mice have been studied, and just a few of them were found to exist in only one species. And yet these unique genes result in all kinds of biological differences ranging from how genes are turned on and off to important qualities like life span. Mice live for two to three years. Their life span doesn't allow them to endure the kind of stress a human does over the course of seventy or eighty years. They're not subjected to inflammation, oxidation, insulin resistance, and vascular assaults in the same way we are. They simply can't replicate the complicated biology of Alzheimer's in the human brain.

The other major problem with genetically engineered mice is that they're designed to express the late-stage pathology of Alzheimer's—amyloid buildup and hippocampal atrophy—not any of the long-term pathways that also contribute to Alzheimer's (inflammation, oxidation, glucose dysregulation, and lipid dysregulation). Mouse models may represent the same disease outcome, but the cause is not likely to be the same. Researchers are well aware that there is no commonality of pathways in genetically altered mice and humans, but they continue to work with a flawed model. This is why so many clinical trials fail: our animal models don't come close to representing the disease we're trying to cure.

In recent years, Alzheimer's models have progressed to some extent, especially with iPSCs (induced pluripotent stem cells). iPSCs are adult cells that have been genetically manipulated to become any type of cell we want to study: heart, liver, pancreas, brain. We can now take nascent cells from patients who had Alzheimer's and turn them into neurons. From these neurons scientists create what are called neuro lattices, minibrains that are grown from actual human tissue. While having a human genetic model is a huge step forward, these neuro lattices still lack the three-dimensionality of the actual brain, as well as all the processes outside of genetics—like diet, exercise, and stress—that we know are so important to chronic diseases like Alzheimer's.

None of the models we currently use are at all accurate representations of this complex disease. In mouse models, false amyloid lesions lead to false results. In neuro-lattice models, an incomplete picture leads to an incomplete treatment. As any scientist will tell you, an inaccurate model will only yield inaccurate outcomes.

Assuming Clearance Equals Restoration

Yet another flawed aspect of Alzheimer's research is the assumption that clearing amyloid and tau will restore cognitive function. Drugs are designed to attack amyloid. Mouse models are designed to express amyloid so we can figure out different ways to remove it. But by the time amyloid and tau have accumulated in the brain, hundreds of thousands of neurons have died. Brain structures have been permanently altered, and the overall volume of the brain has decreased. While removing amyloid and tau may have some minor but temporary effect on cognition, this approach will never be a cure. There's very little chance of restoring significant cognitive function once this much damage has been sustained. In most clinical trials, treatments are given to subjects with mild to moderate Alzheimer's, well after amyloid and tau have accumulated on top of all the other structural damage in the brain. This is why no drug designed to cure Alzheimer's has ever improved cognition. We need to intervene much earlier if we want to influence this disease, and we need to recognize that amyloid and tau are a small part of a larger picture, likely the result of insults that have been mounting for years or even decades.

Given the many limitations of our dominant research model, it's not surprising that Alzheimer's clinical trials have such a staggeringly high failure rate. To date, the only thing that has been shown to affect the curve of decline or slow the progression of Alzheimer's is lifestyle change, which is the basis of the NEURO Plan in Section Two. Not amyloid-clearing medication, not anything developed on a flawed mouse model costing billions of dollars and years of testing—but lifestyle change. We have a solution to Alzheimer's, and we have proof. So why aren't we doing what works? Why is the most hopeful means of preventing and slowing Alzheimer's almost completely ignored by both the research establishment and clinicians?

One simple answer: there's a long-standing belief that an organ as complex as the brain can't be affected by lifestyle. Somehow the brain is outside of the body, subjected to a different set of rules. This couldn't be further from the truth. As we explained earlier in this chapter, the brain is the "end organ" that receives all the stress and trauma—or, conversely, all the resilience and resistance—from other body systems. Each lifestyle chapter in this book will show you how the brain is part of the body, and how when we harm the body with unhealthy lifestyle choices, we especially harm the brain.

The more troubling answer is that the research establishment has given up on lifestyle intervention without ever even attempting it—and this is in spite of many researchers who now acknowledge that lifestyle influences Alzheimer's disease. The NIH, the National Science Foundation (NSF), and similar leading research organizations categorically reject the possibility of lifestyle change. They just don't think it's worthwhile. They claim that interventions are difficult if not impossible for the general public, and that lifestyle protocols invariably fail to create lasting change. Though a small amount of funding is allocated to simple interventions in order to study the effects of lifestyle on cognitive health (a specific diet, for instance, or a basic exercise routine), these interventions are never comprehensive and thus never have a chance of illuminating the power of lifestyle. The real money goes to single molecule studies, which are deeply flawed in all the ways we previously discussed. Even if some researchers wanted to study the disease more broadly, they wouldn't be able to secure funding for multifaceted, multivariable research. The funding, of course, comes from pharmaceutical companies interested in patenting pills, and from grants awarded exclusively to researchers who believe in the single molecule model of chronic disease.

Anyone who's gone to a primary care doctor or neurologist knows that this attitude pervades clinical practice as well. Doctors aren't trained in prevention. They go through twelve years (or more) of advanced training in disease identification and management with perhaps an obligatory lecture or two about prevention. This hyperfocused, myopic approach to overall health teaches doctors not to believe in anything beyond their education, and that's why almost all of them dismiss prevention and behavioral change. Most physicians have never seen an example of a well-designed, effective lifestyle intervention, and the health-care system affords them no time or space in which to attempt it (the average primary care doctor spends between ten and fifteen minutes with each patient). The few doctors who do want to address lifestyle run out of time or simply don't know how. Every patient suffering from cognitive decline should be informed of the many lifestyle risk factors, yet almost none are. And because of doctors' all-knowing, inflexible approach to medicine, patients are often too intimidated to speak up and ask questions.

A few brave scientists have pursued lifestyle research despite the overwhelming barriers, and the data we now have is truly remarkable: proper nutrition and exercise significantly lower your risk of progressing from mild cognitive impairment to dementia and also decrease your chances of developing cognitive decline in the first place. And yet the amount of media coverage and scientific interest is negligible. This is not a conspiracy: it's simply a cultural disconnect. The research is flawed, the clinical application is flawed, and our understanding is flawed. But if we can change our understanding, if we can unpack the myths and misunderstandings about Alzheimer's, we can revolutionize the way we fight this disease.

The Solution in Plain Sight

Despite all the myths and misunderstandings, the failed clinical trials and misguided theories, there is a way forward. Research points unequivocally toward lifestyle intervention as the cure for cognitive decline. We learn more every day about how our behavior impacts the health and resilience of our brains. People are growing frustrated with the conventional approach to health care, especially when it comes to Alzheimer's and dementia. Awareness is growing and the system is changing. Progressive medical practitioners are increasingly interested in finding the cause of a disease instead of merely medicating symptoms and risk factors. For almost every chronic disease, the root cause can be traced back to an unhealthy lifestyle. And when patients change their lifestyles, they experience a decrease in all types of chronic disease.

We also have a precedent for how to study lifestyle change and implement it in clinical settings. Thanks to Dean Ornish's incredible Lifestyle Heart Trial in 1990, we now know that heart disease, America's number one killer, can not only be prevented but also, in most cases, reversed with a plant-based diet, moderate exercise, and stress management. Another study found that people following healthy lifestyles experienced more than a 90 percent decrease in the risk of developing heart disease. The same goes for diabetes. Research now shows that plant-based diets both decrease the risk of developing diabetes and improve blood sugar levels. A landmark study published in the *New England Journal of Medicine* in 2002 found lifestyle intervention was more effective at reducing the risk of diabetes than the standard medical treatment. A follow-up study conducted four years later revealed that participants were able to sustain their lifestyle changes and reduced diabetes risk even after lifestyle counseling had been completed. In other words, they stuck to their new way of living and stayed healthier as a result. New research is also uncovering these same lifestyle effects on cancer treatment and prevention.

There are now hundreds of research projects and plenty of funding to support studies on lifestyle, cardiovascular disease, diabetes, and cancer, and doctors routinely suggest lifestyle changes for patients at high risk for these chronic diseases. It's only a matter of time before we're having the same conversation about lifestyle and Alzheimer's, and in the next chapter you'll learn about the indisputable research that proves this connection.

We see hope in the lifestyle research on cardiovascular disease and diabetes. We see hope in the widespread acceptance of factors other than genetics that put us at a high risk for developing chronic diseases. And most of all we see hope in our patients. We don't agree that people are lazy or incapable of change. The people we meet every day are terrified, and they'll do just about anything they think will help. In our practice in Loma Linda, we've observed a proactive attitude toward this disease: a need to take control and face Alzheimer's head-on. The problem, though, is that our patients exert effort in all the wrong ways. They're convinced they can find a solution through vitamins and supernutrients for the brain. They spend billions of dollars on brain games. They join elaborate, intensive exercise programs when their exercise quotient for the day is only twenty minutes. They take their loved ones to renowned hospitals to consult with the nation's top neurologists, when all the while the solution is at home, in their refrigerators. But no one has told them this. No one has taught them about lasting behavioral change. No one believes that they're disciplined or motivated or intelligent enough to live a truly healthy life.

This book offers a different perspective. We know the current approach isn't working, and we don't have time to lose. Why ignore all the powerful lifestyle research we now have? Why assume that people can't change, that a well-designed lifestyle protocol couldn't usher in a new way of thinking about chronic diseases like Alzheimer's? The NIH is right that lifestyle intervention presents a challenge, but as we'll prove to you in the coming chapters, it's the only solution for brain health, and with the help of our NEURO Plan, it's achievable for everyone.

2.

The Power of
Lifestyle Medicine

The myths and misunderstandings about Alzheimer's disease and dementia can be overwhelming, even devastating when you think of the wasted time and money of countless doctors, patients, and caregivers. But this book is called *The Alzheimer's Solution* for a reason.

In this chapter we'll present compelling data that proves Alzheimer's is deeply influenced by lifestyle factors like what we eat, how often we exercise, and the quality of our sleep. While it may be easier to blame a devastating disease like Alzheimer's on a single gene, this false belief is killing millions. The truth is much harder to accept—that we are bringing Alzheimer's disease into our households through the choices we make every day. But the truth is also liberating because it puts control back in our hands.

Loma Linda

The first thing we noticed was the food. We'd stopped at the hospital cafeteria after our interview at Loma Linda University, expecting to see the usual fare. Anyone who's spent time in a U.S. hospital knows that most cafeteria food is extremely unhealthy. There might be an obligatory salad bar, but you can also order burgers, fries, greasy pizza, sugary desserts, basically your pick of the least healthy food available, and the exact opposite of what you should be eating if you're sick. But at Loma Linda there were roasted vegetables, organic sandwiches, nourishing soups—everything was vegetarian, and the healthiest items were marked "Living Whole" so people could make informed choices.

Across the street we found the Loma Linda Market, which offered a large selection of fresh produce along with bins of nuts, grains, and beans. There was no meat section in the store. A few buildings over stood one of the largest, best-equipped gyms we'd ever seen, and at the very heart of the community was the church. The doors were open, and we could see people of all ages taking a moment out of their day to practice the faith that sustained them.

Then we visited a local nursing home and met Margaret, a 102-year-old woman who walked three miles a day. She didn't just walk—she power walked. She also shopped for her own groceries, volunteered in the Seventh-day Adventist church, and knew the names of all the nurses and other residents. Many elderly people in their eighties and nineties have a noticeable slowness of thinking, but Margaret was as sharp in conversation as a woman half her age. She embodied the totality of a healthy lifestyle—she ate a plant-based diet, exercised regularly, served her community—and she was surrounded by others just like her who led fulfilling lives well into their nineties and beyond.

Loma Linda, California, a small city located sixty miles east of Los Angeles, is widely considered one of the healthiest places in the world. A third of its roughly twenty-five thousand residents are Seventh-day Adventists whose faith is deeply connected to health and wellness. The religion celebrates vegetarianism, regular exercise, stress management, and community service. Smoking, drinking, and even caffeine consumption are discouraged. This unusually healthy lifestyle results in the Adventists' living, on average, ten years longer and healthier than the general population, a statistic that has made them famous worldwide. Since the 1950s organizations like the American Cancer Society and the National Institutes of Health have looked to Loma Linda for answers to the chronic diseases that have exploded elsewhere but seem to have left this community relatively untouched. The research that has emerged over the decades has given us profound insights into the relationship between lifestyle, longevity, and the avoidance of chronic disease:

- A 2007 study found that Adventists who ate a plant-based diet free of eggs and dairy had a lower risk of obesity than both vegetarians who ate eggs and dairy and nonvegetarians. The prevalence of diabetes was 2.9 percent in vegetarians versus 7.6 percent in nonvegetarians. Overall, vegetarians had roughly a 50 percent lower risk of developing diabetes in their lifetime compared to nonvegetarians.

- Another study of the Adventist population found that vegetarians had a lower risk of developing all types of cancer than nonvegetarians. The risk of female-specific cancers was up to 34 percent lower in vegetarians.

- In a 2003 study published in the *American Journal of Clinical Nutrition,* researchers from Loma Linda University compared six studies on low meat consumption and life span with the Adventist Health Studies, a series of long-term studies that look at lifestyle and disease in over 96,000 individuals. They found that people who ate a predominantly vegetarian diet had a longer life span in four of the six studies (and identified no positive or negative associations between meat and longevity in the other two studies).

- A 1993 study titled "The Incidence of Dementia and Intake of Animal Products," found that in a group of over 3,000 individuals, those who ate meat—including those who ate only poultry and fish—had twice the risk of developing dementia compared to vegetarians.

Numerous other studies have found similar associations between the way of life in Loma Linda and the avoidance of some of our most feared diseases.

Loma Linda is also America's only "Blue Zone," a term popularized by Dan Buettner in *The Blue Zones,* his bestselling book about lifestyle and longevity. Blue Zones are communities in which people live measurably longer and healthier lives due to optimal nutrition, exercise, stress management, and social support. As Buettner explains, the nine tenets of healthy living in Blue Zones are: 1) a lifestyle that involves natural movement throughout the day, 2) a deep sense of purpose or meaning, 3) skillful stress management, 4) avoiding overeating and eating late at night, 5) a primarily plant-based diet, 6) enjoying a drink or two with friends (though Adventists abstain from alcohol), 7) connection to a faith community, 8) living near family and finding a lifelong partner, and 9) access to social networks that support healthy living. Communities with such a comprehensive healthy lifestyle are exceedingly rare. There only five in the world: Sardinia, Italy; Okinawa, Japan; Ikaria, Greece; Nicoya, Costa Rica; and Loma Linda, California. Buettner's groundbreaking research on behaviors common to these diverse cultures has since inspired researchers to investigate the underlying science. Cities across the world have adopted features of the Blue Zone lifestyles, hoping that their residents can reduce their risk of chronic disease and experience the same incredible health and longevity.

We were at a crossroads in our medical careers when we discovered Loma Linda. We'd made our way through medical school, knowing that neurology was our calling, and then embarked on residencies and fellowships where we would receive the best clinical training and participate in cutting-edge research. We still believed that the only hope for chronic diseases like Alzheimer's was a pharmacological cure. Both of us were steeped in the individual, mechanistic view of Alzheimer's—the same flawed approach to research we described in Chapter 1—but we were growing increasingly uncomfortable with it.

Ayesha was a research assistant and coordinator for a UC–San Diego study that used functional MRI to look at Alzheimer's-related changes in the brain. Participants with a family history of dementia were tested in their fifties and sixties, and though the implication was that Alzheimer's could be seen as it developed, no interventions or treatment were part of the study. As Ayesha reviewed the brain scans, she would see that some of these individuals had early signs of Alzheimer's, and yet there was nothing she could do. She knew these people would eventually develop the disease, and that it would progress until it took their lives. There was no way to stop it or slow it down. Everyone around her kept repeating what she'd been taught: Alzheimer's disease cannot be prevented.

Dean had a similarly disillusioning experience as a fellow in the Experimental Therapeutics Branch at the National Institutes of Health. Working on numerous clinical trials, he saw a mechanistic approach that didn't consider the whole person, the whole disease, the whole complex process over time. He gave Alzheimer's patients medications that targeted singular pathways, while he and all the other researchers knew the disease was far more complicated than that. He cared for patients suffering from many different types of dementia (including Progressive Supranuclear Palsy, a neurodegenerative disease with Parkinsonian features and dementia) who received infusions directly into their brains. All these trials failed. It didn't matter if the treatment was a pill or an antibody or an invasive brain procedure. Nothing seemed to work.

The research was going nowhere, but it wasn't nearly as frustrating as clinical practice. We could offer our patients little beyond a diagnosis. We had to tell them their disease had no treatment, and with each look of dread on their faces, each family member taking in the horror of what was happening to their loved one, we grew more and more defeated. The realities of the profession started to sink in: we were stuck in a disease-based system that had almost nothing to do with health—and yet we never considered giving up. We'd made it our life's work to search for a cure to this devastating disease. We'd met as young physicians volunteering abroad, and in our first conversation we learned that both of our grandfathers had suffered from dementia. This was the journey we were meant to take, but we kept wondering whether there was another approach, a way to reach people and make a difference before their symptoms emerged and nothing could be done.

One night, while we were still at UC–San Diego, we attended a talk by Dr. Elizabeth Barrett-Connor, the founder and principal investigator of the Rancho Bernardo Heart and Chronic Disease Study. She and her team of researchers had collected data on lifestyle and cognitive function in men and women for over twenty years. They'd found gender differences in elderly populations with cognitive decline and had also discovered associations between dementia and both smoking and alcohol consumption. Listening in the audience that night, we were intrigued by what scientists had learned about habits and behaviors that put us at a high risk for Alzheimer's. We wondered how much literature existed about the risk factors for cognitive decline.

We began doing systematic reviews of publications in peer-reviewed journals, collecting decades of studies on the connection between lifestyle and chronic diseases like heart disease, stroke, diabetes, and cancer, hoping for insights into risk factors that also played a role in Alzheimer's. One study showed that eating nuts lowered the risk of heart disease; another that fruit consumption lowered the risk of lung cancer. The Nurse's Health Study and the Health Professionals Follow-Up Study showed us that every incremental increase in fruit and vegetable consumption lowered the risk of stroke by 6 percent. A separate analysis of the Nurse's Health Study found that women who ate a predominantly Mediterranean diet high in fruits, vegetables, legumes, nuts, and fish had a 29 percent lower chance of stroke compared to those who ate predominantly a Western diet high in sugar and processed foods. The Cardiovascular Health Study revealed that obesity in midlife increased the risk of dementia by 40 percent. Scientists at Columbia University concluded that high insulin levels in elderly people could account for 39 percent of Alzheimer's cases.

All these chronic diseases seemed to be related. What was good for the heart and kidneys also appeared to be beneficial for the brain. A whole-food, plant-based diet was by far the best dietary pattern for fighting each one of these diseases—not a single study showed any benefits of eating meat. The more we thought about it, the more sense it made. The body is a collection of interconnected systems, and the brain is itself a system. Why wouldn't it be affected by what we eat, how much we exercise, our overall state of health? People with healthier lifestyles were often able to avoid other chronic diseases. What if there were also a way to avoid Alzheimer's?

A few months later we read *The Blue Zones* and realized there was an epicenter of healthy living just next door. So much had been published about Loma Linda and heart disease, diabetes, and even cancer, but there were only a few early studies related to dementia. No research on Alzheimer's and the Loma Linda population had been published in nearly ten years. We wondered if anyone had looked further at the association between cognitive decline and lifestyle. Was it possible to replicate the previous results or learn more about which healthy behaviors afforded the most protection? And if there were a clear association, wouldn't we have heard about it by now?

We knew that studying lifestyle would put us at odds with the research establishment. Our mentors warned us that we'd be risking our careers, our reputations as clinicians and researchers. But at the same time, we knew that if we dedicated ourselves to the same myopic approach, we would never contribute something of value or actually help our patients. To us as doctors, it seemed almost irresponsible not to look into this possibility and learn what it might mean for the fight against Alzheimer's. So we took a huge risk. We went to Loma Linda with curiosity but also conservative expectations. We would be objective and unflinching in our research. We would have to be exceedingly convinced of the results to truly believe in the power of lifestyle.

Getting to Work

Our clinic—the Memory and Aging Center at Loma Linda University Medical Center—gave us the chance to do things differently. We'd conduct the standard blood tests, looking at biomarkers like vitamin B12, folic acid, HDL ("good") cholesterol and LDL ("bad") cholesterol, general inflammation, glucose, insulin, glycated hemoglobin (a measure of glucose levels over the past three months), thyroid hormones, and many other labs, as well as comprehensive neuropsychological testing and neuroimaging to determine the extent and nature of a patient's decline. In addition, we would also collect detailed information on our patients' lives, on how they were living day to day and how their lifestyle choices may have affected their risk of developing Alzheimer's. We drew up detailed questionnaires regarding diet, physical activity, sleeping patterns, stress, and general psychological health (including depression).

We also designed our clinic around the family as a system. Everyone who came in had to bring at least two family members, but they were encouraged to bring more. We knew that families were an essential support system for those struggling with Alzheimer's, and also that lifestyle choices often come from the family. If we could learn more about the culture of nutrition and exercise within a family unit, we might gain more insights into the behaviors that influence cognitive health, and maybe even prevent another member of the family from developing Alzheimer's. Spouses were especially important. As we stated earlier, partners of those who develop dementia have a 600 percent greater risk of developing the disease themselves compared to the general matched population, and this isn't attributable solely to stress. Shared lifestyle risks are a major factor in the health outcomes of long-term couples. One of the central aspects of our current research at Loma Linda is the disease incidence in spouses, one or both of whom are suffering from cognitive decline.

We saw elderly people everywhere in Loma Linda. In the early mornings we'd go to the state-of-the-art gym on campus and watch people in their nineties doing more bicep curls than we could. Just looking around town, you can see Loma Linda's longevity statistics playing out in real life. We didn't think we would have any difficulty recruiting patients. When we opened our doors, we were the only dementia clinic in the Loma Linda community, and because the population is well educated and engaged in health care, we assumed they'd come to us. We waited. And we kept waiting.

In those early days we were also studying the existing body of research for more insights into lifestyle and Alzheimer's. We wanted to know about everything that had ever been published. Together we did comprehensive reviews of nutrition and the three most prevalent diseases of the brain: dementia, Parkinson's disease, and stroke. One study by researchers at Columbia University found that participants who adhered to the Mediterranean diet had a 40 percent lower risk of developing Alzheimer's than those who ate a standard American diet high in meat, dairy, processed grains, sugar, and fat, and extremely low in fruits and vegetables.

The same researchers looked at eating patterns and the risk of developing MCI (mild cognitive impairment). Again, a Mediterranean diet reduced the risk of MCI by 28 percent, and those individuals who did develop MCI had a 29 percent lower chance of progressing to Alzheimer's. Another study in our comprehensive review found a similar pattern for Parkinson's disease: a Mediterranean diet high in plant-based foods reduced the odds of having Parkinson's by 14 percent. A 2012 study published in *Movement Disorders* compared 249 people with Parkinson's disease to a normal age-matched population. Researchers found that a higher consumption of foods rich in vitamin E reduced the risk of developing Parkinson's disease by 55 percent. We knew there wasn't a single pharmaceutical agent in the world that could boast these kinds of results.

We were also given access to the Adventist Health Studies database, the source of so many of the incredible lifestyle studies on the Loma Linda community. We looked at a wide spectrum of participants who had taken an exam called the California Verbal Learning Test, a robust neuropsychological test for determining verbal learning and memory. When controlling for age, race, and education, we found that for two of the cognitive variables we tested, individuals who ate a plant-based diet had on average a 28 percent lower risk of cognitive impairment. Vegetarians tested better than both pescatarians (people who eat fish) and omnivores. There appeared to be a spectrum in terms of animal protein intake and its effect on brain function: the less meat you ate, the healthier your brain remained over time.

A pattern began to emerge at the clinic. We were seeing low numbers of Alzheimer's patients in the Adventist population, and the more people we met, the more curious we became about neighboring populations and their cognitive health. We started having conversations with the larger community about healthy aging, our clinic, and our research. One afternoon Dean spoke at a Catholic church in a lower socioeconomic neighborhood on the outskirts of Loma Linda. The crowd was diverse and the church was packed. Afterward a long line formed—everyone had questions. As he met these people one by one, he realized he was seeing the undeniable result of unhealthy living. Alzheimer's or some other form of dementia seemed to have affected almost every elderly person he met. One elderly African American man told Dean that both he and his wife had been diagnosed with dementia. If longevity and wellness were readily apparent in the Adventists' community, this crowd gave him a glimpse of chronic disease run rampant. The stark difference between these populations was staggering: one of the healthiest communities in the United States was living right next door to one of the sickest.

We soon learned that the residents of San Bernardino suffered from diabetes, cardiovascular disease, stroke, and dementia to a much greater extent than their Loma Linda neighbors. They visited hospitals much more often and died a lot younger. There were also clear racial and ethnic differences that played a role in the prevalence of Alzheimer's in this region. In 2010, the Alzheimer's Association found that African Americans were two to three times more likely to have Alzheimer's than Caucasians; Hispanics were nearly twice as likely to have Alzheimer's. As we reached out to more and more churches and community centers, we saw that poor health was the thread connecting local residents. At one Healthy Aging talk we gave at a Baptist church in San Bernardino, we noticed that all the people in leadership roles were women. Dean asked where the men were, and the pastor explained that out of fourteen women, five of their husbands had died from stroke and heart disease, and a couple of them had dementia. Health awareness was low, especially concerning cognitive decline. When it came to lifestyle, the residents of San Bernardino had no resources and no knowledge. The sense of confusion was overwhelming.

Soon we were volunteering every weekend, trying to share what we'd learned about lifestyle with everyone we could. More and more patients came to the clinic, though almost none of them were from the Adventists' community. We mostly saw people from the surrounding communities, those we were meeting through our talks, or residents of Loma Linda who had no connection to the church or its emphasis on healthy living. A lot of our patients had diets high in meat and processed foods. They usually didn't exercise. They suffered from risk factors like hypertension and high cholesterol that we knew were accelerating their cognitive symptoms.

At the same time, we were discovering more and more research that offered remarkable insights into other lifestyle factors that affected the brain:

- The Framingham Longitudinal Study, a famous longitudinal study on the residents of Framingham, Massachusetts, found that daily brisk walks resulted in a 40 percent lower risk of developing Alzheimer's later in life.

- Chronic stress was shown to decrease the level of brain-derived neurotrophic factor, which is the main protein responsible for the production of new brain cells.

- Researchers at Washington University in St. Louis found that sleep-deprived individuals had more amyloid plaques in their brains.

- Several studies from the mid-1990s found an inverse relationship between formal education and the incidence of Alzheimer's, suggesting that sustained, complex cognition protects the brain against normal aging.

We also read a prominent study conducted at Rush University in which researchers compared different dietary patterns. They tested the DASH diet (Dietary Approach to Stop Hypertension, a specialized diet for patients suffering from high blood pressure), the Mediterranean diet, and the MIND diet, which is a hybrid of the DASH and the Mediterranean diets. The results showed that all three diets reduced the risk of Alzheimer's, but that even moderate adherence to the MIND diet improved brain health. This meant that each small step toward lifestyle change had a measurable effect. Ayesha searched other databases to see if she could confirm this same incremental influence of healthy eating on the vascular health of the brain. She analyzed the California Teachers Study, looking at the dietary patterns of nearly 140,000 women and using a diet adherence score to measure the extent to which the participants stuck to a healthy diet (positive scores were given for each fruit and vegetable, for example, and negative scores were given for sweets and foods high in saturated fat, like meat). She found that for every unit of increase in the adherence score, the risk of stroke dropped by 10 percent, proving that daily choices have a major effect on chronic diseases of the brain. This study was such an important contribution to the field of lifestyle medicine that Ayesha received the award for Cardiovascular Disease Research in Women's Health from the American Heart Association.

We kept collecting data on our patients, and as a clear association between lifestyle and dementia was emerging, our practice was also shifting. In addition to tracking the behaviors and lifestyle that had led to dementia, we began experimenting with lifestyle as a treatment. Our own research and the studies from around the world were so compelling that we didn't want to wait for a randomized clinical trial. Lifestyle intervention had been shown to be incredibly effective in the treatment and even reversal of cardiovascular disease. Why not apply the same philosophy to chronic diseases of the brain? We began to think of lifestyle as an off-label treatment for cognitive decline. We figured it would help our dementia patients live healthier and happier lives, and at the very least it would do no harm.

Families, we were learning, were not just useful for emotional support but essential to lifestyle intervention. They could give us insights into the patient's life—a habit of sitting in front of the TV all day, or an unhealthy obsession with pizza—that would help us know where to intervene. The more support our patients had, the better, and every person who came to the clinic would learn how to avoid dementia themselves. We kept encouraging our patients to bring as many people as possible. One woman came in with fourteen family members, and Dean searched the clinic until he found enough chairs.

For each appointment, we were now spending five minutes on the typical neurological exams and the other twenty-five minutes on lifestyle intervention. We made rudimentary packets with the results from our research and other lifestyle studies, showing our patients exactly how to eat, exercise, and live for better brain health. Later on Ayesha added brain-healthy recipes. We were notorious in the clinic for printing out thousands of worksheets to track our lifestyle inventions, the same worksheets that appear in the NEURO Plan in Section Two. Identifying a patient's unique strengths and weaknesses, we learned, was essential to behavioral change. So was follow-up. We'd call insurance companies on our patients' behalf, asking for coverage for more than the standard six-month or one-year appointments. We knew lifestyle change would be almost impossible if we couldn't closely monitor our patients' progress. As we continued to refine our method, the process became more personalized and more precise. Over time we saw that our patients felt empowered instead of doomed, despite their diagnoses. You could often hear laughter in our clinic. We felt like we were inventing a whole new style of practice, a way of reaching people and helping them change their lives.

It also occurred to us that we could help the residents of San Bernardino just like we were helping our patients. Dean researched how to implement lifestyle change in areas where unhealthy living was the norm. He talked with the Alzheimer's Association, shopkeepers, elderly people, family members, senior center directors, nursing home directors, local doctors, and faith and community leaders. He asked each of them what kind of programs would be relevant for the people they served. What kinds of interventions would be useful given the community's unique resources, limitations, and strengths? How could we apply interventions that had at least a chance of being successful? Where did residents go for information and guidance? Whom did they trust and why? The goal wasn't to make everyone live like the Seventh-day Adventists. As Ayesha's research on stroke had shown, every positive step makes a difference in cognitive health. No matter the culture or cuisine, we can all eat more vegetables and reduce our intake of sugar, saturated fats, and fried foods. We can all engage in some form of exercise, often in our own homes. Support and knowledge can come from the communities themselves. Lifestyle intervention can work for everyone, as long as it's precise, personalized, and culturally specific.

To say our findings changed the course of our lives as doctors would be an understatement. What we discovered revolutionized our whole way of thinking about dementia, cognitive health, and the future of Alzheimer's treatment—and we wrote this book to share it with you. Of the approximately twenty-five hundred dementia patients we saw in our clinic, only nineteen—that's less than 1 percent—were vegetarians who followed a strict healthy lifestyle. The way of living intrinsic to the Adventists' community in Loma Linda that had generated groundbreaking research on heart disease, diabetes, and cancer was just as important for the brain. People who ate a plant-based diet, exercised regularly, managed stress, got quality sleep, and belonged to a strong community were protected against

DEAN: STRENGTH IN NUMBERS

After speaking at churches throughout San Bernardino County and seeing the alarming effects of unhealthy living, I decided I needed to do something more. Sharing the insights we were learning in the clinic every day was a good start, but people needed more support than we could offer through community talks. I didn't want to wait around at the clinic doors for sick people to come in—I wanted to reach out to them in the community before they ever got sick. This is one of the central tenets of medical practice at Loma Linda University, and an idea at odds with every other health-care system we've encountered: do your best to keep patients out of the hospital.

At the time I was the director of the Memory and Aging Center at Loma Linda University Health as well as director of research for the Neurology Department. Though I didn't exactly have extra time, I accepted an offer to become community chair in the Department of Aging at San Bernardino County. I knew there was a cognitive health crisis, and if I didn't address it at the community level, there would be tremendous suffering ahead for more people than I wanted to count. I went to meetings every Wednesday and many Fridays

---

cognitive decline by the very behaviors that saved them from other chronic diseases. We had seen it all unfold before our eyes. Altogether, our comprehensive reviews, studies, and clinical data yielded significant findings on nutrition and lifestyle that had not been seen elsewhere in the field of Alzheimer's research. The solution to Alzheimer's, we were now certain, wouldn't come in a pill but in the way we live our lives.

But there were also other findings at the clinic—results that were almost unbelievable. We worked with a patient who had a bad habit of eating cookies and cake. Her glycated hemoglobin level was 13 (as revealed by an HbA1c blood test, which measures average blood sugar over a period of three months); a score of 6.5 or above is considered diabetic. She was beginning to forget names and struggle with simple tasks at her job, both of which were creating great anxiety. We helped her reform her diet and

that lasted late into the night. There I met pastors, business leaders, mayors, and policymakers. I told them how important communities were to healthy living. A city with walking spaces helps encourage exercise. Residents should have access to fresh fruits and vegetables, if not from grocery stores then from community gardens. Stress reduction can be taught in churches and schools. Leaders can support cognitive health by improving the daily lives of their fellow residents.

I realized through attending these meetings that there was a lot of confusion and lack of knowledge, but also many dedicated people who wanted to help. I wondered how best to share information about the importance of lifestyle and the insights from our clinic. After more meetings and passionate discussions, I decided to form the Healthy Minds Initiative. We held our first "Healthy Living, Healthy Aging" conference in Loma Linda in September of 2013 with the objective of spreading awareness about cognitive health and lifestyle. The conference tagline was: "Health care doesn't start in the hospital, it starts in your living room."

after three months, her HbA1c had plummeted to 6. Even more shockingly, she said her brain fog had lifted. Another patient started walking around his neighborhood each morning and reported that he was thinking more clearly than he had in decades. A follow-up neuropsychological test confirmed that his memory had in fact improved. One woman in the early stages of cognitive decline was suffering from white matter disease (deterioration of white matter, a type of brain tissue). One year after she adopted a plant-based diet, an MRI revealed improvements in the size of her hippocampus. Our patients were showing us over and over that lifestyle could not only slow the progression of Alzheimer's disease, but even reverse cognitive symptoms. Lifestyle was not just prevention: it was a potential treatment.

We now have hundreds of these remarkable stories, many of which

AYESHA: THE NEUROLOGIST-CHEF

In working with patients during my stroke and epidemiology fellowship at Columbia University, I realized that behind all the science, behind all the statistical analysis and the papers published year after year in well-respected journals, is the plate of food on the table. The biggest factor in our long-term health is what we choose to eat three to four times per day. Whether I saw patients in the clinic or during a research study, we never discussed how the dietary adherence score was calculated, or the groundbreaking papers by role models and mentors like Nikolaos Scarmeas from Columbia and Walter Willett from Harvard. None of that really mattered when I was trying to convince patients who suffered from stroke or cognitive impairment or Alzheimer's to eat healthy food. They would never stick to a nutrition plan if the food wasn't delicious.

You could say that I'm pretty passionate about food. I used to watch cooking shows and wonder, *How can I make this recipe healthy?* The cholesterol in meat wasn't recommended for stroke patients or people experiencing cognitive decline. The added salt would raise blood pressure. The butter would cause plaques, and the sugar would spike insulin levels. But if I could find a way to make something equally appealing, I might be able to truly affect my patients' health.

Eventually I became curious enough to enroll at the Natural Gourmet Institute, a culinary school that takes pride in its healthy-cooking curriculum. I remember rushing to class, still in my scrubs, eager to start the next lesson. I learned how to make sauces and dressings, and how to properly cut and

we share with you in Section Two of this book, where you'll also find fascinating research on the ways in which our lifestyles promote or prevent neurodegenerative disease. As new lifestyle studies were published, and as we improved our protocol with each patient, each positive behavioral change, we became certain that the following aspects of healthy living are essential for maintaining and optimizing cognitive health:

prepare vegetables—kale is so much more manageable when it's thinly sliced and properly marinated; warm salads are sometimes better than cold salads; nuts make a wonderfully creamy salad dressing. I also enrolled in an online plant-based cooking program called Rouxbe to further my studies.

One of the things I learned early on in my clinical work was that people have a lot of trouble giving up cheese. And yet cheese is one of our main sources of saturated fat, making it dangerous if not deadly for stroke patients. I figured if I could come up with a cheese alternative, it would be a great first step in lifestyle intervention. So after many hours in the kitchen I created a queso blanco sauce to pour over vegetables, mix in macaroni, or use on any dish as a replacement for white or cheddar cheese. My plant-based "cheese" was made with cashews, nutritional yeast, lemon, almond milk, and garlic. It was free of saturated fat but contained healthy fats and other vitamins and minerals from the cashews, and nutritional yeast was a great source of vitamin B12. Most importantly, my patients loved it. I developed some original salad dressings as well, as I knew salads drenched in high-fat, high-sugar, store-bought dressing nullified any health benefits from the vegetables. I experimented quite a bit in the kitchen as I continued developing recipes. There were definitely a few failures along the way, but they motivated me to make healthy food even more delicious without compromising the ingredients. Healthy living starts with what you eat, and I've found that prescribing recipes is often much more effective than prescribing medication.

- Eating meat is bad for your brain. A whole-food, plant-based diet rich in vegetables, fruits, beans, whole grains, and healthy fats is what the brain requires to thrive.

- Physical exercise increases both the number of brain cells and the connections between them.

- Chronic stress puts the brain in a state of high inflammation, causing structural damage and impairing its ability to clear harmful waste products.

- Restorative sleep is essential for cognitive and overall health.

- Higher education and other complex cognitive activities protect your brain against decline, even late in life.

- Social support and meaningful, constant engagement with your community has an undeniable influence on the way your brain ages.

The latest lifestyle research supports our comprehensive approach to brain health. In the Finnish Geriatric Intervention Study to Prevent Cognitive Impairment and Disability (FINGER), published in 2015, participants who adhered to a diet with a greater focus on plant-based foods, exercised regularly, engaged in cognitively challenging activities, and addressed metabolic and vascular risk factors like diabetes, hypertension, and high cholesterol had a significantly higher score in overall cognitive performance than participants who received standard medical care. This was the first large clinical trial to prove that we can prevent cognitive decline using a comprehensive protocol, even in individuals at a high risk of developing Alzheimer's. Interventions like this are not only essential for long-term cognitive health but also possible for each and every one of us.

A Plan for Success

Through all these endeavors, and through working together, we've completely reenvisioned our approach to Alzheimer's. We are now conducting the most comprehensive research to date that explores lifestyle risk factors and the development of neurodegenerative disease. Our lifestyle program at Loma Linda University is one of the most sophisticated in the world—we have the most advanced imaging techniques, the latest biomarker and neuropsychological tests, and a behavioral intervention protocol more thorough and personalized than anything ever developed. Ayesha has become a recognized expert in nutrition, stress management, and restorative sleep, while Dean specializes in exercise, optimizing the brain's infinite power through cognitive and social activities, and bringing these habits into both the home and community.

The following aspects of a healthy lifestyle form the heart of our unique NEURO Plan:

Nutrition: A whole-food, plant-based diet low in sugar, salt, and processed foods.

Exercise: An active lifestyle that incorporates movement every hour—not just a stop at the gym after an otherwise sedentary day.

Unwind: Stress management in the form of meditation, yoga, mindful breathing exercises, time spent in nature, and the support of strong communities.

Restore: Seven to eight hours of regular, detoxifying sleep through intensive sleep hygiene, treatment for sleep disorders, and management of medications and foods that adversely affect sleep.

Optimize: Multimodal activities (like music) that challenge and engage many of the brain's capacities, as well as meaningful social interaction.

Using these five factors, we create highly personalized lifestyle plans—as we'll teach you to do in the upcoming chapters—instituting one or two changes at a time based on your individual resources and capacity for change. As you'll soon see, the comprehensive nature of our approach brings about a nearly foolproof process of personalized, incremental change.

How to Use This Book

Before you start implementing the NEURO Plan in your own life, we want to share with you some of the fundamental principles of lifestyle change that we've found are incredible tools for achieving success with our protocol.

Whole Body Synergy: Brain health can only be achieved through whole body health. When you address vascular risk factors like high blood pressure, high cholesterol, and microvascular disease, you protect not only your heart and kidneys but also your brain. When you work to achieve metabolic and hormonal balance to prevent diabetes, nutrient deficiencies, and immune disorders, you also decrease the risk of cognitive decline. Health is synergistic: anything that's good for the rest of the body is good for the brain, and vice versa. As you'll learn throughout Section Two, knowing your personal health risks is essential to protecting and optimizing your brain.

Personalization Is Key: A personalized program is the future of Alzheimer's treatment. We are moving toward precision medicine, an emerging specialty for disease treatment and prevention that takes into account the interplay between genes, environment, chronic wear-and-tear, protective factors, and lifestyle for each individual. Alzheimer's prevention based on these individual differences, an approach exemplified in the NEURO Plan, will be the standard of care in the future. As you read through Section Two, keep looking for ways to personalize this program based on your unique needs. Use the upcoming information in the Seven Stages on the Road to Dementia section and The Alzheimer's Solution Risk Assessment to determine where best to begin.

Keep Yourself Accountable: Lifestyle change requires focus and effort; it can only work if it's constant and intensive and results in habit formation. We work closely with patients in our clinic, keeping them accountable through personal messaging, monthly evaluations, and comprehensive workups every three months. You can do all this on your own by using the tools and techniques we offer in Section Two. Making your progress visible—on a whiteboard in your living room, for instance—can help keep you focused and motivated.

Find a Community: The most effective way to prevent Alzheimer's is by paying close attention to the way you and the people around you live. What do you eat together? How do you stay physically active together? How do you encourage a healthy lifestyle together? As you begin the NEURO Plan, we recommend that you enlist the support of your family and friends. They will help you achieve success and also learn how to protect themselves against cognitive decline in the process. Faith communities, community centers, volunteer groups, and online groups are also wonderful sources of support. We know one woman who didn't have family or friends to help her. Instead, she decided to start a healthy aging group at her church. She was so successful at developing a supportive community that we were able to implement her plan in dozens of other churches. If you're unable to find or start a community, there are countless communities online, including our own, which you can find at TeamSherzai.com.

In our years of research and clinical work, perhaps the most profound thing we've realized is this: the pursuit of cognitive health is about so much more than just avoiding Alzheimer's. Getting old doesn't have to be about mental decline. The brain can actually expand as we get older, giving us the capacity to see the world more complexly, to truly understand ourselves and the people around us. Aging can be a beautiful, fascinating process. In fact, studies have shown that when elderly individuals are in good health, they report greater happiness and contentment than any other age group.

Our goal is to reclaim the concept of wisdom. We want everyone to approach their later years with curiosity instead of fear. We want to use lifestyle not just as a shield against neurodegenerative disease but as a way of living better for longer. Our patients, and our own lives, have shown us that all this is possible. *The Alzheimer's Solution* will teach you how.

The Seven Stages on the Road to Dementia

Alois Alzheimer observed in his now famous patient some of the classic symptoms of advanced Alzheimer's: paranoia, outbursts, confusion, withdrawal. But what are the first signs of the disease? In the great majority of cases, the earliest symptom of Alzheimer's is difficulty with short-term memory (though in some variants of Alzheimer's, the earliest symptoms are predominantly visuospatial, language oriented, or behavioral). Over time the disease progresses into mood swings, disorientation, difficulty with language, and the inability to carry out basic activities like bathing, putting on clothes, and in later stages even walking and swallowing. By

THE SEVEN STAGES ON THE ROAD TO DEMENTIA

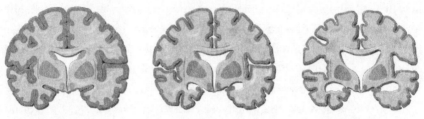

STAGE 1   **STAGE 4**   **STAGE 7**

Physical manifestations of the changes in the brain from Stage 1 through Stage 7.

STAGE 1: PRECLINICAL
Can last 20 or more years
- Appears normal with occasional forgetfulness

STAGE 2: MILD DECLINE
Can last 20 years
- Occasional forgetfulness; others may notice
- Can still do daily activities

STAGE 3: MILD COGNITIVE IMPAIRMENT
Lasts 1 to 3 years
- Forgetfulness noticed by others
- May be anxious; difficulty at work
- Can still do daily activities

STAGE 4: MILD TO MODERATE DEMENTIA
Lasts 2 to 3 years
- A formal diagnosis is often made
- Difficulty with driving
- Anxious, aggressive, or withdrawn
- May have difficulty with finances

STAGE 5: MODERATE TO SEVERE DEMENTIA
Lasts 1½ to 2 years
- Now has difficulty with finances
- Unable to drive
- Anxious, aggressive, or withdrawn
- Confusion pronounced; often forgets address and numbers
- Hygiene is now often affected

STAGE 6: SEVERE DEMENTIA
Lasts 2 to 2½ years
- Unable to do any daily activities
- Professional care is needed
- Personality changes (aggression or silence)
- Sometimes doesn't recognize close family
- Completely bound to one caregiver
- Sleep cycles severely affected

STAGE 7: THE FINAL STAGE OF DEMENTIA
Lasts 1 to 2 years
- Now needs help with all daily activities
- May become unresponsive
- Often refuses to eat
- Difficulty walking
- Little or no language
- Often loses control of urine and bowel movements
- Often experiences less anxiety

definition, a person has developed dementia when he or she has difficulty with one or more daily activities such as driving, taking medication, making phone calls, cooking, and finances.

The common denominator of all stages of dementia is anxiety. Even people in the early stages experience significant anxiety because they fear further decline. Anxiety often diminishes in the final stage, perhaps an indication of declining awareness of one's condition, or even one's self. Some researchers believe that psychological changes in midlife like increased anxiety, stubbornness, sadness, and aggression can also be early indicators of cognitive decline. Oftentimes these conditions are diagnosed as neuropsychiatric disorders, while the root cause may be brain changes associated with early neurodegenerative and neurovascular pathology.

Though the development and speed of the disease are unique to each individual, dementia generally progresses through the following seven stages. Changing the course of your health requires understanding where you fall on this spectrum. Before taking the Risk Assessment at the end of this chapter, we recommend you review the stages of dementia, as we'll refer to them throughout Section Two and the NEURO Plan.

Stage 1: Preclinical

A person in this stage has no impairment, no memory disorder or cognitive deficits, though amyloid plaques and tau tangles may be accumulating in the brain (Alzheimer's and other dementias begin to form years—and often decades—before they manifest). There may also be inflammation, vascular changes, and atrophy in certain parts of the brain, but not enough to cause symptoms.

This stage can last twenty years or longer. Preclinical individuals experience significant benefits from all aspects of the NEURO Plan. Proper nutrition will slow down the inflammatory, oxidative, and vascular damage that may have already started. Exercise will help regrow neuronal connections and increase blood flow to the brain. Both nutrition and exercise will reduce insulin resistance. Stress reduction allows the brain to heal itself, and sleep is the brain's ultimate detox. Optimizing cognitive activities will also restore and further reinforce connections.

Stage 2: Mild Decline

Some mild memory changes begin to emerge in Stage 2. A person can still do everything they've always done. Their finances, driving, and work responsibilities are not yet affected, and family members haven't noticed any changes.

This early stage can also last up to twenty years before symptoms worsen. Individuals with mild decline will experience the same benefits from the NEURO Plan as preclinical patients. Many individuals at this stage are able to reverse their symptoms if lifestyle change is implemented early on.

Stage 3: Mild Cognitive Impairment (MCI)

A person's friends and family may begin to notice changes in memory and thinking in this stage. The individual may actually be in denial and claim he or she is only experiencing mild short-term memory problems. People with mild cognitive impairment experience more forgetfulness, lose things more often, and struggle to perform tasks they could easily do before. When neurologists conduct a cognitive exam, they notice some changes as well. Word finding, planning and organizing, and visuospatial skills tend to present difficulties.

There are two types of MCI: amnestic MCI disproportionately affects short-term memory (which is processed in the hippocampus) compared to long-term memory (which is more diffusely stored in the brain and thus more resilient in earlier stages), and is closely associated with Alzheimer's disease; multidomain MCI simultaneously affects several cognitive domains (specialized aspects of cognition that control language, attention, executive function, behavior, and other cognitive functions) and is associated with vascular dementia. It is thought that each year about 10 to 15 percent of patients with MCI convert to dementia, and that ultimately up to 50 percent will convert to dementia. It's entirely possible to reverse course at this stage, even for the 50 percent of people who would have otherwise proceeded to dementia.

On average, this stage lasts between one and three years. Individuals with mild cognitive impairment will experience all the benefits from the NEURO Plan as patients in Stages 1 and 2.

Stage 4: Mild to Moderate Dementia

Patients now have more difficulty with cognition and memory. They forget some of their life histories and are unable to remember what they did over the last week. Short-term recall is significantly affected. In a neurologist's office, a person at this stage will fail to recall a list of five words. Often they're more tense when driving (avoiding the highway is common), and they've made some mistakes with their finances. At this stage, by definition, a person is having difficulty with one or more daily activities like managing finances, cooking, or taking medication on their own. A formal Alzheimer's diagnosis is most often made during Stage 4. Many of these patients withdraw, either consciously or unconsciously, because of how they're struggling with memory and managing conversations. This stage is especially dangerous because most patients are still in denial and want to maintain control of their daily lives.

Stage 4 lasts an average of two to three years. Patients with mild to moderate dementia will also benefit from all aspects of the NEURO Plan. Stress management is especially important for reducing anxiety, which is present in some form in all individuals at this stage. Restorative sleep is also very helpful for these patients as sleep patterns may start to change dramatically. By far the most important factor during Stage 4 is social activity: if patients aren't actively engaged with the people around them, their rate of decline will increase.

Stage 5: Moderate to Severe Dementia

Patients at this stage need assistance. Confusion is now pronounced, with an increasing inability to recall details like phone numbers and addresses. Hygiene begins to be affected as well: patients need to be reminded to shower, brush their teeth, and use the toilet. Sometimes anxiety in this stage can manifest as frustration and anger.

Stage 5 often lasts one and a half to two years. Just as in Stage 4, anxiety reduction is extremely important for these patients. They also benefit from cognitive and social activities that can help them maintain and strengthen neuronal connections. Regular exercise is crucial. Beginning with Stage 5 and throughout the remainder of the disease, Alzheimer's patients have three times the risk of falls and hip fractures. There is evidence that maintaining muscle strength and balance through exercise significantly reduces the chance of injury, and interestingly, even increases cognitive health.

Stage 6: Severe Dementia

Professional care is needed in Stage 6. Patients are confused, unaware of their environments, and also experience major personality changes—sometimes aggression emerges, other times a person completely withdraws. People in this stage may not recognize close family members. There's often one very close family member, usually a spouse or child, that the patient depends on for a sense of security. If this person leaves the room, the patient instantly grows anxious. In this way, the Stage 6 patient is completely bound to the caregiver. Other times, however, patients suffer from Capgras syndrome, where they believe that a familiar person is an imposter. Sleep cycles are also severely affected. Wandering can occur during this stage if the right safeguards are not instituted ahead of time (bracelets, identification, locked doors).

This stage lasts roughly two to two and a half years. Patients with severe dementia can still benefit from a diet low in sugar and saturated fats, though they will need someone to oversee their dietary plan. A simple walking routine, or exercise in the home, is an excellent way of slowing down the disease process, which usually accelerates at this stage due to general frailty. Because the sleep-wake cycle is often erratic in patients with severe dementia, sleep hygiene techniques can be especially helpful. Stress management can also help reduce anxiety, though at this stage the focus should be on creating a familiar and relaxing environment (rather than on meditation or yoga).

Stage 7: The Final Stage of Dementia

The patient's appetite is poor, and he or she has problems swallowing, difficulty walking, and little to no language—though there can be flashes of lucidity that are often connected to a patient's strongest memories and associations (more on this in the "Optimize" chapter). Thankfully, many patients at this stage experience less anxiety and aggression, which seems to be an indication of diminished consciousness, the awareness of one's self in an environment. Patients at this stage require assistance with all activities of daily living.

The final stage of the disease can last anywhere between one and two years. Anxiety reduction and functional sleep patterns still help patients in Stage 7. Even in the final years of Alzheimer's, patients benefit greatly from social interaction in a familiar environment.

Though learning about the stages of dementia may at first be overwhelming, it's important to know where you or a loved one falls on this spectrum so you can tailor the NEURO Plan to your individual needs. Knowledge really is power. And as we'll prove throughout Section Two, you can often reverse your symptoms entirely if you're in the early stages of cognitive decline, and even once dementia has started, there are many things you can do to significantly slow down the progression—often for years or decades.

OTHER TYPES OF DEMENTIA

Traditionally, dementia is broken down into reversible and nonreversible types, which are then further divided into neurodegenerative and nonneurodegenerative dementias. These categories have created a fair amount of confusion and also fail to account for the influence we have over the so-called nonreversible types of dementia. Instead, we prefer to categorize dementias →

according to the degree to which we can influence them. We do in fact have influence over every type of dementia, though the degree of influence varies.

Dementias over which we have considerable influence are associated with depression, certain medications (like those for seizures, headaches, and psychiatric diseases), vitamin and mineral deficiencies (especially vitamin B12 and folic acid), hormonal dysfunction (especially thyroid disease), infections (bacterial, viral, and fungal), delirium (due to medical conditions, dehydration, or extreme environmental effects), and drug and alcohol abuse (those due to vitamin deficiency can often be reversed; those due to significant structural brain damage and environmental toxins [lead and PCB exposure] can often be irreversible).

While Alzheimer's disease accounts for 60 to 80 percent of dementia cases and is the focus of our protocol, there are many other types of dementia that will also benefit from the NEURO Plan.

Vascular Dementia: Vascular dementia often manifests after a major stroke, but it can also be caused by multiple smaller strokes throughout the brain, or even one stroke in a critical area like the hippocampus or thalamus. Cognition, memory, and thinking are affected, and patients also seem to struggle with daily activities. Many people exhibit a slowness of thinking and movement. Vascular dementia presents one of the best opportunities for healing through lifestyle change—that is, if it's caught at the predementia stage (called "vascular cognitive impairment"). A large proportion of the population suffers from this kind of dementia, especially those with diabetes, high cholesterol, and high blood pressure.

Lewy Body Dementia: This form of dementia damages the visuospatial system, induces hallucinations in up to 30 percent of patients, and causes cognitive deficits and extreme emotional vacillation. Parkinsonian symptoms are also common, including abnormal gait, tremor, and stiffness. Robin Williams was found to have had Lewy body dementia before his death. His wife, Susan Schneider Williams, described his debilitating symptoms in a letter published by the journal *Neurology*: "His left hand tremor was continuous now and he had a slow, shuffling gait. He hated that he could not find the words he wanted in conversations. He would thrash at night and still had terrible insomnia. At times, he would find himself stuck in a frozen stance, unable to move, and frustrated when he came out of it. He was beginning to have trouble with visual and spatial abilities in the way of judging distance and depth. His loss of basic reasoning just added to his growing confusion." Williams had always been fascinated with diseases of the mind. Sadly, in the end he succumbed to one.

Parkinson's Dementia: A significant proportion of Parkinson's patients develop dementia. Several studies have investigated the connection between these two neurodegenerative diseases. One study found that 48 percent of Parkinson's patients had been diagnosed with dementia after a period of fifteen years; another concluded that Parkinson's patients experience a sixfold increase in the risk of developing dementia. Muhammad Ali, who suffered with Parkinson's for over thirty years, also developed dementia later in life, which affected both his memory and reasoning skills.

Frontotemporal Dementia: This is one of the more common forms of dementia in which the frontal and temporal lobes are predominantly affected. There are three main types of early symptoms in frontotemporal dementia: behavior (patients are often more obstinate, argumentative, and inclined to act out of character); language (patients either can't understand language or have trouble producing language); executive function (difficulty with multitasking and complex behavior). Memory decline is common in all cases. Inhibitions are lowered as the frontal lobe is affected, and sometimes artistic capacities emerge in patients who have been discouraged from creative activities earlier in life. In other patients, disinhibition can lead to drastic personality changes, including unexplained anger, emotional outbursts, and even violent behavior. This form of dementia is associated with ALS (amyotrophic lateral sclerosis), a fatal motor neuron disease: as many as 50 percent of patients with ALS have frontotemporal behavioral changes, and as many as 10 percent go on to develop frontotemporal dementia.

Normal Pressure Hydrocephalus: This is a potentially reversible type of dementia caused by a slow increase of cerebrospinal fluid (CSF) in the brain. The CSF pushes against the ventricle walls of the brain and usually causes a cluster of symptoms, including urinary incontinence, imbalance, and cognitive decline. A lumbar puncture can be used to diagnose this form of dementia. Upon drainage of a fairly large amount of CSF (40–60 cc), patients often see improvement in their gait and balance and even cognition. This form of dementia must be detected early enough to relieve symptoms before permanent damage occurs.

The Alzheimer's Solution
RISK ASSESSMENT

Now that you've learned about the progression of Alzheimer's, it's crucial that you understand your nonmodifiable and modifiable risk factors for neurodegenerative disease. We all have them, and knowing your specific risks will shed light on why you're experiencing symptoms, how you can manage or reverse your symptoms, and how to change the trajectory of your health. The goal of the following assessment is to give you a sense of how much risk you have based on your age and genetic profile (nonmodifiable risk). We'll also assess the many risk factors that you can adjust at any age (modifiable risk). We believe this second score—the result of your lifestyle choices—is much more significant than the first. Please note that a higher (positive) score indicates a greater risk for Alzheimer's, while a lower (negative) score indicates greater protection against Alzheimer's. The numbers assigned to each element below are not representative of true risk or risk reduction. We're still years away from knowing the relative weight of each of these variables in a given individual. This assessment is our attempt at weighing the risks and benefits of lifestyle choices based on our research and clinical experience. While not a perfect representation of risk, it's still a very useful tool for learning about the many factors that contribute to neurodegenerative disease.

The following questions will give you an excellent idea of where your risk lies, and how best to use our program.

NONMODIFIABLE RISKS

Age and Genetic Profile make up the nonmodifiable risks for Alzheimer's disease. Please use the information below to calculate your score for each category.

Age

The older you get, the greater your risk of developing Alzheimer's. Use your current age to determine your risk.

Age	Points
<65	1
65–69	2
70–74	4
75–79	8
80–84	16
>85	32

Our Example: You're seventy-three years old. Your risk for this age is calculated as 4 points.

_____ TOTAL

Genetic Profile

Your Genetic Profile is calculated by adding up the points for each question below. Please note that first-degree family members include mother, father, sister, and brother.

Family Members with History of Alzheimer's or Dementia at Sixty-Five Years of Age or Older

_____ Father (+4)

_____ Mother (+4)

_____ Other First-Degree Family Members (+2 for each)

Family Members with History of Alzheimer's or Dementia Before Sixty-Five Years of Age

_____ Father (+8)

_____ Mother (+8)

_____ Other First-Degree Family Members (+2 for each)

Family Members with Vascular Disease (Stroke, Heart Disease, Peripheral Vascular Disease)

_____ Father (+2)

_____ Mother (+2)

_____ Other First-Degree Family Members (+1 for each)

Genotyping (for those who have completed genetic testing; otherwise, skip this section)

_____ 1 APOE4 Gene (increases risk by as much as 3 times), (+6)

_____ 2 APOE4 Genes (increases risk by as much as 10 to 12 times), (+24)

_____ 1 APOE2 Gene (reduces risk by 40%), (-24)

_____ 2 APOE2 Genes (reduces risk by 60%), (-34)

_____ PSEN 1, PSEN 2, or APP (each increases risk, PSEN 1 most significantly), (+30 for each)

Add up all points to calculate your Genetic Risk.

Our Example: Your father was diagnosed with Alzheimer's after the age of sixty-five (+4), your mother has been diagnosed with heart disease (+2), and your genetic testing revealed that you have 1 APOE4 Gene (+6). Your Genetic Profile score is 4 + 2 + 6 = 12.

_____ **TOTAL**

To calculate your Nonmodifiable risk score: Add your Age score to your Genetic Profile score.

Our Example: Age score (4) + Genetic Profile score (12) = 16.

This number is your nonmodifiable risk, the measure of those risk factors over which you don't have control.

_____ **GRAND TOTAL**

MODIFIABLE RISKS

Modifiable risks are composed of your scores for Nutrition, Exercise, Stress, Sleep, Mental Activity, Social Activity, and Medical History of Modifiable Diseases. These risk factors are under your control and amenable to lifestyle change.

Nutrition

Select the food and drinks you have consumed daily within the past two years and add up the corresponding points.

_____ Beans, 1 cup (-2)

_____ Berries, ½ cup (-2)

_____ Green Vegetables, 2–3 cups (-2)

_____ Other Vegetables, 2–3 cups (-2)

_____ Fruits, 1–2 cups (-2)

_____ Nuts, ½ cup (-2)

_____ Seeds, 1–2 tablespoons (-2)

_____ Whole Grains, 2–3 servings (-2)

_____ Sugar, 6 teaspoons or more per day (+4); if you consume more than 6 teaspoons of sugar per day, add 1 for each additional teaspoon (1 teaspoon equals 5 grams of sugar; add 4 points if you consume more than 25 grams of sugar per day)

_____ Meat, more than once a week (+3)

_____ Dairy (1 cup of milk or yogurt, or 4 ounces of cheese or butter) and/or Eggs (more than one per week) (+4)

_____ Processed Packaged Foods (+2)

_____ Supplement: DHA/Omega-3 (-2)

_____ Supplement: Turmeric (-2)

_____ Alcoholic Drinks, 12 ounces (+2 if you have more than four drinks per week)

_____ History of Alcohol Abuse, as diagnosed by CAGE criteria or others (+6)

_____ **TOTAL**

Exercise

Evaluate your level of physical activity to determine your Exercise risk.

_____ Exercise (lifelong), at least 120 minutes per week of strenuous aerobic exercise that makes you short of breath (-10)

_____ Exercise (in the last year), at least 120 minutes per week of strenuous aerobic exercise (-5)

_____ Exercise (in the last month), at least 120 minutes per week of strenuous aerobic exercise (-2)

_____ 3 Hours or More Per Day Spent Sitting (in the last five years) (+5)

_____ **TOTAL**

Stress

Evaluate your level of stress to determine your Stress risk.

_____ At least 20–30 minutes of meditation or mindful relaxation/ breathing every day for the last 10 years (-10)

_____ At least 20–30 minutes of meditation or mindful relaxation/ breathing every day for the last 2 years (-5)

_____ Long walks (at least 120 minutes per week) in the last 10 or more years (-10)

_____ Long walks (at least 120 minutes per week) in the last 2 years (-5)

_____ Stress (lifelong) (+10)

_____ Stress (in the last five years) (+8)

_____ Stress (in the last few months) (+2)

_____ **TOTAL**

Sleep

Evaluate the quality of your sleep to determine your Sleep risk.

_____ Restorative Sleep for 7–8 hours per night for the last 10 years (-10)

_____ Restorative Sleep for 7–8 hours per night for the last 2 years (-5)

_____ Multiple years with sleep apnea without use of CPAP (+16)

_____ Multiple years with sleep disorder (+4)

_____ Multiple years using sleep medications (+4)

_____ **TOTAL**

Mental Activity

Evaluate your level of mental activity to determine your Mental Activity risk.

_____ Significant mental activity (daily mental challenges) throughout life (-20)

_____ Complex job (not merely repetitive but challenges thinking and reasoning) for more than 10 years that is for the most part enjoyable (-16)

_____ Challenging mental activity for several hours daily or daily brain games for the last 10 years (-10)

_____ Lack of mental activity in the last 10 years or more (+10)

_____ Lack of mental activity in the last 2 years (+4)

_____ **TOTAL**

Social Activity

Evaluate your level of social activity to determine your Social Activity risk.

_____ Significant level of social activity (three or more extensive conversations per week, on separate days, with one or more people) for the last 10 years or more (-16)

_____ Significant level of social activity in the last 2 years (-6)

_____ Minimal social activity (less than three extensive conversations per week, on separate days, with one or more people) for the last 10 years or more (+10)

_____ Lack of satisfying close relationships (those that result in positive emotions) in the last 2 years (+2)

_____ **TOTAL**

Medical History of Modifiable Diseases

Add up the points for modifiable medical conditions for which you do not receive treatment.

_____ Long history of diabetes (poorly controlled) (+10)

_____ Uncontrolled diabetes in the last 2 years (+6)

_____ Current hyperglycemia or borderline diabetes (+4)

_____ High cholesterol (+4)

_____ History of minor stroke (+4)

_____ History of transient ischemic attack (+2)

_____ History of heart disease/coronary artery disease (+4)

_____ History of atrial fibrillation (+1)

_____ History of chronic obstructive pulmonary disease (COPD)/ lung disease (+4)

_____ Long history of depression (+6)

_____ Depression in the last 2 years (+2)

_____ Long history of anxiety (+6)

_____ Anxiety in the last 2 years (+2)

_____ Thyroid disease (+4)

_____ Currently smoking cigarettes (+2)

_____ Smoking for more than 10 years (+4)

_____ B12 deficiency or levels in the lower range (+2)

_____ Body mass index is greater than 30 (+4)

_____ **TOTAL**

Add up your points for each category. The highest number indicates the lifestyle factor that puts you most at risk. We recommend starting your personalized NEURO Plan with this factor, and then adding the others as you progress.

To calculate your total Modifiable risk, add all subscores together.

_____ GRAND TOTAL

Now compare your nonmodifiable and modifiable risks. A high non-modifiable risk means that lifestyle intervention is especially important. A high modifiable risk means you have many opportunities to reduce your chances of developing Alzheimer's or dementia.

For a much more in-depth interpretation and discussion of your risk, please visit our website: TeamSherzai.com.

SEEING A DOCTOR

You don't need a doctor to start making healthy changes in your life, but if you're exhibiting symptoms of cognitive decline or mild cognitive impairment, we recommend that you see a neurologist. The following symptoms accompany cognitive diseases like Alzheimer's, normal pressure hydrocephalus, Parkinson's dementia, Lewy body dementia, metabolic disorders leading to cognitive decline, depression, or simply anxiety. Having two or more of these symptoms consistently means you should meet with a specialist as soon as possible.

- ☐ Difficulty finding words
- ☐ Difficulty finishing sentences
- ☐ Difficulty remembering names
- ☐ Repeating questions
- ☐ Repeating stories
- ☐ Easily distracted

☐ Forgetting to turn off lights/TV/water, forgetting to close doors, closing the cupboard more than a couple times

☐ Forgetting appointments or plans more than a couple times

☐ Having to rely on others to make appointments and plans for you much more than before

☐ Having to take notes much more than before

☐ Losing or misplacing things much more than before

☐ Forgetting where you parked your car

☐ Losing your train of thought in conversation more than a couple times in the last few months

☐ Difficulty orienting in less familiar places (more than one place in the last year)

☐ Difficulty orienting in familiar places

☐ Difficulty doing things that once came easily to you, such as cooking and driving, on more than one occasion

☐ Attention span is worse than it was ten years ago

☐ Skipping meals without realizing it

☐ Minor or major car accidents

☐ More aggressive, obstinate, and argumentative without cause

☐ Less talkative in the last few months to years

☐ Protracted periods of sadness

☐ Periods of nervousness and anxiety that affect your activities and/or sleep

☐ Balance or dexterity problems (tripping, falls, and dropping items)

☐ Loss of or diminished sense of smell or taste in the last few years

☐ Unusual movements of the limbs

☐ Paranoia (thinking people are after you or trying to steal things from you, excessive fear, or similar unwarranted beliefs that have no basis in reality)

☐ Hallucinations (seeing or hearing things that are not there)

☐ Difficulty with visuospatial skills (taking longer to process visual cues, or having difficulty with driving and even walking—despite normal visual acuity)

☐ Change in appetite (loss of appetite, inadvertent weight loss, much easier weight loss than before, increased appetite, weight gain, or an excessive sweet tooth)

☐ Difficulty with delayed gratification

☐ Urinary incontinence in the last few years

☐ Unable to do complex tasks

☐ Life seems without purpose

If you aren't experiencing two or more of these symptoms consistently but are at high risk (either nonmodifiable or modifiable), then speak with your primary care specialist about lowering your risk. Create a personalized lifestyle intervention program with the help of this book, and consider visiting the Brain Health and Alzheimer's Prevention Program at Loma Linda University, and participating in our Brain Health Workshops, retreats, and clinical intervention programs throughout Southern California.

The NEURO Plan

Now that you've taken the risk assessment and determined where you fall on the spectrum of dementia stages, it's time to support the health of your brain and, simultaneously, the health of every system in your body. The next five chapters will guide you on the road to recovery and prevention, and include the most up-to-date research on the choices you make every day and how they affect your risk of developing Alzheimer's.

As we revealed in Chapter 2, the five key lifestyle factors for preventing Alzheimer's and cognitive decline are Nutrition, Exercise, Unwind, Restore, and Optimize. Put briefly: you need to eat well, move in the right ways, manage chronic stress, create a restful, restorative sleep pattern, and optimize brain function. While this might sound like a significant life transition, we promise you a brain-healthy lifestyle will be worth the effort. Imagine never having to worry about succumbing to Alzheimer's disease. Imagine doing the things you love well into your seventies, eighties, and beyond. Imagine never forgetting names, losing your keys, repeating yourself, or relying on loved ones to take care of you. Imagine reversing the symptoms you've begun to experience, and helping someone you love ease their own symptoms of cognitive decline. We've seen hundreds of patients use our NEURO Plan to reverse what seemed to be an imminent Alzheimer's diagnosis.

Personalization is the foundation of the NEURO Plan. As the assessment showed, your risk for Alzheimer's disease, dementia, and cognitive decline is as individual as your fingerprint, and your lifetime of experience has created a brain with a now unique set of challenges, symptoms, and protective factors. The only way for you to prevent Alzheimer's is by understanding exactly what a healthy lifestyle is for *you*. To that end, here is how our program is designed:

The chapters begin with an in-depth discussion of each lifestyle factor ("Nutrition," "Exercise," "Unwind," "Restore," "Optimize") and its impact on cognitive health. We've included the latest research, important findings from past studies, remarkable stories of patients we've seen in our clinic, and intervention strategies you'll need in order to start the program. At the end of each chapter is the program itself, which features a self-assessment, detailed lists for daily success, best practices, strategies to overcome obstacles and propel you forward, and more. We recommend beginning with Nutrition, as it is the single most important lifestyle factor (but if the risk assessment revealed that another factor is important for you to address, please start there). Together, the NEURO Plan's five essential lifestyle programs will help you regain your health and keep your brain sharp and resilient well into old age.

3.

Nutrition

Food determines the fate of our bodies—how we grow, how we age, and how we die. What we eat every day creates and re-creates both our cells and their supporting structures. What we fail to eat causes deficiencies that stress and traumatize the body. Though the brain comprises only 2 percent of the body by weight, it uses up to 25 percent of the body's energy, and because food is energy, our brains are especially vulnerable to each nutritional choice we make.

We can think of food as a type of environmental exposure through which we set up the potential for health or the potential for disease. What you choose to eat creates either an environment in which the brain can thrive and repair itself, or an environment that promotes decline. Some researchers have argued that Alzheimer's is essentially a garbage disposal problem, the brain's inability to cope with what we feed it over a lifetime. Poor nutrition damages the brain in so many ways: it causes inflammation and the buildup of oxidative by-products, clogs blood vessels, and deprives your brain of the nutrients it needs to strengthen neurons, their connections, and critical support structures.

Because of its fundamental role in sustaining and regenerating the body, food is the single greatest tool we have in the fight against Alzheimer's. As lifestyle physicians and researchers, we cannot overstate the importance of food for brain health: it is by far the most important lifestyle factor. The dietary choices we make every day influence the prevention, delay, or progression of cognitive decline. Our clinical research has shown again and again, with patients of all ages and degrees of neurodegenerative disease, that adhering to a brain-healthy diet results in better cognition. It's that simple.

Or is it? We all know we should eat "healthy." We know that vegetables are a better choice than cake, that we should avoid sodas and sugary drinks and anything called "fast food." Most of us know that the steady increase in our consumption of processed foods over the past fifty years has led to an epidemic of obesity, heart disease, and diabetes. But many of us don't understand the direct connection between food and the brain. As we stated in Chapter 1, there is an assumption—perpetuated by scientists, researchers, and even doctors—that the brain is too complex to be influenced by our daily actions, that it's somehow not part of the physical body. Many of our patients accept that diets heavy in saturated fat contribute to cardiovascular disease. Alcohol consumption poisons the liver. Studies have proven that smoking causes lung cancer. Yet most patients have trouble accepting that the cognitive symptoms they're experiencing could be the result of something as simple as food. Clearly articulating the connection between food and brain health is the main goal of this chapter and the personalized plan that follows. As we'll argue in the coming pages, the brain is damaged exponentially by poor nutritional choices, more so than all other bodily systems given how hard it works, how much energy it consumes, and how much waste it's responsible for clearing. This chapter will prove that cognitive health is intrinsically linked to overall health, and when we fail to nourish our bodies, we also fail to nourish our brains. The inverse is true as well: giving our bodies the right foods protects and strengthens our brains.

Nutrition is unique in that it creates more anxiety and confusion than any other lifestyle factor in the NEURO Plan. With all of the overwhelming and contradictory information about nutrition, it might seem nearly impossible to come up with a plan that you feel confident is contributing to your overall health, let alone your brain health. One website tells you to cut out carbohydrates. Your doctor, in a hurried appointment without much time for questions, says you should eat less meat—but how much is "less"? Then you read a book that says some, but not all carbohydrates, are essential. A good friend tells you that fat is now considered healthy.

A magazine article claims that vegetarian diets don't provide all the protein you need. Despite your frustrations and your very busy life, you do the best you can. You adopt a heart-healthy diet. You try to lose weight. You make a concerted effort to eat more vegetables and buy fewer prepackaged foods, and hope that will be enough. If you're in the midst of this struggle yourself, you've come to the right place. This chapter offers a clear, science-based approach to brain-healthy eating that has helped our patients prevent and reverse the debilitating symptoms of cognitive decline. Though current research points to an ideal diet for brain health—a whole-food, plant-based, low-sugar diet with little meat and dairy—numerous studies have also proven that incremental steps toward brain-healthy eating have tremendous benefits. Please keep this important concept in mind as you read. The goal is not necessarily to eat perfectly for the brain but to figure out the best, most sustainable diet for you based on verified research and your unique circumstances.

Evelyn

The unfortunate reality when it comes to nutrition is that few of us are eating in a way that maximizes the health and resilience of our brains. When we encounter patients who know they have a poor diet—fast food, pizza, pastries, prepackaged desserts, and soda, one of the most common offenders—our work is fairly straightforward. These patients accept that their diet has some room for improvement and is likely affecting their health. More often than not, however, we meet people who've done their own research on nutrition and have made conscious decisions about what to eat every day. They've read books and articles and consider themselves well informed. They go vegan, Paleo, or gluten-free. They think their diets are healthy, that they're making the right nutritional choices for their bodies, and yet they're still experiencing cognitive decline and other health issues. In these cases, our work as physicians is twofold: we first need to inform these patients as to why their chosen diet isn't supporting their cognitive health, and then show them how to adopt the dietary patterns that are proven to protect the brain against decline and disease.

Take Evelyn, for instance. She came to see Ayesha after experiencing depression, anxiety, and memory impairment. The memory decline had taken place over a two-year period but had accelerated recently. Evelyn was a sixty-one-year-old attorney whose work required her to travel frequently, meet many new people, and engage in high-energy conversations. She had always been authoritative, in control, and extremely capable. But lately she felt a nagging sense of confusion and exhaustion. She was more irritable than she'd ever been. She was second-guessing her decisions, tacking notes on her refrigerator so she wouldn't forget meetings and phone calls. She lost her first house key, then her second house key, which she later found in the freezer. Remembering names had always been a source of pride for Evelyn—she knew that learning people's names was one of the most powerful skills in business. But in the past few months she'd forgotten the names of two important clients. Then there was a big presentation she gave to a group of colleagues from London. She prepared diligently, as she always had. Despite the stress and anxiety she felt, Evelyn knew how to stay both focused and calm. The presentation got off to a great start, but about halfway through she blanked and couldn't find her place. She struggled through her notes and, after a very tense minute, regained her composure. A few minutes later it happened again: a total blank. Evelyn had never experienced anything like this before. It wasn't anxiety—she was used to high-pressure environments. Something else was going on.

In the office that first afternoon, Ayesha noted that Evelyn looked listless and weak. She sat next to her daughter and did her best to answer questions about her family history of Alzheimer's, but she had great trouble focusing. Evelyn had been diligent about her yearly physicals. She'd been told by her primary care physician that she had fluctuating blood pressure (but didn't have hypertension), borderline diabetes, and cholesterol that was high but didn't yet require medication. Her doctor's recommendation was to reduce carbohydrates and eat more protein. Ayesha asked about her diet, what an average breakfast, lunch, and dinner looked like. Both Evelyn and her daughter seemed dismayed. "I know my diet," Evelyn said flatly. "I'm doing well with food."

This is the kind of reaction we see almost every time we ask about nutrition. Patients don't want to talk about their diets, especially if they've done some research and are convinced they're eating well. Instead, they arrive at our clinic hoping for a pill that can cure their cognitive symptoms. They want some kind of medication and routinely come to appointments armed with lists of drugs and supplements they've found online. What they don't know at the time, but what we teach them through our program, is that the best medication for your cognitive symptoms is lifestyle, and in particular, nutrition. The effects of nutrition are exponentially greater than any pill, especially for chronic diseases of aging like Alzheimer's. Lifestyle, with nutrition foremost, is the only kind of medicine that has been proven to reduce and even reverse cognitive decline. This is why food is an integral part of our unique approach, and the first lifestyle factor we present in the NEURO Plan.

Evelyn reluctantly agreed to go through her diet with Ayesha. Based on the research she'd done, Evelyn had adopted a high-fat, low-carbohydrate Paleo diet. This dietary pattern stems from the hypothesis that our Paleolithic genes aren't compatible with modern living. Therefore, the Paleo theory goes, we should eat what our ancestors ate (a diet rich in vegetables, fruits, nuts, roots, and meat), and avoid dairy, grains, legumes, processed oils, sugar, alcohol, and coffee. While we agree that anyone can benefit from eating more whole, unprocessed foods, especially vegetables, fruits, and nuts, the reality is that many people following the Paleo diet eat large quantities of meat and other foods laden with saturated fats. This misinterpretation of the original Paleo philosophy is something we encounter almost daily. In Evelyn's case, she mainly ate red meat, fish, chicken, eggs, vegetables, and "once in a while" she had dessert. She ate little fruit because she was concerned about the sugar affecting her blood glucose levels. She had also cut out potatoes and other high-carb vegetables as well as legumes like beans and lentils. Evelyn was a very disciplined person. She'd stuck to her eating plan religiously for the last three years and even lost fifteen pounds. She had made such an investment in time and lifestyle change that she was convinced her diet was helping and that her problems were being caused by something else. Despite her best intentions and efforts, Evelyn was wrong.

Meat Consumption and the Brain

Here is the truth about diets high in meat: they unequivocally contribute to cognitive decline. A 1993 study at Loma Linda University called "The Incidence of Dementia and Intake of Animal Products," the same study that first led us to investigate the Loma Linda population over a decade ago, found that in a group of over 3,000 subjects, those who ate meat—including those who ate only poultry and fish—had twice the risk of developing dementia compared to vegetarians. This same troubling association between meat and chronic disease has been found repeatedly for heart disease, cancer, and diabetes. Meanwhile, numerous epidemiological studies have shown that minimizing animal products has the opposite effect: people who consume a diet rich in leafy greens, vegetables, fruits, and nuts (with minimal red meat and dairy) are at the lowest risk for Alzheimer's compared to people who consume fewer plants and more fatty animal products. In a new study published in 2017, researchers at Columbia University found that participants who ate a plant-based diet had a lower risk of cognitive decline over a span of six years compared to those who ate a standard American diet.

Why are the differences in health outcomes so stark? What about meat could be causing these effects?

Research over the years has shown that both cholesterol and saturated fat in meat, eggs, and dairy are closely associated with the degeneration typical of Alzheimer's disease. Below are some of the most important findings:

- The Chicago Health and Aging Project, a longitudinal study of chronic disease, found that in a group of 2,500 older adults, those who consumed higher amounts of saturated and trans fatty acids over a six-year period had a higher risk of developing Alzheimer's, while those who ate fats derived from plants had a lower risk.

- Scientists looked at nearly 9,900 patients in the Kaiser Permanente Northern California Group and determined that individuals with high cholesterol during midlife had a 57 percent higher risk of developing Alzheimer's disease later on. Even borderline high cholesterol increased the risk of Alzheimer's by 23 percent.

- Researchers for the Women's Health Study at Harvard looked at a group of roughly 6,000 women over a four-year period and found that higher saturated fat intake was associated with a poor trajectory of cognition—specifically a faster decline in memory. Women with the highest saturated fat intake had nearly a 70 percent higher risk of negative change in brain function. Women with the lowest saturated fat intake had the brain function of women six years younger.

Along with these powerful studies that directly connect cholesterol and saturated fat intake with Alzheimer's, we also have evidence that meat consumption increases many risk factors for Alzheimer's, including high blood pressure, high triglycerides, high inflammation, and high LDL ("bad") cholesterol. As you may have realized, these risk factors are also associated with cardiovascular disease. This means that research investigating diet and cardiovascular health can also provide insights into how certain foods influence cognitive health. In one such landmark study published in the *Journal of the American Medical Association* in 2016, researchers looked at the dietary patterns of 131,342 participants from the Nurses' Health Study (conducted from 1980 to 2012) and the Health Professionals Follow-Up Study (conducted from 1986 to 2012). They found that substituting plant protein for animal protein resulted in a lower risk of both cardiovascular disease and type 2 diabetes. Specifically, they concluded the following: increasing animal protein intake by 10 percent was shown to increase overall mortality by 2 percent and cardiovascular mortality by 8 percent; increasing plant protein intake, however, resulted in a 10 percent decrease in overall mortality and a 12 percent decrease in cardiovascular mortality. The Iowa Women's Health Study also found an inverse association between plant protein intake and cardiovascular mortality—that is, eating more plants meant less vascular disease. When subjects substituted plant protein for animal protein, they experienced substantially fewer deaths as a result of cardiovascular disease. Additionally, a 2003 study published in *Metabolism* found that subjects who swapped vegetables for meat experienced, on average, a 61-point drop in LDL ("bad") cholesterol within a matter of weeks. These studies and more show that animal protein intake, and specifically cholesterol and saturated fat, damages the cardiovascular system via the same pathways that damage the brain.

But not all fat is bad. Fat is actually essential for brain health. More than 60 percent of the brain is composed of fat, and the brain uses fats constantly in the process of rebuilding cells and other support structures. What matters is the type of fat you're consuming. Saturated fat from animals clearly increases your risk for Alzheimer's, as the previous studies prove. But plant-based fats, like the mono- and polyunsaturated fats found in nuts, seeds, avocados, and olives, have been associated with a lower risk of Alzheimer's and other dementias. Omega-3 fatty acids (found in nuts, seeds, marine algae, and fish) are especially critical for brain health. These molecules are integral to brain growth and neurotransmitter synthesis and are the foundation of anti-inflammatory and anticoagulation pathways. Alzheimer's patients tend to have lower levels of omega-3s in their blood. A 2014 study conducted by researchers at UCSF found that subjects with higher blood levels of omega-3s had less shrunken brains after a period of eight years. The Framingham Longitudinal Study, the highly regarded longitudinal study overseen by researchers at Boston University, found that when individuals have higher levels of omega-3s, the process of cognitive decline is much slower. Another randomized controlled trial showed that omega-3s improved cognitive function, caused less brain shrinkage, and maintained better brain structure (specifically in white matter) among healthy older adults after only six and a half months of omega-3 supplementation.

Given all the convincing studies about the relationship between animal products, neurodegenerative disease, and vascular risk factors, as well as the research on foods like omega-3s that have been shown to improve cognition, you might be wondering why your doctor hasn't told you about any of these findings. As we explained in Chapter 1, there's a certain cynicism in medical practice when it comes to prevention and behavioral change. Not only do doctors not study prevention and lifestyle intervention, but they're taught that it's impossible. Many of them don't know about the latest nutritional research, nor do they understand how to implement those findings in clinical practice. This chapter—and the entire book— assumes the opposite. You deserve to be informed about the consequences

THE BEST SOURCE OF OMEGA-3 FATTY ACIDS

While it's true that fish are rich in omega-3s, farmed fish and large predatory fish (like albacore tuna, swordfish, halibut, red snapper, Spanish mackerel, pike, marlin, and sea bass) are also high in mercury, polychlorinated biphenyls (PCBs), and other industrial chemicals that are toxic to the brain. For this reason we recommend limiting your consumption of fish. If you must consume fish, always choose wild (not farmed) sources of smaller, less contaminated fish like anchovies, sardines, and salmon. Plant-based sources of omega-3s include walnuts, chia, flax, and hemp seeds, and green leafy vegetables like kale, brussels sprouts, and spinach. However, the short-chain omega-3s in nuts, seeds, and greens are not as easily absorbed by the body. Therefore, the best source of highly absorbable, toxin- and pollutant-free omega-3s is marine algae. Look for a high-quality algal supplement that contains both DHA and EPA (two types of long-chain omega-3s). We recommend taking at least 250 mg of DHA per day.

of your daily choices, and you deserve access to the techniques and strategies than can help you transform your life.

The existing research on the cognitive effects of consuming meat was persuasive enough for us to start recommending a whole-food, plant-based diet in our clinic, but it was when we conducted our own lifestyle research at Loma Linda University that we became utterly convinced of this connection. The striking results told a similar story about the direct relationship between animal products and cognitive decline. You'll remember from Chapter 2 that less than 1 percent of the dementia patients at our Loma Linda clinic lived according to the lifestyle practices we recommend in this book—whole-food, plant-based eating; regular exercise; stress management; quality sleep; and meaningful cognitive and social activity. This again showed us that lifestyle, and especially nutrition, could dramatically lower the risk of Alzheimer's. Ayesha's study of dietary patterns and stroke in 140,000 women also illuminated the clear benefits of each incremental step toward a healthier diet. This was an important finding as it proves that even minor dietary changes have discernible positive effects, and that each step toward better health is worth the effort. Our formal study of the California Verbal Learning Test (CVLT), also described in Chapter 2, revealed that individuals who ate a plant-based diet had on average a 28 percent lower risk of cognitive impairment. This research, along with our clinical work, provided further evidence that dietary choices could either prevent or promote neurodegenerative disease.

———————

Given Evelyn's meat-heavy diet, it's not surprising that her test results showed evidence of critical risk factors for dementia. Her cholesterol was elevated, as were her C-reactive protein and homocysteine levels (both biomarkers of inflammation). Her fasting blood sugar was so high that she had borderline diabetes, despite the fact that she had cut most of the sugar from her diet. Many patients don't realize that meat spikes insulin levels because the saturated fat overwhelms our insulin receptors. That is, meat can raise our blood sugar just as much as pure sugar. Ayesha also conducted a neuropsychological assessment and found that while Evelyn's short-term memory was impaired, her focus and attention were even worse.

"But what about the books I read?" Evelyn asked after Ayesha shared these results. "I thought I was doing something good for my brain," she said, clearly frustrated.

Ayesha explained that popular books, like those about the Paleo diet, can be persuasive, despite the overwhelming evidence we have for the benefits of whole-food, plant-based diets. The most important thing is to look carefully at the research and claims. Historically, the Paleo diet was consumed at a time when the average human life span was twenty to thirty years. For millions of years, and for more than 99.99 percent of our existence, the goal was to pass on your genes early and then die so that the ecosystem, which had limited resources, would be sustained for the next generation. There was no incentive to live past the point of reproduction, and there was certainly no incentive to live well into your nineties without developing chronic diseases of aging. Yet we're now pushing the boundar-

COCONUT OIL

Many of our patients ask us whether coconut oil is healthy for the brain. Our answer is no. Coconut oil is a rare plant oil that contains saturated fat. It also increases LDL ("bad") cholesterol. Because vascular health is so critical to cognitive health, we strongly recommend plant and nut fats, which are packed with monounsaturated fatty acids that actually decrease cholesterol levels. Several years ago there emerged some anecdotal evidence for coconut oil's ability to slow the progression of Alzheimer's. Dr. Mary Newport, a pediatrician, decided to give coconut oil to her husband who was suffering from Alzheimer's. She claimed, through observation, that the oil helped, but this claim has never been validated in any legitimate scientific studies. Researchers are currently studying the effects of medium-chain fatty acids (a component of coconut oil) on the brain, but again, we have yet to find strong evidence. If you're eating for brain health, it's best to choose mono- and polyunsaturated fats from nuts, seeds, avocados, olives, and other plants, all of which have been scientifically proven to protect against cognitive decline in numerous studies.

ies of longevity and seeing the unfortunate consequences of lifelong diets high in cholesterol and saturated fat. While meat may provide us with a quick burst of energy, we simply aren't designed to process it in a way that protects our long-term health. Back in the Paleolithic period, we weren't great hunters—there are many animals that can outrun us, and we're not terribly skilled at climbing trees. Plants were much easier for us to harvest and eat, and so we evolved to digest plants much more efficiently than animal fats. Researchers have also pointed out that the original Paleo diet looked at eating patterns of humans within the last two million years—but we've been evolving for twenty-five million years. When you consider the other 90 percent of our evolution, it turns out that 95 percent of our diet was plants. We're all plant eaters by design. Because we didn't evolve to eat meat two or three times per day, we are especially vulnerable to cholesterol and saturated fats.

Landmark studies on Inuit populations have also dispelled long-standing myths about the purported health and longevity of meat eaters. The popular misconception is that Eskimos live longer and have lower rates of heart disease despite a low-carbohydrate diet comprised almost exclusively of meat and fish. But researchers from the National Institute of Public Health in Greenland teamed up with Canadian scientists and discovered something different. Autopsy analyses showed that the Inuits suffered significantly from atherosclerosis and heart disease. In the groundbreaking paper published in the *Canadian Journal of Cardiology*, these researchers concluded that the Inuit had a greater incidence of mortality from heart disease than other Western populations, and that a more modern diet and lifestyle actually reduced their heart disease mortality rates. Numerous other studies confirm these findings: a long-term diet heavy in meat both makes us sick and shortens our lives.

After hearing all this, Evelyn was more open to dietary change—but she didn't know where to start. Ayesha told her that part was easy, thanks to the remarkable research we have on diets that are scientifically proven to prevent cognitive decline. Plants are the foundation of all healthy diets that have been studied and evaluated for brain health, and a whole-food, plant-based diet is the gold standard. Plant-centered diets first captured the attention of the scientific community in the 1950s when epidemiologist Ancel Keys studied populations in Spain, France, Italy, and Greece and found that people who lived near the Mediterranean Sea had a very low risk for diseases of aging (heart disease, cancer, and dementia), often living well into their eighties and nineties. Keys looked at other lifestyle practices but concluded that diet was by far the biggest contributing factor to their overall health. The diet in the Mediterranean region was composed of mostly vegetables, legumes, fruits, whole grains, nuts, and seeds. The main source of fat was olive oil. Fish was consumed roughly once a week; meat was consumed only once or twice a year.

Now, nearly seventy years later, we have dozens of publications attesting to the Mediterranean diet's effects on dementia and cognitive decline, and this research shows that most, if not all, of the diet's benefits are attributable to its plant components. Higher adherence to the Mediterranean diet is associated with a reduced risk of Alzheimer's disease in multiple studies;

IS ORGANIC PRODUCE BETTER?

Organic fruits and vegetables may be somewhat healthier than nonorganic produce in terms of nutrient density and pesticide levels, but the data so far doesn't appear to be very significant for cognitive health. If you can find and afford organic produce, by all means make it a large part of your diet. But under no circumstances should you drastically cut down on produce just because organic options aren't available. Fruits and especially vegetables are the foundation of a brain-healthy diet—no matter how they were grown.

---

the higher the adherence to the diet, the lower the risk of dementia. In one study, Columbia University researchers examined the effects of the Mediterranean diet in patients with mild to moderate Alzheimer's. They found that those who adopted the Mediterranean diet had lower mortality and better quality of life. The chance of dying from Alzheimer's was up to 73 percent lower among those who strongly adhered to the diet, as opposed to 35 percent lower for those who only moderately adhered to the diet. After ten years, 90 percent of the people in the low-adherence group had died. At the end of the twelve-year study, researchers found that those who adhered to the diet lived an average of four more years.

Two other diets—both variations on the original Mediterranean diet—have also been shown to decrease the risk of cognitive decline. In the 1990s, the National Institutes of Health developed a diet for people suffering from hypertension. It was called DASH: the Dietary Approach to Stop Hypertension. This low-sodium diet stressed a high intake of plant foods, fish, poultry, whole grains, and low-fat dairy products. When the DASH diet was evaluated in a clinical trial with 124 subjects who had high blood pressure, researchers found those on the diet had better memory, reasoning, planning, and problem-solving skills compared to those eating a Western diet. The MIND diet is a hybrid of the Mediterranean and DASH diets and was developed by an epidemiologist at Rush University in Chicago. It features brain-healthy foods like green leafy vegetables, berries, nuts, beans, whole grains, and olive oil and restricts red meat, butter, margarine, cheese, sugar, salt, and any fried or fast food. According to the MIND diet, whole grains should be eaten three times a day; berries at least three times a week; and beans every other day. In a study that involved almost a thousand people between the ages of fifty-eight and ninety-eight, strict adherence to the MIND diet resulted in a 53 percent reduction in risk for Alzheimer's. Even moderate adherence to the diet was associated with a 35 percent risk reduction, proving yet again that each step toward a healthy diet protects you against cognitive decline. Participants who showed high adherence to the diet had cognitive functioning equivalent to a person who was seven and a half years younger. This dramatic reduction in Alzheimer's risk didn't even include exercise or any of the other lifestyle factors implicated in cognitive decline. There's also growing evidence that the MIND and Mediterranean diets are associated with slower progression of cognitive decline. Recent studies have concluded that the two most critical aspects of these diets in terms of brain health are high vegetable consumption and the ratio of unsaturated to saturated fats (plant fats to animal fats). Overall, research shows that a whole-food, plant-based diet has the greatest effect on cognitive health.

POULTRY VS. RED MEAT

Some people think that switching from red meat to poultry will afford them the benefits of a vegetarian diet. White meat is much healthier than red meat, right? It turns out that poultry is one of our main sources of saturated fat and cholesterol. One study showed that when people switch from red meat to white meat, there is no significant lowering of their LDL ("bad") cholesterol. Another study found that people who ate roughly 20 grams of chicken per day (the amount of meat in one chicken nugget, or the equivalent of a single chicken breast once every two weeks) had a significantly greater increase in their BMI (Body Mass Index). Poultry, just like red meat, increases your risk for both vascular disease and dementia.

Evelyn agreed to try the MIND diet, but she needed Ayesha's help in reducing her intake of meat. Together they made a list of the meat products Evelyn consumed on a daily basis. She ate eggs with bacon for breakfast, chicken breast or a chicken sandwich for lunch, and usually a plate of cheese, some vegetables, and sandwich meats for dinner (most often ham and turkey). Though bacon is a processed meat that Ayesha knew should be removed from Evelyn's diet, it was also Evelyn's favorite food. Cutting favorite foods right away can be frustrating to the point where a patient might abandon the diet altogether. So Ayesha started by eliminating sandwich meats instead, knowing that intervening step by step would make the process sustainable and also yield results. In their place, Evelyn was asked to add a serving of beans or lentils, which are high in both protein and fiber, and a cup of whole grains (brown rice, barley, quinoa, or any whole grain she liked). She was also encouraged to eat low-glycemic vegetables as much as possible—cauliflower, broccoli, carrots, asparagus, kale, artichokes, and sweet potatoes. Evelyn had lost one food item, but she'd gained three others. This is one of our main philosophies when it comes to dietary change: don't just take things away—add healthy and tasty replacements. If after several weeks Evelyn found it relatively easy to adjust to this initial change, she could then cut out chicken breast, again swapping in beans, grains, and vegetables in its place. She was to move slowly and methodically so that she could measure her progress.

Ayesha also gave Evelyn the following list of twenty scientifically proven brain-nourishing foods and ten foods we know increase your risk for Alzheimer's. She was encouraged to refer to this list as she took steps to reform her diet.

Top Twenty Brain-Nourishing Foods

Avocados: This fruit is packed with monounsaturated fats that support brain structure and blood flow.

Beans: Beans are high in antioxidants, phytonutrients, plant protein, iron, and other minerals, and have been shown to increase longevity and reduce the risk of stroke (one of the four most common neurodegenerative diseases that shares risk factors with dementia). Beans can lower cholesterol and regulate blood glucose even many hours after being consumed—hence the phrase, "second meal effect" (where certain foods affect blood sugar and insulin levels during subsequent meals).

Blueberries: In a Harvard longitudinal study conducted on 16,000 nurses, the consumption of berries, especially blueberries and strawberries, was associated with a lower risk of cognitive decline. Specifically, the study suggested that regular consumption of berries delayed cognitive decline by two and a half years.

Broccoli: Rich in lutein and zeaxanthin, carotenoid antioxidants that can cross the blood-brain barrier and reverse damage caused by free radicals and normal aging. A large study at Harvard Medical School of over 13,000 women found that those participants who ate more cruciferous vegetables like broccoli had less age-related memory decline.

Coffee: The caffeine in coffee is an adenosine receptor antagonist, which stimulates the production of acetylcholine, a known neuroprotective agent in the brain. Coffee also contains potent antioxidants in the form of polyphenols and chlorogenic acid.

Dark Chocolate: Dark unprocessed cocoa or cacao nibs, the purest forms of chocolate, are incredible sources of flavanol phytonutrients that have been shown to relax arteries and help supply oxygen and nutrients to the brain. In fact, people who eat dark chocolate have a lower risk of stroke.

Extra-Virgin Olive Oil: In small amounts as a replacement for saturated fats, excellent source of monounsaturated fatty acids and polyphenols.

Flax Seed: Contains the highest amount of plant-based omega-3 fatty acids that have been shown to decrease inflammation and reduce LDL ("bad") cholesterol levels. Flax also contains lignans, chemical compounds that protect blood vessels from inflammatory damage.

Herbal Tea: Mint, lemon balm, and hibiscus teas are the three most anti-inflammatory beverages available. Iced herbal tea (with added stevia or erythritol for sweetness) can easily replace sugary drinks in the summer.

Herbs: Fresh or dried herbs like cilantro, dill, rosemary, thyme, oregano, basil, mint, and parsley contain ten times the antioxidants of nuts and berries. Even a small amount boosts your daily antioxidant consumption.

Leafy Greens: A rich source of polyphenols (plant-derived antioxidants that fight free radicals), folic acid, lutein, vitamin E, and beta carotene, all nutrients that are associated with brain health.

Mushrooms: Whether they're fresh, dried, or powdered, mushrooms improve overall immunity and reduce inflammation in the blood vessels of the brain. Cremini mushrooms are an excellent plant source of vitamin B12, which is linked to a lowered risk of Alzheimer's disease.

Nuts: Nuts provide the highest source of healthy unsaturated fats, which have been shown to reduce the risk of Alzheimer's in multiple studies.

Omega-3 Fatty Acids (derived from algae): High-powered, plant-based omega-3s that reduce inflammation and boost the immune system.

Quinoa: One of the most nutrient-rich foods. Quinoa is the only grain that's a complete protein source (most grains lack the amino acids leucine and isoleucine). It also contains ample fiber, vitamin E, and minerals like zinc, phosphorus, and selenium, all essential building blocks for brain cells and their supporting structures.

Seeds (Chia, Sunflower): High in vitamin E and other brain-boosting minerals.

Spices: Spices contain the highest amounts of antioxidants per ounce compared to any other food and are excellent at supporting the brain's innate detox systems. Both spices and herbs like cinnamon, cloves, marjoram, allspice, saffron, nutmeg, tarragon, and others should be a regular part of our diet, not just a once-in-a-while addition.

Sweet Potatoes: Packed with phytonutrients, fiber, vitamins A and C, and minerals, this tuber actually has the ability to regulate blood sugar. Its anti-inflammatory effects have also been documented in numerous studies.

Tea: Green tea contains green tea catechin, another polyphenol that activates toxin-clearing enzymes.

Turmeric: Curcumin, an extract of turmeric, is an antioxidant, anti-inflammatory, and antiamyloid powerhouse. In studies of both animals and humans, curcumin has been shown to have a direct effect in reducing beta-amyloid.

Whole Grains: Packed with cholesterol-lowering fiber, complex carbohydrates, protein, and B vitamins. The starch in whole grains like oats, buckwheat, millet, teff, sorghum, and amaranth is the most beneficial type of complex carbohydrate: it both feeds good bacteria in the gut and provides an excellent source of sustained energy for the brain.

Top Ten Foods to Avoid

Processed Foods: Chips, cookies, frozen dinners, and white bread are all high in salt, sugar, and saturated fats that clog the brain's arteries and directly damage brain tissue.

Processed Meats: Meats like pastrami, salami, bacon, and hot dogs are filled with preservatives, salt, and saturated fats that promote inflammation and damage blood vessels in the brain.

Red Meat: Farmed or grass-fed beef and wild game meat are high in inflammatory saturated fats. They may cause less inflammation than processed meats, but they still result in considerable damage at the vascular and cellular levels.

Chicken: The main source of cholesterol in the standard American diet. Chicken contains three times more fat than protein and is a major contributor to obesity.

Butter and Margarine: High in saturated and trans fats that clog arteries and shrink the brain.

Fried Food and Fast Food: High in trans fats that reduce brain volume, contributing to cognitive decline.

Cheese: High in saturated fat. Damages blood vessels in the brain.

Pastries and Sweets: High in sugar. Cause inflammation and brain burn-out.

Sugary Drinks: The main source of sugar in the standard American diet. Causes inflammation and neuronal damage.

Excessive Alcohol: Alcohol is neurotoxic and directly damages brain cells.

When Evelyn returned to Ayesha's office two months later, she was a completely different woman. She was more energized, and her focus and attention had improved significantly. A second set of labs revealed that Evelyn's blood pressure had dropped and her LDL cholesterol had plummeted by 50 points. Her inflammatory markers (C-reactive protein and homocysteine) had also gone down significantly, and her HbA1c (a measure of average blood sugar over a period of three months) had dropped by 20 percent. As a result of her new diet, she'd also lost 10 pounds. Her daughter said that the whole family had noticed Evelyn's improvement. Evelyn herself was shocked by how much energy she had. She told Ayesha she'd been worried that eating less meat would make her tired and weak, but she felt better than she had in a decade.

Her neuropsychological results reflected the same improvement Evelyn reported in her cognitive symptoms: her short-term memory score increased by 30 percent and her attention score increased by 50 percent. She had been firmly on the road to dementia, but through nutrition was able to reverse her symptoms. These results were truly remarkable given Evelyn's condition when she first came to see Ayesha, and were a welcome sign of the potential reversal of early Alzheimer's pathology. After three more months of healthy eating, Evelyn was even more focused and alert. She said she'd never felt so healthy and mentally strong.

Evelyn kept referring to her progress as a "miracle." Ayesha explained that it wasn't a miracle at all—it was the simple consequence of nourishing the brain and allowing it to heal itself. People seem to think that the brain is somehow beyond our reach, and that affecting it for the better must be *magic* or even *miraculous*. But just the opposite is true: we make choices every day that determine our cognitive fate. It's a simple message that so many of us seem to have missed.

Sugar: The Poison of the Twenty-First Century

If we had to name a single food that plays the biggest role in the development and progression of Alzheimer's, it would be sugar. Sugar consumption has been associated with cognitive impairment and Alzheimer's disease in numerous studies as well as with many other chronic diseases and disorders including cancer, diabetes, depression, anxiety, and stroke. Sugar is often called empty calories, meaning that it contains no micronutrients, nothing of value for the body to digest and utilize other than raw, refined energy. But we don't consider sugar "empty." It has severe consequences in every part of the body. Sugar robs us of our cognitive and vascular health. It induces and aggravates all the diseases associated with metabolic syndrome, a group of risk factors for heart and brain disease (hypertension, high triglycerides, insulin resistance, and diabetes). Sugar's toxic effect on the liver is akin to the damage caused by alcohol. It also accelerates the aging process by damaging lipids, proteins, and even DNA. Sugar is one of the most destructive compounds we can ingest, and we're consuming more of it now than at any other point in human history.

In the year 1900, we consumed an average of five pounds of sugar annually. Our main source of sugar at that time was fruit, and even then we only ate what was available seasonally—and in much smaller amounts. But by 2010 our annual sugar consumption had skyrocketed to 190 pounds, most of which is in the form of refined added sugar, the most dangerous kind.

Food Trends in 1900 and 2010 by Average Annual Personal Consumption

Food	1900	2010
Sugar	5 lbs	190 lbs
Oils and Fats	4 lbs	74.1 lbs
Cheese	2 lbs	30 lbs
Meat	140 lbs	210 lbs
Fruits and Vegetables	131 lbs (homegrown)	11 lbs (homegrown)
Soft Drinks	0 gallons	53 gallons
Average Daily Calories	2,100	2,757

Source: USDA, Food Review, Major Food Trends: A Century in Review

This staggering shift in sugar consumption is a direct result of the amount of processed food in our diet—food that affords us far more calories than we're accustomed to, and far less nutritional value. Sugar is the foundation of the standard American diet, disguised as high-fructose corn syrup, crystal dextrose, sucrose, and many other scientific-sounding names. Because our food is so highly processed and refined, and because we've become so estranged from how real food looks and tastes, oftentimes we don't even realize we're eating sugar. Pasta sauce, yogurt, salad dressing, granola bars, coleslaw, and even ketchup all contain added sugar. It's virtually everywhere.

Barbara

Barbara, like so many of us, was in the dark about how much sugar she consumed on a daily basis. She was fifty-eight, the mother of two grown children, and also a proud grandmother. She worked as a research coordinator for an academic hospital and had started to notice memory problems in the past year. Suddenly she was losing notes, files, and folders. She confused patients she'd known for years. Multitasking seemed almost impossible. Her husband had noticed these changes as well. He would tell Barbara a story, and after a few hours Barbara had no recollection of their conversation. All these changes had made Barbara depressed. She felt increasingly insecure at her job and defeated in the face of an illness she believed was untreatable.

As always, Ayesha started her inquiry by asking about Barbara's diet. In the mornings Barbara had a twelve-ounce glass of orange juice, oatmeal with a brown sugar topping, or breakfast sandwiches with eggs and sausage. Lunch was usually chicken salad or a sandwich. For snacks she ate granola bars, yogurt with fruit, or low-fat cookies. At night she ate a chicken dish, pasta with cheese, or sometimes a frozen dinner that

---

THE MANY NAMES OF SUGAR

Sugar may be lurking in your favorite foods. Here are some of the many forms to look out for:

agave syrup	invert sugar
brown sugar	lactose
corn sweetener	maltose
corn syrup	malt syrup
dextrose	maple syrup
fructose	molasses
fruit juice concentrate	raw sugar
glucose	sucrose
high-fructose corn syrup	sugar
honey	

Source: https://www.nia.nih.gov/health/publication/whats-your-plate/solid-fats-added-sugars

she could toss in the oven and prepare in fifteen to twenty minutes. Cooking was difficult with Barbara's busy work schedule. She ate out three to four times a week—mostly Chinese, Thai, or diner food. A couple times a week she splurged on dessert (a slice of cake, ice cream, or pudding).

Ayesha had Barbara fill out a Food Frequency Questionnaire to get a sense of how much of these foods she was eating. When Ayesha calculated the grams of sugar per food, she discovered that Barbara was consuming a tremendous amount of sugar every day:

Orange juice (1 12-oz. glass) = 28 g

Brown sugar oatmeal topping (1 tablespoon) = 13 g

Unrefined raw cane sugar in coffee (1 packet) = 5 g

Thousand Island dressing (2 tablespoons) = 4.6 g

Granola bar (1) = 8 g

Fruit-on-the-bottom yogurt (1 container) = 17 g

Low-fat cookies (2) = 14 g

Pasta sauce (½ cup) = 5 g

Chinese takeout = 10–14 g (mostly in sauces)

Cheesecake (1 medium slice) = 35–40 g

Carrot cake (1 medium slice) = 12–15 g

The American Heart Association has set the limits for daily added sugar at 38 grams (9 teaspoons) for men, and 25 grams (6 teaspoons) for women. On a typical day (without dessert and takeout), Barbara's added sugar intake was a shocking 95 grams. That's almost 24 teaspoons of sugar a day—four times the recommended amount. If Barbara ate Chinese food, her sugar consumption shot up to 104 grams (26 teaspoons). If she ate dessert, she'd have consumed between 105 and 130 grams (27 to 32 teaspoons). And if she ate both takeout and dessert, her sugar total was 119 to

144 grams (30 to 36 teaspoons), raising her daily consumption to nearly six times the recommended intake.

Neuropsychological testing showed that Barbara had MCI (mild cognitive impairment)—the type that disproportionately affects short-term memory and puts people at a high risk for Alzheimer's disease. Ayesha also administered the Montreal Cognitive Assessment during which Barbara was asked to remember a five-item list. A few minutes later, she could only recall one item. Her blood tests revealed high fasting blood sugar, high triglycerides, and high blood pressure. Barbara had known she had elevated blood pressure and was trying to control it with salt restriction in place of medication. An MRI showed white spots around the ventricles in the center of her brain, which are caused by long-term high blood pressure, blood vessel inflammation, high cholesterol, and diabetes. Barbara was clinically diabetic despite never having been diagnosed. It seemed as if her doctor hadn't followed her blood sugar levels closely enough and had failed to identify when Barbara passed from prediabetes into clinical diabetes. As you learned in Chapter 1, both conditions put us at a high risk for dementia.

How did sugar cause all this damage? Put simply, sugar forces us to operate on too much energy, stressing and overwhelming us on a cellular level. Again, it comes down to how our bodies have evolved, and how drastically our diet has changed in the last fifty years. As a species, humans have never had access to sugar the way we do now. We can get any fruit we want in any season. We can stop at the gas station and buy a candy bar that provides us with more sugar than we're designed to eat in a month. We can start our days with processed cereal and end our nights with ice cream. All this is a far cry from the amount of sugar our bodies have evolved to process.

Sugar is nature's ultimate stimulant. It gives us quick, efficient energy. When the dopamine centers in our brains see sugar, they positively light up with activity. They recognize quick energy that sustains the human body to the point of reproduction. But quick energy isn't healthy, especially over the long term. Quick energy is for survival, the energy to stay alive through a drought, to run away from a bigger animal, to roam the land in search of food. A surge of quick energy causes systemic inflammation, which we know is linked to cognitive decline. Sugar also causes an increase in the harmful lipids that contribute to arteriosclerosis (the hardening and thickening of the artery walls), which in turn diminishes the blood supply to critical areas of the brain. A dose of sugar leads to increased oxidation as well, resulting in free radicals that steal electrons from proteins and fats, and in doing so, damage cell walls and even DNA. Our mitochondria, which produce cellular energy, are completely overwhelmed in the presence of sugar. Sugar has also been shown to disrupt our sirtuins, biological compounds that affect a number of cellular processes like aging, programmed cell death, and altered metabolism in a way that increases our risk for Alzheimer's and many types of cancer. Perhaps most important, sugar alters our insulin-resistance systems to the point that the cellular response to glucose is severely impaired. This is why many prominent scientists have called Alzheimer's "type 3 diabetes" or "diabetes of the brain."

Here's how sugar drastically alters brain function: It all starts with insulin, a hormone made in the pancreas that is critical for the healthy function of all cells in the body, including neurons. After we eat a meal, the digestive system breaks down our food into glucose. Once this glucose reaches the bloodstream, the pancreas reacts by releasing insulin to help all different kinds of cells take in and use glucose. Insulin resistance occurs when the pancreas makes enough insulin, but the cells fail to respond appropriately because their receptors have become desensitized to insulin and reduced in number. As we explained in Chapter 1, there's no way for the insulin to pass through the cell membrane and facilitate the transfer of glucose. The pancreas works overtime, but no matter how much insulin it produces, glucose continues to build up in the blood, eventually causing hyperglycemia (high blood glucose levels). When a certain threshold of high insulin and high blood glucose is crossed, a person is diagnosed with type 2 diabetes.

In the brain, insulin resistance causes neurons to starve from lack of glucose and also initiates a cascade of inflammatory stress and oxidative damage. The resulting by-products have four main effects on brain function: 1) They damage organelles (small structures inside cells) like mitochondria; 2) They impair the communication within and between

CHEESESTEAK AND CHOCOLATE—
HOW WE TRANSFORMED OUR DIET

About twelve years ago, when we first met, we weren't exactly healthy lifestyle models. Dean was a serious meat eater. He had convinced himself that a protein-heavy diet was the healthiest option, and he ate meat at every meal. His go-to breakfast was a sausage, egg, and cheese sandwich. He'd eat any kind of steak or cheeseburger he could find. When he lived in Pittsburgh, he'd drive all the way to Philadelphia just to have a cheesesteak sandwich. Ayesha, on the other hand, was obsessed with candy and chocolate. Not dark chocolate, but sweet milk chocolate—the sweeter the better. Sweets were everywhere in her parents' home when she was growing up, and during her years as a student she'd gotten into the habit of stashing chocolate in her backpack and the glove compartment of her car. She was never without it.

It's amazing to look back now and realize just how unhealthy we were and how little we understood the connection between what we were eating and how we felt. Dean was experiencing migraines at least once a week. These were severe headaches that caused vomiting and even shimmering light in the periphery of his vision. Long-term migraines are associated with cognitive decline and vascular disease in the brain, and Dean had suffered with them for decades. Ayesha knew she had an addiction to sweets. She then learned that her blood sugar was slightly elevated, putting her at great risk for developing diabetes in the future. She was also light-headed at times, another sign of distress in her glucose metabolism.

Through our work as physicians we learned more about nutrition, about the effects of sugar on the brain and the fact that cured meats, cheeses, and high-fat foods are some of the main triggers for migraines. Together we decided it was time to change. For Dean this meant eliminating red meat. When he first started, he gave himself one day a week when he could have some form of red meat or cheese because they were some of his favorite foods.

Over a period of several months, he was able to eliminate red meat altogether by adding more fish, turkey, veggie burgers, mushrooms, and other savory foods. None of these tasted like his beloved steak, but they were close enough to get him through this transition. Within the first few months, his LDL cholesterol dropped by forty points and he was experiencing far fewer migraines. Eventually he cut out all poultry and his migraines disappeared. Ayesha systematically identified all the sources of sweets in her life—everywhere she kept chocolate and cookies, the restaurants and stores she'd visit to buy sweets, the habit she had of turning to sugar at the end of a stressful day. She traded sweet milk chocolate for darker chocolate with much less sugar. It wasn't the same, but again, it was enough of a replacement in sweetness and texture to help her reform her diet. She changed her daily commute so that she wouldn't be tempted to stop for dessert. She also added more snacks throughout the day so she wouldn't be vulnerable to cravings at night. She discovered that berries offer a touch of satisfying sweetness and are packed with healthy antioxidants. Over a period of several months, she was able to eliminate chocolate altogether. When she tested her blood sugar again, it was within the normal range. She'd lost weight, too, something she'd been struggling to do since her teenage years.

Reforming your diet isn't about losing things—it's about gaining things, swapping in healthy but delicious choices for the foods we know put us at greater risk for neurodegenerative disease. For us, success with one element—red meat, chocolate—gave us the motivation to completely transform the way we ate. Do we fail occasionally? Of course. Is Ayesha sometimes tempted to eat chocolate? Absolutely. Dean still occasionally succumbs to a tall stack of fried onion rings. But we feel healthy every day, and we know we're taking the right steps to optimize our brains now and protect them against decline in the future.

neurons; 3) They prompt an exaggerated inflammatory response; and 4) They cause amyloid proteins that are normally soluble to become insoluble. Insoluble amyloid proteins can't be easily degraded and washed away like the proteins in soluble form. The result is the formation of sticky amyloid plaques, the hallmark pathology of Alzheimer's.

This phenomenon is strongly associated with cognitive decline. Remember that amyloid protein is a normal part of aging. For people with normal glucose metabolism, the protein can be broken down and removed. For people with high insulin and high blood sugar, the protein aggregates in plaques. Enzymes also play a role in plaque formation. Insulin-degrading enzyme (IDE) is responsible for breaking down both insulin and amyloid. When we have high insulin levels in the body, this enzyme develops a functional defect and can't properly do its job. It becomes overwhelmed by the amount of insulin and fails to clear any amyloid, which is its secondary function.

Numerous studies have found direct links between glucose dysregulation, insulin resistance, and Alzheimer's disease. A 2017 report on the Framingham Longitudinal Study found that high sugar consumption was associated with low hippocampal and total brain volumes. Individuals who consumed more sugar also experienced a greater loss of brain volume over the course of two years. Another study published in 2015, this one by scientists at the University of Iowa, looked at the relationship between insulin resistance and cognitive function. They found that higher insulin resistance was associated with lower use of glucose in the brain overall, and specifically in the left medial temporal lobe, a brain region strongly associated with memory. Those individuals who had the lowest glucose uptake in this brain region also had the lowest scores in immediate and delayed memory performance. In our own analysis of a large national sample—the National Health and Nutrition Examination Survey (NHANES)—we demonstrated that for every unit increase in insulin resistance, elderly individuals experienced impaired cognitive function.

It was clear to Ayesha that Barbara's sugar consumption had to be drastically reduced—and fast. Barbara was shocked to learn that she had been eating so unhealthily, despite her efforts to eat healthy snacks at work and avoid desserts on most nights. Not only was she scared by the results, but because she was suffering from MCI, she feared she wouldn't be able to make big changes in her diet. Ayesha reassured her that they would come up with an easy-to-follow daily plan. They would set her up for success, and each step she took would help her fight the process of cognitive decline.

Ayesha suggested that Barbara focus on two critical areas. The first was adding vegetables to every meal. Diets rich in vegetables have been shown to reduce the risk for type 2 diabetes. Fiber seems to be particularly

---

THE BRAIN'S GLUCOSE REQUIREMENTS

A healthy brain runs on glucose; an unhealthy brain is damaged by a diet high in added sugar. How much sugar do we really need? For optimal cognitive function, the human brain needs up to six servings of complex carbohydrates per day. Not white sugar, but natural carbohydrates bound with fiber so that the sugar is released and processed in a way that doesn't cause dangerous spikes in blood sugar.

Healthy Sources of Complex Carbohydrates

Whole grains like oats, quinoa, and barley

Fiber-rich vegetables like leafy greens, squash, and bell peppers

Fruits, especially berries

Root vegetables like sweet potatoes, carrots, and rutabaga

Unhealthy Sources of Carbohydrates

All refined sugar

Fruit juices: Juices are pure sugar without the fiber of whole fruit.

"Natural sugars": Agave, honey, and maple syrup may have a lower glycemic index than refined sugar, but the spike in glucose is similar in the brain. If our patients absolutely need a sweetener in their diets, we recommend stevia or erythritol, which don't cause the same energy surge that burns out the brain over time.

important for glucose metabolism and balancing blood sugar levels. It has also been shown to lower inflammation throughout the body. The Nurses' Health Study and the Health Professionals Follow-Up Study, both introduced in the beginning of this chapter, concluded that diets high in unprocessed plant foods (and low in animal foods) were associated with nearly a 20 percent reduction in the risk for diabetes. By increasing Barbara's daily consumption of vegetables, Ayesha hoped to reverse some of the damage caused by her high-sugar diet.

The second part of Barbara's plan was to incrementally reduce added refined sugar. The goal was simple: eliminate as much sugar as possible by using the swap method (eat this, not that). The specific instructions for Barbara were as follows:

Avoid orange juice: 28 grams of sugar eliminated. Instead, drink water, coffee, or tea.

Avoid adding sugar to your coffee: 5 grams of sugar eliminated. Use a packet of stevia or erythritol instead.

Avoid adding brown sugar to oatmeal: 3 grams of sugar eliminated. Use berries or bananas instead.

Eliminate processed salad dressing: 4.6 grams of sugar eliminated. Use lemon and olive oil for salad dressing, or a nut- or seed-based dressing (like the Lemon Tahini Dressing that begins on page 298).

Avoid granola bars: 5 grams of sugar eliminated. Instead eat a handful of unsalted roasted nuts.

Avoid fruit-on-the-bottom yogurt: 17 grams of sugar eliminated. Instead eat a banana or cup of blueberries (or any other berries).

Avoid "healthy" cookies: 14 grams of sugar eliminated. Instead eat an apple.

Avoid bottled pasta sauce, or check the label to make sure it's sugar-free: 5 grams of sugar eliminated. Instead make homemade sauces once every two weeks and freeze, or try the Red Lentil Bolognese (recipe on page 311).

Avoid Chinese food with heavy sauces: 10–14 grams of sugar eliminated. Ask for brown rice and steamed or stir-fried veggies with tofu. If you need sauce, choose lemons, low-sodium soy sauce, or sugar-free hot sauce (check labels / ask the chef).

Avoid cakes and desserts as much as possible: 12–40 grams of sugar eliminated. Opt for a bowl of fruit, or the Blueberry Crisp (recipe on page 304).

What was added:

¼ cup nuts: antioxidants, healthy fats, and vitamins

1–2 cups berries: antioxidants, vitamins, polyphenols

1 apple or 1 banana: antioxidants, vitamins, polyphenols

What was taken away in addition to added sugar:

Saturated fats in desserts and cookies

Extra salt in salad dressings, pasta sauce, and Chinese food sauces

This new plan would bring Barbara's added sugar intake down to almost zero. She left the office determined but nervous. The first two days she didn't notice any difference. On the third day, she had a headache and felt anxious and upset. She was also experiencing a mild tremor in her body, and when her brain fog was unbearable in the afternoon, she called Ayesha and said she was ready to quit. Ayesha explained to her what was happening: Barbara's body was going through withdrawal as it readjusted to a healthier sugar intake. This is common and a vital part of the body's healing process. For some, the discomfort lasts only a day, and for others it can last up to a week. She recommended that Barbara take Tylenol for her headache, drink lots of water, and go to bed early that night. The fourth and fifth days were the same. Barbara persevered despite these difficulties.

Day seven was different. Her headaches suddenly went away. She felt alert and refreshed. Barbara noticed that her attention had improved as well. It was a strange sensation, focusing on her own breathing, how her bracelet clinked against her keyboard as she typed. These sounds and sensations had always been part of her workday, but she was just now noticing them.

From day seven to day twenty, Ayesha was unable to reach Barbara by phone. She left messages every other day and wondered whether she'd pushed Barbara too far. Was dietary change just too overwhelming for Barbara? She seemed motivated but also afraid and insecure. Ayesha had a sinking feeling that she had failed Barbara.

Then the phone rang. There was a new energy in Barbara's voice. "I feel this new awareness of what's around me," she told Ayesha. "I feel clearer, and I don't feel so tired in the afternoons." She said she still had trouble remembering stories and names, but if she paused and tried her best to concentrate, she could often recall what she'd forgotten.

Over the weekend she'd been to a boutique on Long Beach Pier and had a conversation with the owner about some beautiful shawls imported from India. She was telling her husband about the shop that night and realized she never would have been able to do that a few weeks ago. She even remembered the shopkeeper's name. Her husband was equally surprised. Though Barbara missed her desserts at night, she'd found that she was sleeping better, too. The late-night sugar had been negatively affecting her ability to get quality rest. Cutting out processed food had also improved her constipation, which she'd suffered from for the past twenty years.

Barbara's labs after two months showed definite improvements: her fasting blood sugar had dropped from 124 to 93; her triglycerides from 189 to 154; and her blood pressure from an average of 145/95 to an average of 130/79. She had also lost eight pounds, which was not the goal but a fortuitous side effect of healthy eating. When Ayesha repeated the Montreal Cognitive Assessment during a follow-up appointment, Barbara remembered all five items. Even more important, she was once again comfortable at work. In fact, when her supervisor gave her an additional project to manage, she eagerly accepted the challenge. Barbara was so motivated by these changes that she started making other healthy changes in her life, like cooking more of her own food and taking meditation classes.

A year later Ayesha evaluated Barbara's memory with a neuropsychological test. Several areas of her cognition had improved, especially executive function (planning, judgment, and problem solving). Her recall scores—with and without cuing, or hints that prime the memory—had improved by 65 and 75 percent, respectively. This clear reversal of symptoms was the exact opposite of the decline we typically observe a year after patients have been diagnosed with MCI. While she still had white matter lesions in her brain, they had not progressed and her brain structure had been maintained (in the absence of lifestyle intervention, the brain

---

OBESITY AND COGNITIVE HEALTH

How closely is obesity tied to cognitive decline? A 2016 study published in the *Neurobiology of Aging* found that obese participants had reduced white matter volume in their brains. White matter is the superhighway of the brain— decreased levels mean slower signaling and processing, a prominent aspect of cognitive decline. Perhaps most alarmingly, researchers found that an overweight person had the white matter volume of a lean person ten years older. Obesity appears to dramatically accelerate the process of cognitive decline because of the stress it puts on the brain and the entire body.

Obesity also follows a counterintuitive pattern as we age. Brain changes related to Alzheimer's start twenty to thirty years before symptoms manifest, and some of the earliest areas to be affected are brain regions that regulate appetite and hunger. As a result, some people who were obese in midlife gradually start to lose weight as they enter the pre-Alzheimer's stage of cognitive decline, usually a decade before they show signs and symptoms. We rarely see Alzheimer's patients in the later stages of the disease who are obese. By that point, changes in the brain have caused them to be disinterested in food. Though a lower body weight later in life may help prevent other chronic disease like cardiovascular disease and diabetes, unfortunately the brain doesn't benefit because the underlying cause of weight loss, a cascade of inflammation, oxidation, vascular disease, and neurodegeneration, far overshadows any benefits that may accompany weight loss.

continues to shrink and the lesions continue to grow). Barbara and Ayesha worked together on a more comprehensive lifestyle plan—including daily exercise and social activities—and are checking Barbara's memory each year to monitor her progress.

Nutrition Myths

Coconut oil is good for the brain: Coconut oil is high in saturated fat. While researchers are currently investigating the potential cognitive benefits of coconut oil, given what we know now, it's best to avoid it.

Carbs are bad for you: Complex carbs are essential for the body and especially the brain, which runs on glucose. Simple carbs (sugars) create harmful spikes in energy, but complex carbohydrates—like those found in vegetables, beans, nuts, and whole grains—are good choices for promoting brain health.

A vegetarian diet is automatically a healthy diet: Not if you're eating processed soy foods, chips, and refined carbohydrates in place of meat. Data from China and India shows that diets high in unhealthy fats, fried foods, and sugar not only negate the benefits of a vegetarian diet, but can also cause serious harm.

Fruits have too much sugar: The sugar in fruits is bound to fiber, which allows it to be slowly released into the body. Fruit in its whole form is a wonderful source of fiber, vitamins, minerals, and antioxidants. Fruit juices, on the other hand, are stripped of fiber and have an effect similar to that of refined sugar. Keep in mind that some fruits are naturally higher in sugar (mangoes and grapes), while others have less sugar (berries, lemons, and limes).

Fat is bad for the brain: Not all fat is bad—it depends on the source. Animal fats are composed almost entirely of harmful saturated fats, whereas the fats in olive oil, nuts, seeds, and avocados are necessary for brain function.

Yogurt and cereal are healthy: Often these packaged products are filled with sugar, saturated fats, and harmful preservatives. In fact, one popular yogurt cereal mix contains an artificial coloring that has been linked to hyperactivity and attention deficit disorder.

Fat-free salad dressing is healthy: Salad dressing fools many people. Regular salad dressing can have more calories from fat and sugar than many of the supposed unhealthy foods it was meant to replace. The fat-free versions aren't much better: they're usually made of water, sugar, simple starches, and artificial color and flavoring. The sugar and additives can have a significant negative effect on the brain—especially on our attention centers.

It's okay to have cheat days: everything in moderation: Moderation is a subjective term—it means something different for everyone. If you were eating pizza five times a day and you decreased your consumption to three times a day, that's eating in moderation. But that much pizza is still going to make you very, very sick. What we argue for is an approach that measures each person against optimal health, knowing that each step in the right direction yields results. Often we think we're being moderate (ice cream only a few times a week, cutting back on red meat), but we need to understand what a brain-healthy diet truly is before deciding how to define moderation.

The Truth About Pills

Thomas came prepared. When he walked into Ayesha's office he was holding a large bag of vitamins that he took daily to fight cognitive decline. He reported that he was fairly healthy, though he had marginally high cholesterol and had been taking medication for the past six years. Thomas was sixty-four; his father had been diagnosed with Alzheimer's at sixty-five. He didn't notice any problems with his memory, other than some occasional forgetfulness and an inability to multitask as well as he once could. He was always the one forgetting his glasses or pen in the conference room at work. Sometimes he left his cell phone in the restroom, or his jacket on his chair overnight. He had never been good at remembering names. People at the office jokingly called him "Spacey Tom" and "Mr. Scatterbrain." Thomas played along at first, but lately he had started to believe something was wrong with him. He told his wife he was afraid he would end up just like his dad.

As his anxiety about Alzheimer's grew, Thomas searched online and found several supplements that were touted as memory enhancers. He figured they couldn't hurt, and if there was a chance they'd help his brain, they were worth the cost and effort. Each supplement said its results were based on "research," but Thomas hadn't looked at any of the sources. One of his friends also recommended a supplement he'd learned about through a commercial. This particular supplement was supposedly used by billionaires and was described in several magazines as a "revolutionary" brain-power pill. It contained specially formulated fatty acids and powder from a rare South American superfood. Thomas decided to take it in addition to his other supplements, which included vitamins A, B complex, C, D, E, K; iron, copper, and other minerals; and tryptophan, L-carnitine, phosphatidylserine, and other so-called natural antioxidants for improving memory. Initially he was energized and better able to focus, but after a month he felt jittery. He had a hard time falling asleep and would wake up several times at night to use the bathroom. He also had indigestion and stomach pain. Some of the focus he had gained was now wearing off.

Thomas seemed to be experiencing a lot of anxiety the day he met Ayesha. He told her he distrusted doctors and hospitals after what had happened to his father. The doctors did nothing for his father's disease, and Thomas feared ending up in the same situation. Still, his wife had convinced him to find out what was going on, what might be causing his forgetfulness. Ayesha assured him that she would do her best to figure out the reason for his symptoms.

Blood tests revealed that Thomas's cholesterol, while on the high end, was still in the normal range, but his C-reactive protein and homocysteine (markers of inflammation) were exceptionally high. His blood pressure had shot up twelve points since his last measure. His neuropsychological test results were normal, but he was "barely normal" in the domains of attention and complex executive function. Testing also revealed that Thomas had stomach ulcers.

Ayesha researched the "revolutionary" pill he was taking and found out that the main ingredient was caffeine (equivalent to five cups of coffee). The supplement also contained a large dose of ginkgo biloba. Thomas's jitteriness, lack of good sleep, and stomach pain were almost certainly due to the large amount of caffeine in the pills. She urged him to stop taking the supplement and instead work on cleaning up his diet.

Ayesha explained to Thomas that if he ate well, not only would he be consuming antioxidants that are better tolerated and absorbed by the body, but he would also be able to lower his cholesterol naturally to the point where he didn't need medication. She then showed him the latest research on vitamins: though some smaller studies have found a potential benefit for certain micronutrients, a recent meta-analysis revealed that no vitamins or supplements had any significant effects on normal brain aging, MCI, or dementia. In Thomas's case, Ayesha was particularly concerned about vitamin toxicity. As she told Thomas, some vitamins and supplements can be harmful. For instance, large doses of vitamin E can sometimes cause muscle weakness, fatigue, nausea, and diarrhea, and on rare occasions even bleeding and stroke. Green tea is good for brain health, but green tea extract can increase your risk for liver cancer. Vitamin A can cause dizziness, double vision, headaches, irritability, and confusion in extreme cases, and vitamin K can interfere with blood coagulation. Further testing revealed that Thomas's vitamin D levels were elevated, which can cause a buildup of calcium in the blood as well as nausea, vomiting, and poor appetite. His vitamin A levels were also high. But his B12 levels, though within the normal range, were on the very low end of the spectrum.

Ayesha decided to prescribe a B12 supplement (5,000 mcg per week) along with an omega-3 supplement, two micronutrients that have been shown to work together in the body to benefit brain health. In one recent study, a group of 266 people with MCI were given either high-dose B vitamins or a placebo for a period of two years. Researchers found that when a subject's blood had low concentrations of omega-3 fatty acids, the vitamin B treatment had no effect on cognitive decline. But for individuals who had omega-3 fatty acids in the upper range of normal, the vitamin B treatment slowed the progression of cognitive decline. In this study the relationship between micronutrients was cooperative—the presence of omega-3s enhanced the effects of the B vitamins. But this isn't always the case. Sometimes micronutrients compete for absorption, as when even a minor overconsumption of manganese can increase iron deficiency. The main point is that micronutrients are incredibly complex. We don't have nearly enough research to understand how they're absorbed in the body and utilized by the brain. But we do know that the natural combination of nutrients is critical, and that whole foods are much more important than individual vitamins in pill form. That's why eating a whole-food, plant-based diet is the best way to ensure you're getting the nutrients and vitamins you need.

Ayesha also told Thomas about prescription medications that may have negative cognitive effects. Proton pump inhibitors (PPIs), for instance, are among the most commonly prescribed medications in the United States. They're used to treat ulcers, dyspepsia, gastritis, and acid reflux, and they work by making the stomach less acidic. Though proton pump inhibitors improve the gastric function of many patients, they have also been shown to increase the chance of developing dementia by 40 percent. Some researchers speculate that PPIs affect the proteins associated with beta-amyloid plaques. Though a recent meta-analysis called this finding into question, we still believe that any medicine that affects acid production or alters the gastrointestinal environment must affect digestion and absorption of nutrients, which will ultimately affect brain function.

Statins, which lower LDL ("bad") cholesterol and are used by over 40 percent of people in the United States, may also have a deleterious effect on the brain. Despite a recent guideline claiming there is insufficient evidence that statins contribute to cognitive impairment, some studies indicate that both short- and long-term usage of statins may be associated with harmful cognitive effects. Statins reduce cholesterol systemically, a process that may strengthen the arteries and protect against cardiovascular disease but can be problematic for the brain. Cholesterol is vital to the myelin sheaths of neurons, facilitating the transmission of neural

PROBIOTICS AND THE BRAIN

A new study from Iran looked at the effects of drinking fermented yogurt rich in lactobacillus probiotics. Researchers found that drinking yogurt resulted in slower cognitive decline over a period of one year. Though this single paper hasn't yet been validated, it is no surprise to us that the gut microbiome directly affects the brain, as we know that the health of the body dictates the health of the brain. At our clinic, we're waiting for more definitive research to give us insight into this important connection.

Given what we know now, our recommendation is again to focus on whole foods rather than pills. A plant-based diet high in vegetable fiber naturally increases the level of healthy bacteria in the gut. Kimchi and other fermented vegetables are also a great source of natural probiotics without the saturated fats and sugars in yogurt and other dairy products.

---

impulses. Treatment with statins, however, reduces cholesterol synthesis and interferes with myelin formation and function. For patients at a high risk of vascular disease, statins will likely reduce the risk of Alzheimer's disease because they affect the vascular pathology that we know greatly contributes to cognitive decline. But for the general population, those who don't have a high risk of vascular disease at midlife and are able to lower their cholesterol through lifestyle change, we believe it's always more beneficial to choose lifestyle over pharmaceuticals.

Thomas admitted that despite all the research he'd done, he'd never thought to research the medications his doctor had prescribed. He was also intrigued by the discussion of micronutrients and how many of the pills he was taking hadn't been proven to have any effect on cognition. With Ayesha's guidance, he agreed to stop taking everything except for the B12 and omega-3 supplements.

Reforming Thomas's diet presented somewhat of a challenge. He didn't have a lot of time to prepare healthy meals. In fact, he had never cooked in his life. He liked eating deli sandwiches and big plates of spaghetti. He also loved macaroni and cheese and any meat-based pasta dish. There were only a few foods he ate on a regular basis: sandwiches, chips, soda, pasta, and pizza. Though he realized these selections weren't the healthiest, he wasn't motivated to make big changes in his diet.

Ayesha decided to make a list of his favorite foods. Her goal was to expand Thomas's horizons by asking, "If not pizza, then what?" She searched for alternatives that he could reasonably eat three or four times a week. Alternative meals needed to be both hearty and easy to prepare in twenty to thirty minutes. She explained to Thomas that it would be difficult to find healthy versions of his favorite foods unless he went to specialty restaurants and stores. But with a little practice, preparing everything at home

---

MORE ON MEDICATION AND THE BRAIN

The following medications have also been connected to cognitive decline:

Androgen Deprivation Therapy: Recent studies have found that androgen deprivation therapy, which is widely used in the treatment of prostate disease (hypertrophy and cancer prevention), is associated with an increased risk of Alzheimer's disease.

Benzodiazepines: A 2016 study in *Neuroepidemiology* concluded that benzodiazepine, an antianxiety medication, is significantly associated with dementia risk. More research is needed to determine the exact cause and mechanism.

Antidepressants: These common medications have also been associated with cognitive impairment. However, having a diagnosis of depression may significantly increase the risk of cognitive impairment. Therefore, the decision to take antidepressants should be made on a case-by-case basis, and further research is needed to understand this association.

If you're taking one of these medications, be sure to ask your doctor about the possibility of cognitive side effects.

---

would actually be much easier and more time efficient. Eventually they settled on three main alternatives, each with fewer than ten ingredients:

Bean and Lentil Chili in place of pizza: All Thomas needed were three types of canned beans, chili spices, and tomato sauce (low-sodium, without added sugar; recipe on page 282).

Brain-Boosting Caesar Salad in place of deli sandwiches: This salad uses antioxidant-rich kale and spinach. Instead of store-bought dressing, Thomas learned how to make a plant-based Caesar dressing with cashews and tahini (both filled with vitamin E and other minerals) blended with a bit of garlic, lemon juice, and capers. Instead of croutons, Thomas baked chickpeas once a week and used them for a protein boost (recipe on page 296).

Mindful Mac and Cheese in place of macaroni and cheese: White beans make a wonderful replacement for cheese, even for cheese lovers like Thomas. This dish was simple to prepare in under thirty minutes (recipe on page 302).

Ayesha gave Thomas a detailed grocery list so he could easily buy the ingredients he would need each week. She also recorded videos of how to make these simple recipes. He agreed to give the new plan a try.

After several months Thomas returned. He reported that at first the recipes took a little longer than he'd hoped, but after a few weeks he was able to make them all in under twenty minutes. He'd always assumed you needed special tools and appliances and a lot of time to cook something that tasted good, but this plan had changed his mind. He admitted that he actually enjoyed the recipes Ayesha had given him, and over time he was able to move further away from his meat- and dairy-centered diet. His inflammatory markers were now in the normal range, and he was able to halve the dosage of his cholesterol medication for three months, and then quit it completely after six months. In terms of cognitive health, his focus was much better at work and the side effects he'd been experiencing were gone. He had just taken on a complex marketing campaign that would have been unthinkable six months earlier. When Ayesha repeated the neuropsychological test, Thomas's scores in attention and executive function improved dramatically. This was the first time that we had seen results so striking in terms of attention and dietary intervention. By steering Thomas toward whole foods and away from saturated fats and sugar, and by optimizing his supplements, we likely averted the onset of neurodegenerative disease.

Conclusion

Nutrition is a source of confusion for so many people, but it's also our greatest resource in the fight against Alzheimer's. Whole-food, plant-based diets have been shown again and again to protect the brain against decline and disease—and they're healthy for your entire body. Cutting out refined sugar is one of the most important actions you can take as you're reforming your diet. It's also important to remember that no amount of medication or supplements can make up for a poor diet, especially over the long term. With effort and commitment, you can learn to eat in brain-healthy ways. As always, it's a matter of setting clear, attainable goals and marking your progress over time.

Your Personalized
NUTRITION
Program

As you now know, nutrition is by far the most important lifestyle factor. The following program will show you how to design your own brain-healthy diet and also offers suggestions and strategies for implementing long-term dietary change. Begin with the self-assessment below and then proceed through the program with your unique goals, challenges, and symptoms in mind. All of the recipes referenced here can be found in the Recipes section in the back of this book.

SELF-ASSESSMENT

Vision, Strengths, and Weaknesses: Assess your vision for a brain-healthy eating plan, and identify factors that might help or hinder your efforts.

Vision: What is the ideal diet for brain health? What symptoms will a new diet help relieve? What do you hope to experience as a result of a brain-healthy diet? What foods will be most difficult for you to cut from your diet, but what would you gain by removing them?

Strengths: What strengths and resources will help you achieve your vision?

Weaknesses: What are the obstacles to your vision?

1. How will you benefit from better nutrition?

Examples: I will lower my blood pressure. I'll have lower cholesterol and blood sugar levels. My short-term memory will improve. It will be easier for me to stay focused. I will have more energy.

2. What are the most important areas for you to work on?

Examples: I want to eliminate fried foods. I need to eat more fruits and vegetables. I want to eat less meat. I need to clean my pantry and fill it with healthier foods. I need some new recipes so I can learn how to cook in healthier ways. I need to come up with a plan for eating healthy at restaurants and parties. I want to eat healthy lunches at work.

3. What obstacles might prevent you from eating healthier?

Examples: My husband/wife keeps ice cream in our freezer. I travel and am forced to eat at restaurants several times a week. I often have to eat on the run and don't have healthy options. It's hard for me to decline food at parties. There isn't a health food store or co-op near my home.

4. What might help you eat healthier? What are your resources?

Examples: I can prepare a healthy breakfast at night. My husband/ wife can go grocery shopping with me and help me find healthy foods. I can take a healthy lunch to work. I can prepare vegetables in batches so they're easy to eat with each meal. I can search my neighborhood for fresh, reasonably priced produce.

5. Who can help you and how?

Examples: My spouse is willing to join me in this effort. Several of my colleagues at work are interested in eating healthier. There is a healthy eating group at my church. I found some online forums where people like me are sharing recipes and strategies.

6. When will you start?

Our Recommendation: You should start as soon possible, but only once you have identified your resources and prepared yourself for success (cleaning your pantry, for instance, or bringing your own lunch to work so you can avoid eating cafeteria food). Begin your new nutrition plan when you don't have holidays, vacations, or major celebrations. These kinds of events can present big challenges when you're embarking on a significant life change.

CLEAN YOUR FRIDGE AND PANTRY (AND STOMACH!)

Work Toward Eliminating and Replacing:

Sweets: Get rid of any sweets, sugary syrups, regular or diet sodas, processed fruit juices (without pulp or fiber), ice cream, and other frozen desserts.

Replace with erythritol, stevia, applesauce, or whole dates for sweetness without spiking your blood sugar. Try the Brain-Healthy Chocolate Chip Cookies (recipe on page 292) for an alternative dessert.

Processed Junk Food: Processed foods have been modified so that beneficial components are minimized and harmful components are added in their place. These foods are usually high in salt, sugar, and saturated fats. As Michael Pollan said, "If it comes from a plant, eat it. If it's made in a plant, don't."

Replace with nuts, fresh fruit, bean dips, and sliced vegetables for an instant snack.

Sugary Cereals: Throw away any cereal that has more than six grams of sugar per serving.

Replace with Oatmeal Amaranth Porridge (recipe on page 283).

THE NEURO PLAN NUTRITION SPECTRUM

Herbs:
Parsley, Oregano, Cilantro, Dill, Basil, Rosemary, Hibiscus, Garlic, Mint, Thyme, Sage

Black Beans, Pinto Beans

Kidney Beans, Navy Beans

Cannellini Beans

Squash

Pumpkins

Whole-Wheat Pasta and Bread

Nut Milk

Berries*

Greens**

Carrots

Celery

Beets

Artichokes

Bell Peppers

Sweet Potatoes

Seeds (Sunflower, Pumpkin)

Walnuts, Pistachios

Almonds, Cashews, Pecans

Tofu

Seitan

Tempeh

Sea Vegetables

BENEFICIAL

Lentils

Bok Choy

Cabbage

Millet

Flax, Chia Seeds

Kale

Cauliflower

Quinoa

Corn

Mushrooms (Portobello, Shiitake, Cremini, Oyster)

Teff

Broccoli

Peas

Brown Rice

Brussels Sprouts

Kohlrabi

Sorghum

Oats

Wild Rice

*Berries:
Blackberries, Strawberries, Blueberries, Goji Berries, Indian Gooseberries (Amla), Cranberries, Kumquats, Mulberries

Buckwheat

**Greens:
Watercress, Chard, Spinach, Arugula, Mustard Greens, Collard Greens, Romaine Lettuce

Spices:
Turmeric, Cloves, Cinnamon (Ceylon), Coriander, Black Pepper, Saffron, Cumin, Ginger, Mustard, Allspice, Curry

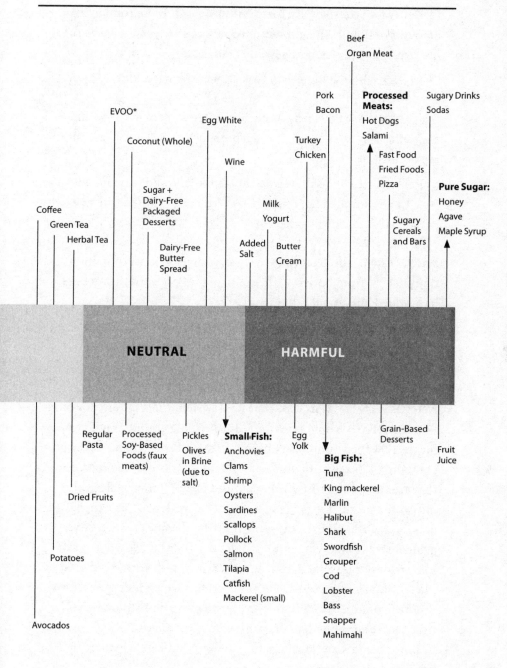

Beef
Organ Meat

Pork
Bacon

Processed Meats:
Hot Dogs
Salami

Sugary Drinks
Sodas

EVOO*

Egg White

Turkey
Chicken

Coconut (Whole)

Wine

Fast Food
Fried Foods
Pizza

Pure Sugar:
Honey
Agave
Maple Syrup

Sugar +
Dairy-Free
Packaged
Desserts

Milk
Yogurt

Coffee

Green Tea

Herbal Tea

Added
Salt

Butter
Cream

Sugary
Cereals
and Bars

Dairy-Free
Butter
Spread

NEUTRAL

HARMFUL

Regular
Pasta

Processed
Soy-Based
Foods (faux
meats)

Pickles

Olives
in Brine
(due to
salt)

Small Fish:
Anchovies
Clams
Shrimp
Oysters
Sardines
Scallops
Pollock
Salmon
Tilapia
Catfish
Mackerel (small)

Egg
Yolk

Grain-Based
Desserts

Fruit
Juice

Dried Fruits

Big Fish:
Tuna
King mackerel
Marlin
Halibut
Shark
Swordfish
Grouper
Cod
Lobster
Bass
Snapper
Mahimahi

Potatoes

Avocados

*Extra-Virgin Olive Oil

Cookies, Cakes, Cereal Bars, and Baked Packaged Goods: These contain high amounts of sugar, salt, and saturated fats and are generally low in fiber, high in calories, and devoid of nutrients.

Replace with the Blueberry Crisp (recipe on page 304).

Chips, Crackers, and Other Salty Snacks: These items are high in sodium and unhealthy fats. Again, if you like crunchy snacks, find a healthier replacement.

Replace with low-salt, veggie chips (like kale and plantain chips) with no saturated fat, crispy baked fruit chips, or the Chickpea Sandwich (recipe on page 281).

Buttery Popcorn: These products have shocking amounts of sodium and saturated fat from butter. It's better to opt for popcorn that doesn't have added butter and salt.

Replace with freshly popped, unsalted, unbuttered popcorn seasoned with dried parsley and garlic powder (or any other dried herb or spice).

Processed White Bread Products: Your pantry shouldn't contain anything that isn't "100% whole wheat" or "100% whole grain." Whole wheat means that the wheat hasn't been milled and refined and still contains all its constituent parts—like the endosperm and bran— that are full of vitamins, minerals, and fiber. "100% whole grain" means the product is made of unrefined cereals such as rice, barley, oats, and wheat. These grains are healthy (the fiber is protective against stroke and dementia), as long as they're 100% whole grains. Beware of phrases like "100% wheat," which means that the product likely contains refined wheat; "multigrain," which means that the product contains more than one type of grain and still may be processed and refined; or "heart-healthy," which usually means low in saturated fats and sodium, but does not indicate whether the bread or baked good is processed.

Replace with 100% whole-wheat bread.

Dairy and Eggs: Throw away milk, creams, yogurts, cheeses, eggs (that's right—no eggs, as one egg carries more than your daily limit of cholesterol, up to 235 mg), butter and buttery spreads, mayonnaise (full fat or low fat), and any other dairy-based products. Replace with nut/soy milk and nut cheeses or dairy- and egg-free mayonnaise for similar textures and flavors.

Replace with the Tofu Turmeric Scramble (recipe on page 288), Lemon Tahini Dressing (recipe on page 298), and Caesar dressing from the Brain-Boosting Caesar Salad (recipe on page 296).

Meats, Processed Meats, and Poultry: There should be little to no room for these items in your fridge because they are heavy in saturated fats and nitrates. Fish is a better choice of protein because of its omega-3 fatty acids, which reduce inflammation in the brain and throughout the body. However, farmed fish and large predatory fish can be high in mercury, PCBs, and other pollutants that are toxic to the brain. For this reason, if you must eat fish, we recommend reducing your consumption of larger fish like swordfish, albacore tuna, halibut, lobster, red snapper, Spanish mackerel, pike, marlin, and sea bass and choosing wild (not farmed) sources of smaller, less contaminated fish like anchovies, sardines, and salmon. An algal DHA and EPA supplement is also an excellent plant-based source of omega-3s.

Replace with beans, tofu, tempeh, or seitan, or try the Bean and Butternut Squash Enchiladas (recipe on page 279), or the Stuffed Bell Peppers (recipe on page 285).

Alcoholic Beverages: A few studies have found that drinking wine may have cognitive benefits, but these claims are often overstated. Those who drink socially may have better cognitive function not because of the resveratrol or other ingredients in wine, but because drinking is often done in a social context that both challenges the brain and reduces stress and anxiety. In general, alcohol is harmful to the brain. Under no circumstances should it be consumed in large quantities or on a consistent basis. Two glasses of wine per week is a good rule of thumb, but we recommend eliminating alcohol entirely if you're experiencing significant memory problems or taking medications that may have side effects when combined with alcohol.

Replace with herbal and green teas, and fruit-infused water.

Canned Soups and Noodle Packets/Cups: One serving could contain a day's worth of sodium! If you must have packaged soups, please opt for those that contain no more than 300 mg of sodium per serving.

Replace with the Tomato Bisque (recipe on page 307).

Tropical Oils (Coconut and Palm): These oils are high in saturated fats (coconut oil contains 92% saturated fat; palm oil contains 50% saturated fat).

Replace with extra-virgin olive oil, safflower oil, or sunflower oil.

Work Toward Increasing:

All Kinds of Fresh and Frozen Vegetables

Artichokes • Asparagus • Bell peppers • Broccoli • Brussels sprouts • Cabbage • Carrots • Cauliflower • Collard, mustard, and turnip greens • Corn • Cucumbers • Eggplant • Garlic • Ginger • Herbs (cilantro, parsley, rosemary, sage, mint, chives) • Kale • Mushrooms • Onion • Peas • Salad greens • Spinach • Squash • Sweet potatoes • Tomatoes • Yams • Zucchini

Fresh and Frozen Fruits (Frozen fruits are sometimes better because they're picked ripe, have fewer preservatives, and last longer. Just make sure there is no added sugar.) These fruits are presented in order of sugar content (low to high). People with diabetes or high blood sugar should always choose low-sugar fruits.

Avocados (Yes, they are fruits!) • All kinds of berries (especially darker berries like blueberries and blackberries) • Lemons • Limes • Papaya • Watermelon • Peaches • Nectarines • Apples • Plums • Oranges • Kiwi • Pears • Pineapple • Grapes • Bananas • Mangoes

Beans and Lentils (canned, preferably with no added salt or low sodium, or better yet, raw beans)

Black beans • Black-eyed peas • Cannellini beans • Chickpeas • Fava beans • Kidney beans • Lentils • Navy beans

Other Canned Goods

Artichokes (in water, low sodium) • Tomato sauce (low sodium) • Water chestnuts • Whole tomatoes

Sugar-Free Nondairy Plant Milk

Almond • Cashew • Hemp • Oat • Rice • Soy

100% Whole-Wheat Bread and Tortillas

Pasta

Brown rice • Quinoa • 100% whole wheat

Organic, Non-GMO Sprouted Tofu

100% Whole-Grain Cereals

Bulgur (cracked wheat) • Grits • Steel-cut or rolled oats

Whole Grains

Barley • Brown rice • Kamut • Quinoa • Rolled oats • Wheat berries

Seeds

Chia • Flax (whole or ground) • Pumpkin • Sunflower

Nuts (unsalted, raw, or roasted)

Almonds • Brazil nuts • Cashews • Hazelnuts • Macadamias • Pecans • Pistachios • Walnuts

Brain-Healthy Oils (in small amounts; ideally a whole-food plant is best)

Avocado • Canola • Grapeseed • Olive • Safflower • Sunflower

Low-Calorie, Plant-Based Sweeteners

Date sugar (whole dried, powdered dates) • Erythritol • Stevia

In general, work to reduce items that have too many ingredients, especially ones you can't pronounce. Consume whole foods whenever possible.

GROCERY SHOPPING TIPS

1. **Prepare your list:** Don't leave the house without it! Use the above list and *The Alzheimer's Solution* recipes to plan your meals for the week.

2. **Get in and get out:** Don't linger, don't spend time reasoning that a slice of bologna won't kill you, etc. It's easy (almost inevitable) to become illogical when surrounded by tempting foods. Figure out how much time it will take you to find the items on your list and don't stay a minute longer.

3. **Never shop on an empty stomach:** You're more likely to buy high-calorie/-fat/-sugar/-salt foods if you're hungry.

4. **Ask a trusted friend to accompany you:** He or she can keep you accountable.

5. **Head to the produce area first:** When your cart is filled with colorful veggies and fruits, you will have a sense of accomplishment and be less likely to buy junk food.

6. **Avoid the snack aisles:** Out of sight, out of mind.

10 TIPS FOR EATING AT RESTAURANTS

1. Drink water, unsweetened tea, or coffee.

2. Choose meals with large servings of vegetables or plant-based meals, such as grilled vegetables, legume-based dishes, or salads. Avoid meat whenever possible. Ask for alternatives like mushrooms, tofu, or beans.

3. Ask the server not to add cheese to your dishes.

4. Opt for a touch of olive oil and vinegar or lemon as dressing. If these aren't available, ask for the dressing to be served on the side. That way you can use less of it.

5. Stay away from foods that are drenched in cream-based sauces and gravies.

6. Order items that are steamed, grilled, or boiled—not fried.

7. Opt for brown rice or whole-wheat pasta instead of white rice and regular pasta. Choose whole-wheat bread or tortillas instead of white bread or regular tortillas for sandwiches and wraps.

8. Choose a small- or medium-portion dish. Do you need to eat an entrée? You might order two or three side dishes instead. Grilled/sautéed vegetables, rice, and beans are great choices.

9. Order fresh fruit for dessert. Ask for no sugar to be added.

10. Call ahead. Find out if the kitchen can modify menu items. Ask what kind of oil the cooks use. Most restaurants are willing to replace butter with olive oil, or suggest menu items with no oil or saturated fats.

BEST BRAIN-HEALTHY SNACKS

1. The best snacks are fruits and vegetables. Always keep cut slices of fruits and vegetables in your refrigerator in a closed container.

2. Hummus, bean dips, vegetable-based dressings, and purees. Great for adding flavor to vegetable slices.

3. Iced/hot green tea or coffee sweetened with erythritol can be enjoyed regularly.

4. A handful of nuts or seeds.

SUGGESTIONS FOR EATING HEALTHY WHILE TRAVELING

1. **Book a hotel room with a refrigerator or kitchenette:** Stock the fridge with fruits, vegetables, nut milk, and hummus. Also buy nuts, cereal, and dry bean soups low in sodium.

2. **A simple hotel breakfast:** Oatmeal or cereal with almond milk, berries, and bananas.

3. **A simple hotel lunch or dinner:** Dry bean soup made with hot water from your coffee maker (high in plant protein, low in sodium, free of cholesterol and saturated fats). Add lemon, a handful of salad greens, and some hot sauce for extra flavor.

4. **Simple snacks:** Nuts, fruit, and carrots can be purchased at airports and even gas stations.

5. **When in doubt:** Avoid meat and sugary, processed foods, and plan ahead as much as possible.

COMMON OBSTACLES

Lack of Access to Healthy Foods: Plan ahead. Don't be caught hungry and without anything healthy to eat. It's easy to carry celery sticks, baby carrots, an apple, or a handful of nuts.

Inconvenience (making healthy meals is complicated, it's hard to plan): Healthy eating is much simpler than you think. You can use far fewer ingredients to make flavorful meals. Fresh produce, beans, nuts, and whole grains can be used to make many different meals and snacks.

Temptation: Our entire brain is built around food as a reward. Dietary change isn't easy for anyone, but people who successfully change their diets plan ahead. Temptation arises from poor planning. Keep healthy food easily accessible. You can set yourself up for success by having a bowl of fresh fruit on the kitchen counter, or by bringing a healthy lunch to work.

Falling for Dietary Gimmicks: Don't fall for the next fad diet or superfood. Instead, make healthy eating a fun and sustainable lifestyle.

OUR PERSONAL APPROACH TO NUTRITION

We Make Healthy Eating Convenient

Our motto is: Plan, plan, plan. Here's what we eat on an *Ideal Day*:

An Ideal Day starts the night before! After we've put the kids to bed, we always head to the kitchen. Our workdays are busy, so we make breakfast and lunch ahead of time. It's important to prepare and plan for the next day after you've eaten dinner. Planning while hungry may lead you to make unhealthy choices.

Breakfast: We prepare oatmeal at night that we can easily heat up in the morning. We like to eat ours with blueberries, a teaspoon of almond butter, and a packet of stevia mixed in for a little sweetness. Other go-to breakfasts are Spelt Pancakes with Chia Berry Sauce (recipe on page 289) and Wholesome Blueberry Muffins (recipe on page 305).

Morning Snack: A handful of nuts or fruit. A crunchy snack goes a long way on a busy morning at the hospital.

Lunch: A Chickpea Sandwich that we've made the night before (recipe on page 281). Quick, easy, delicious. Other standards are the Black Bean Burger Lettuce Wraps with Chipotle Sauce (recipe on page 290) and the Brain-Boosting Caesar Salad with Roasted Chickpea Croutons and Nut Parmesan "Cheese" (recipe on page 296).

Afternoon Snack: An apple, or carrot sticks with hummus. In the past we would sometimes skip afternoon snacks, but then we were much more likely to drive to an unhealthy restaurant on our way home from work. A quick snack around 3:00 P.M. easily solved this problem.

After Work: This is a critical window when we have to set ourselves up for success. We're tired and hungry after work. If we don't have prepared, healthy food in the house, we'll eat something we regret. You have to know your triggers, and postwork exhaustion is one of ours. For this reason we always keep washed lettuce and sliced vegetables like tomatoes, cucumber, green peppers, and onions in our refrigerator. The dressing is simple: salt and pepper, or a nut/seed-based dressing, such as the Lemon Tahini Dressing (recipe on page 298). Dean realized the reason he previously disliked salads was because the lettuce leaves were too big, but he loves eating salad greens and other vegetables that are finely chopped. This might seem like a small detail, but small details can make a big difference when creating healthy patterns. We fill our large salad bowls and enjoy this healthy, satisfying after-work meal. It's a great way to add more vegetables to our diet.

Dinner: About two hours later we eat dinner as a family. We cook healthy food together, tell stories, or sometimes watch a video and discuss it. For us, meals are an occasion to relax, be together, and support one another in our efforts to lead a healthy lifestyle. Favorite dinner dishes include the Buddha Brain Bowl (recipe on page 298), and Zucchini Pasta with Red Lentil Bolognese (recipe on page 311).

Dessert: We make sure not to eat for roughly three hours before bed. Whenever we feel like having dessert, we eat a handful of fresh berries or a square of low-sugar dark chocolate.

We Prepare for Distractions Ahead of Time

One of our main temptations is family dinner parties. Family gatherings, especially those around the holidays, elicit very strong emotions. Whether those emotions are positive or negative, they increase our risk of giving in and eating foods we know may be harming our health. We both grew up with a tradition of beautiful family meals accompanied by less-than-healthy food. Dean's family would eat deer, rabbit, or whatever else could be hunted at the family lodge outside of Charlottesville, Virginia. Side dishes included mashed potatoes with heavy cream, freshly baked white bread, sugar-drenched cranberries, and elaborate cheese platters. Ayesha's family was focused on sweets: candy, cakes with buttercream frosting, and especially chocolate. We know there is nothing more powerful than the memory of celebrating with family and eating unbelievably decadent food. Overcoming this sensory memory would be impossible without organization and planning. Here are some of our secrets for surviving family gatherings with our healthy-eating plan intact:

Eat before you go: If you're not hungry, you'll be much more in control.

Find support: We rely on each other. Ayesha stands next to Dean as he takes in a heaping serving of three-cheese lasagna, quietly reminding him of why he has chosen a brain-healthy diet. Dean supports Ayesha when the cakes and cookies appear. He knows sweets are one of her triggers.

Bring something healthy and delicious that you can eat and share: We always bring one of our favorite plant-based dishes so we know we'll have something healthy to eat. We've been pleasantly surprised to watch our family cultures evolve over the years. The meals are still decadent, of course, but now there are many more vegetables and fresh fruits. There's even a bit of a competition to see who can make the tastiest, healthiest version of classic family dishes.

Gatherings are about family: We try to remember that the point of these elaborate meals is simply spending time with loved ones.

We Stay Informed

Research moves very quickly in the fields of nutritional and lifestyle science, though the basics of a healthy diet—whole-food, plant-based, free of cholesterol, and low in sugar and saturated fats—are well established. If you're still following the eating habits you picked up as a kid, it's probably time to do some research. Don't fall for gimmicks or blindly accept what someone else tells you. Look for validated scientific studies and use what you learn to continually improve your diet.

WEEKLY NUTRITION PLAN

Enjoy these recipes and simple snacks for a week's worth of delicious, brain-healthy food.

Monday

Breakfast:
- Oatmeal Amaranth Porridge (page 283)
- MIND Smoothie (page 284)
- Coffee with almond milk, or tea

Snack:
- Veggies (carrots, lettuce, radishes) with hummus

Lunch:
- Tomato Bisque (page 307)
- Chickpea Sandwich (page 281)

Snack:
- Apple slices and peanut butter

Dinner:
- Buddha Brain Bowl with Lemon Tahini Dressing (page 298)
- Berries for dessert (or any seasonal fruit)

Tuesday

Breakfast:
- Tofu Turmeric Scramble (page 288)
- Coffee with almond milk, or tea

Snack:
- Walnuts and grapes

Lunch:
- Bean and Lentil Chili (page 282)

Snack:
- Pear slices and almond butter

Dinner:
- Cauliflower Steaks with Cremini Mushroom Gravy (page 293)
- Sweet Potato Mash (page 294)
- Kiwis and grapes for dessert (or any seasonal fruit)

Wednesday

Breakfast:
- Wholesome Blueberry Muffins (page 305)
- Coffee with almond milk, or tea

Snack:
- Kale chips

Lunch:
- Brain-Boosting Caesar Salad with Roasted Chickpea Croutons and Nut Parmesan "Cheese" (page 296)

Snack:
- Almonds and grapes

Dinner:
- Mindful Mac and Cheese (page 302)
- Seasonal fruit for dessert

Thursday

Breakfast:
- Spelt Pancakes with Chia Berry Sauce (page 289)
- Coffee with almond milk, or tea

Snack:
- Steamed edamame

Lunch:
- Black Bean Burger Lettuce Wraps with Chipotle Sauce (page 290)

Snack:
- Goji berries and macadamia nuts

Dinner:
- Stuffed Bell Peppers (page 285)
- Blueberry Kamut Salad (page 303)
- Seasonal fruit for dessert

Friday

Breakfast:
- Chocolate Chia Pudding (page 306)
- Coffee with almond milk, or tea

Snack:
- Banana and almond butter

Lunch:
- Roasted Butternut Squash and Brussels Sprouts Salad (page 310)

Snack:
- Hazelnuts and dark chocolate

Dinner:
- Bean and Butternut Squash Enchiladas (page 279)
- Seasonal fruit for dessert

Saturday

Breakfast:
- MIND Smoothie (page 284)
- Coffee with almond milk, or tea

Snack:
- Veggies (carrots, lettuce, radishes) with hummus

Lunch:
- Mediterranean Brain Bowl with Roasted Sweet Potatoes and Chickpeas, Turmeric-Infused Quinoa, and Lemon Tahini Herb Sauce (page 315)
- Creamy Sweet Pea Soup (page 317)

Snack:
- Almonds and blackberries

Dinner:
- Roasted Spaghetti Squash with Pasta Sauce and Nut Parmesan "Cheese" (page 309)
- Wine

Dessert:
- Brain-Healthy Chocolate Chip Cookies (page 292)

Sunday

Breakfast:
- Wholesome Blueberry Muffins (page 305)
- Coffee with almond milk, or tea

Snack:
- Walnuts and dried berries

Lunch:
- Portobello Steaks with Argentinian Chimichurri Sauce (page 300)

Snack:
- Turmeric Milk (page 318)

Dinner:
- Roasted Vegetable Lasagna (page 312)

Dessert:
- Blueberry Crisp (page 304)

4.

Exercise

Jerry sat in Dean's office with his hands carefully folded in his lap. His wife, Rose, read from a small notebook as she described his lengthy medical history. Dean asked Jerry his age. For a moment Jerry was silent. He squinted his eyes as if he hadn't heard or understood the question. He answered, but only after a long pause.

Jerry was fifty-four, African American, and overweight. He had recently received a diagnosis of vascular dementia from his primary care doctor, and Dean could tell during the initial appointment that both Jerry and Rose were distressed. As the interview continued, Dean learned that Jerry worked at an insurance company and spent most of his time sitting at a desk. He said his job was repetitive, and because he'd been doing it for so many years he no longer found it challenging. Both he and Rose worked far from home, and because they spent so much time in traffic, they rarely had the opportunity to cook. They ate fast food at least once a week, and when they did cook, their meals always included large portions of meat. Neither of them exercised.

Rose reported that Jerry's thinking had become much more labored over the past several months: he was struggling to remember names and answer questions, and she'd seen him staring into space, confused and lost, the same behavior Dean observed in the clinic that morning. Jerry stiffened as his wife described his symptoms. He tried to downplay what she'd said, but he admitted that he'd also been noticing changes.

"I'm just slow," he said. "Everything is slow, even the way I move." Jerry felt as if time were passing without his awareness or recognition. He would lose hours and have no idea what happened or where he'd been. This is a common symptom for patients in the early stages of dementia, a kind of cognitive lag where information is delayed on its way to the brain's processing centers. This lag is exacerbated in patients like Jerry with vascular risk factors such as high blood pressure and high cholesterol. Jerry first noticed the problem when he was playing card games with friends. He realized he was falling behind when he needed to make a decision. He'd look at the cards but was too slow to act. His friends would joke with him about his slowness, but lately he'd started to feel self-conscious. For a lot of people with early symptoms of dementia, this cognitive delay creates a dissonance in social settings that is so uncomfortable it causes them to withdraw.

Jerry's body mass index (BMI)—a standard measure of body weight calculated by multiplying body mass (in pounds) by 703 and dividing by the square of body height (in inches)—was 35, which meant that he was clinically obese. A BMI below 18.5 is considered underweight; a BMI between 18.5 and 24.9 is normal; 25.0 to 29.9 is overweight; 30.0 to 40.0 is obese; and a BMI above 40 is considered morbidly obese. An MRI of Jerry's brain revealed white matter changes, implicating persistent high blood pressure or high cholesterol—or both—and a history of small strokes called lacunes. Another brain scan, an FDG-PET that uses fluorodeoxyglucose to identify damaged tissue, found patchy areas of diminished metabolism in the anterior hippocampus and subcortical regions, areas important for memory and speed of processing. Together these images showed that Jerry was suffering from mild vascular dementia. There was no evidence of thyroid disease, or any deficiencies, vitamin or otherwise, that might be causing Jerry's cognitive decline. Though his blood pressure and cholesterol had been elevated in the past, both were now being treated with medication. Still, his cognition continued to worsen. Dean knew lifestyle was the major contributing factor to Jerry's symptoms.

"Is there some medicine that can help me?" Jerry asked halfway through the interview. Dean told him that we do have a medicine that boosts and optimizes the brain's immune system and actually increases the size of its most important memory structure, a medicine that increases neurotrophic factors in the brain, which then grow new brain cells and

strengthen the connections between existing cells. A medicine that reduces anxiety and depression, lowers your BMI and risk of developing
diabetes, and even helps with sleep. Jerry leaned forward, looking hopeful. This medicine, Dean said, also reduces amyloid in cerebrospinal fluid
along with your chances of developing Alzheimer's—and its effects are
seen almost immediately.

"So what is it?" Jerry asked. Rose turned to a new page in her notebook.

"It's exercise," Dean said. Jerry's face fell. He sat back in his chair. Like
so many of our patients, Jerry was accustomed to being prescribed medication. He figured exercise was a healthy thing to do, but it was hard for
him to accept that it could have any effect on the cognitive symptoms that
plagued him.

"Exercise is crucial for every system in your body," Dean told him, "but
especially your brain. We're not designed to sit all day. We're supposed to
move, and move a lot."

The problem is that so many of us live lives void of movement. Many
of our patients don't know how to be active after so many years without exercising, especially when the companies they work for, the cities
they live in, and the many responsibilities of adulthood don't allow them
to prioritize exercise. And when they do try to incorporate an exercise
program, they get overwhelmed by the options and perceived difficulty
of something that should be second nature. What we taught Jerry, and
what we want to share with all of you, is that exercise doesn't have to be
a burden. It can be simple, even enjoyable. You just need to learn how to
make it work for you.

When embarking on behavior change—like beginning an exercise
program—we need to remember that our brain has evolved over millions
of years. Immediacy is the driving force of all our behavior. We're fixated
on survival. Long-term planning isn't one of our strong suits as humans,
especially when we experience any amount of stress, urgency, or desire.
Our brain was designed to worry about the saber-toothed tiger behind a
nearby tree, not figure out how to systematically capture all saber-toothed
tigers in the area over a period of five years. In much the same way, if
you're tired early in the morning when you planned to exercise, the desire to sleep will override all your best intentions, all your planning and

strategizing. This is why it's hard for us to develop long-term healthy habits. We're always susceptible to the immediate want, the immediate gain. The trick is to use these immediate gains and build a program around them, essentially giving the brain what it craves. Immediate gains need to be personally relevant, measurable, and visible. For many of our patients this means understanding that exercise both decreases and reverses cognitive decline, as well as tracking their progress on a whiteboard placed prominently in the home—either in the living room or on the refrigerator. Daily accomplishments help motivate you to continue with your program. You also need to see the clear connection between these immediate gains and your long-term goal. We work with patients to organize their long-term goals into small, achievable steps: if you want to be able to run five miles within six months, you should work on one-tenth of your goal during the first month. Once you've achieved success with that first half mile, you add on, visibly tracking your progress each day.

Searching for a positive emotional connection is another way of reinforcing new patterns. Toward the end of the medical history, Dean learned that Jerry had been an athlete when he was younger. He'd even played college basketball, but after college he quit sports altogether, and since then he'd been slowly gaining weight and becoming less and less active. Dean could sense that despite Jerry's skepticism, he had a desire to regain his physical fitness. Jerry could remember what it was like to be in a strong, capable body. This positive memory and the way it activated the brain's dopamine reward centers was a kind of stimulant that could be used to help Jerry return to exercise. Success built around personal history would be the foundation of Jerry's new plan.

"Can I really start exercising now?" Jerry asked as Dean introduced the idea of a daily exercise regimen. He thought he might be too old for exercise to really make a difference. Dean told him that while lifelong exercisers are healthier overall, multiple studies have shown the benefits of starting exercise later in life. For both children and the elderly, exercise is associated with better executive function (multitasking, planning, self-control), increased brain volume, and improved cognitive performance. People who start exercising early in life seem less likely to experience cognitive decline, but those who pick up exercise later in life are much better off than those who remain inactive. In other words, it's never too late to start. Dean

WHAT WE CALL "NORMAL AGING"

Dr. Ellsworth Wareham, our colleague at Loma Linda University, participated in open-heart surgeries until he was ninety-five. At the age of sixty-four, Diana Nyad broke a human record when she swam from Cuba to Florida. It's now considered "normal" for people in their sixties and even seventies to run marathons. Our expectations about aging have changed drastically over the last century, and even more drastically over the past few decades. Human capacity—both physical and mental—is constantly being reevaluated. Normal physiology is capable of remarkable things at age sixty, seventy, and eighty, and the mind can flourish and expand even in our later years.

If you've been inactive for a while and are resigned to the limitations of midlife or late life, we urge you to challenge your assumptions. Don't settle for an outdated expectation of "normal aging." Don't blindly accept inactivity and decline. Methodical change through small increments can lead to dramatic mental and physical gains. The stories in this chapter serve as proof, and the personalized plan that follows will show you exactly how to get started.

---

told Jerry about a patient he'd had at UC–San Diego, a former veteran who started running marathons in his fifties and kept running into his nineties. With small steps and a clear long-term objective, anything is possible.

But at the same time Dean recognized that Jerry had some specific limitations. He didn't have a lot of time for exercise, and he had balance issues and knee pain because he was overweight. He was always tired at night and had a long-standing habit of sitting in his beloved recliner and watching his favorite shows. Dean knew that any one of these factors could easily become a reason for Jerry to quit his exercise plan—and if Jerry failed with Dean's plan, he wasn't going to try lifestyle intervention again for a while, maybe ever. It's incredibly difficult for people to change after maintaining the same unhealthy patterns for years or decades, and we've designed our lifestyle protocol accordingly. An effective lifestyle intervention must address a patient's unique capacity, resources, strengths, and limitations. Most physicians recommend diet and exercise plans with no understanding of these nuances. They never teach patients how to succeed, and their plans almost invariably fail. For years we've committed ourselves to working differently: we set people up for success with a program that will work in their lives, and we support them every step of the way.

This was Jerry's personalized exercise plan: Dean asked Jerry and Rose to purchase a recumbent bike for their living room. Jerry already spent time relaxing in the living room at night. If he could just switch from his recliner to the bike, he'd have convenient access to exercise right in his home. The seat needed to be comfortable so that Jerry's biking was at least somewhat comparable to his existing routine. At first Rose wasn't thrilled about having exercise equipment in their living space, but Dean made it very clear that a recumbent bike was Jerry's lifeline. It was absolutely necessary for his physical and cognitive health, and therefore the most important piece of furniture in the house. Dean also created a detailed exercise schedule for Jerry to follow each day. He was to pedal slowly as he watched TV every night for two hours. Whenever he had the energy, he would do two quick sessions of rapid pedaling for five minutes each. He needed to pedal hard and tire himself out, but only for those two short bursts. He was encouraged to exercise at least three hours before bedtime so he wouldn't have trouble falling asleep. If everything went well, Jerry could slowly increase the duration of his rapid pedaling sessions by one minute each week. It was critical that exercise was done in a way that allowed Jerry to both see and feel the success. To that end Dean asked Jerry to use a whiteboard to keep a conspicuous record of his progress at home. He would also record how he felt after each session in a small notebook. Tracking his progress would help make Jerry aware of his efforts, and sharing the record with Dean would keep him accountable, which is another key element in behavior change. They agreed to meet again in three months.

Aerobic Exercise

One of the clearest relationships between exercise and brain health has to do with blood flow. You know that feeling when you're doing aerobic exercise—the way your heart pumps as you climb the stairs, blood flowing through your veins as you take your morning walk, your whole body active and engaged and alive. Aerobic exercise is vital for the heart, but it's also vital for the brain. Anything that reduces blood flow (vascular stiffness, plaques in our arteries, high cholesterol, long periods of inactivity) also reduces cognitive function, especially in the medial temporal lobe, which governs short-term memory. Conversely, anything that causes blood to circulate—like intensive aerobic exercise—maintains the health of the brain and the entire body. Many studies have shown that regular aerobic activity (defined as roughly 150 minutes per week of a moderate-intensity activity like brisk walking) significantly reduces the risk of cardiovascular disease, type 2 diabetes, high blood pressure and high cholesterol, anxiety and depression, and obesity, all risk factors for cognitive decline.

There are also numerous studies that directly link aerobic exercise with cognitive health. A 2010 meta-analysis of fifteen studies and nearly 34,000 people found that a high level of physical activity could lower the risk of cognitive decline by 38 percent. Those participants who engaged in a less intensive, more moderate form of exercise still had a 35 percent lower risk of cognitive impairment. Researchers at the University of Lisbon looked at the effects of exercise on 639 elderly subjects whose cognition and vascular health were tested every three years. They found that those who exercised had a 40 percent lower risk of cognitive impairment and dementia, as well as a 60 percent lower risk of vascular dementia. The 2010 Framingham Longitudinal Study, a comprehensive long-term study that began in 1948 and is now tracking the third generation of subjects, confirmed that daily brisk walks led to a 40 percent lower risk of developing Alzheimer's or any kind of dementia later in life. In another study at Harvard of more than 18,000 women, researchers found that ninety minutes a week of brisk walking (for approximately fifteen minutes a day) delayed cognitive decline and significantly reduced the risk of developing Alzheimer's. Researchers at the University of Pittsburgh found that when older people had a habit of walking, they had both larger brain volumes and better cognitive function.

In 2016, several new studies further illuminated the effects of aerobic exercise on the brain. Scientists at Wake Forest University compared stretching versus intensive exercise in individuals with mild cognitive impairment for forty-five minutes a day, four days a week, over a six-month period. Intensive exercise was defined as participants reaching 70 to 80 percent of their maximum heart rate. The results were astounding. In the intensive exercise group, researchers found increased blood flow to the

---

BLOOD PRESSURE

High blood pressure in midlife is clearly associated with cognitive decline later on. We recommend that you check your blood pressure frequently and stay on top of any changes you experience. If you have high blood pressure, moderately high blood pressure, or even borderline high blood pressure, you should take medication to reduce damage to blood vessels throughout the body and brain. Medication lowers blood pressure by temporarily loosening vessels that have grown stiff with cholesterol and smooth muscle injury after years of unhealthy living. The problem is that medication causes a forced, precipitous drop in blood pressure without addressing any of the underlying problems. If you don't improve your lifestyle with nutrition and especially exercise, cholesterol continues to build up, which makes the vessels even stiffer and narrower. Eventually you'll require two medications to widen the blood vessels, and if you still fail to address the lifestyle factors causing your hypertension, you'll reach the point where no amount of medication can maintain normal blood flow. Exercise, in contrast to medication, not only pumps blood to your brain but actually affects the underlying pathology that causes hypertension. It even reverses damage by rejuvenating the blood vessels and increasing angiogenic chemicals that grow new vessels. Exercise also improves the homeostasis of blood pressure, helping to naturally regulate the entire circulatory system. This is why we always prescribe exercise—everyone needs it. Those with high blood pressure must address the underlying pathology; those with normal blood pressure should work to maintain their health; and those with low blood pressure (which has been linked to cognitive decline later in life) need to increase the amount of blood being pumped to the brain.

---

frontal lobe (the brain region dedicated to planning, organization, judgment, and self-control), increased brain size, improved executive function, and protection against cognitive decline despite these subjects' strong genetic risk for Alzheimer's. The stretching group, on the other hand, experienced brain shrinkage and decreased executive function due to the normal course of dementia. The major conclusion was that exercise should be aerobic and intensive. You can't be content with walking at a normal speed or being "active" around the house. Only intensive aerobic activity yields these startling results, which were also confirmed by another study at the Wisconsin Alzheimer's Disease Research Center at the University of Wisconsin. This study looked at lifetime recreational activity and found that occupational and household activities resulted in no improvement in Alzheimer's biomarkers. Jogging and swimming, by contrast, were shown to modulate the brain changes common to Alzheimer's.

The vascular effects of aerobic exercise are critically important for long-term cognitive health and preventing Alzheimer's, but this form of exercise also has many other proven benefits.

Enhancing the Brain's Connectivity: As we age, we lose neurons and the important connections between them. There is evidence, however, that aerobic exercise can enhance connectivity throughout the brain—and this can occur well into the ninth decade of life. Improved connectivity yields better cognitive performance and also protection against dementia in general and Alzheimer's in particular. It works something like this: Imagine a memory of a trip to Italy—like eating a piece of incredibly delicious pizza in Naples. Your brain has made a few connections to this memory file, but as you age, one of these connections gets cut off by a microvascular lesion (blockage of a small blood vessel). Another connection is cut off by an amyloid plaque. If yet another connection is cut off, you'll lose the memory forever. That's why multiple connections—the brain's inherent redundancy—are so important as we age. Aerobic activity seems to boost not just the number of connections, but the strength of each of them.

Improving the Integrity of White Matter: The brain has dozens of tracts that act as superhighways connecting different regions with specific functions. There are tracts that connect the hippocampus (the brain's memory center) with the amygdala (the brain's emotional center), and other tracts that connect the hippocampus and amygdala with the frontal lobe, where executive function and problem solving take place. These tracts are composed of millions if not billions of white matter fibers that connect cell bodies and facilitate rapid communication. White matter appears to be damaged by amyloid plaques, the pathology associated with Alzheimer's disease, but studies have shown that increased blood flow during aerobic exercise can improve the integrity of white matter. The overall effect is faster and more efficient communication between brain regions.

Promoting the Growth of Brain Cells: For over a century scientists believed that the adult human brain was incapable of developing new neurons: you were born with a certain number of neurons, and that number decreased as cells died off during your lifetime. The same was thought to be true about the heart. But we now know that the heart is capable of new growth, and groundbreaking research in the 1990s showed us that the brain can also regrow cells. Aerobic exercise has been directly linked to neurogenesis in critical memory structures like the hippocampus. By contrast,

WHITE MATTER DISEASE

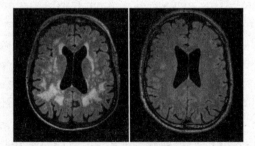

This image illustrates the difference between a brain with white matter disease (left) and a normal brain (right). The brain with white matter disease shows whitening of the inner brain, which indicates damage to the white matter (the main type of tissue in the inner brain). White matter damage results from lifestyle risks like diabetes and smoking, both of which promote vascular disease and inflammation, as well as long-term high blood pressure that can harm small arteries supplying oxygen and nutrients to the brain. White matter disease is associated with vascular and other types of dementia. Exercise has been shown to reduce the risk of white matter disease, and in some cases can even reverse it.

bedridden patients have shown signs of suppressed neurogenesis in the hippocampus. Exercise appears to be the most significant lifestyle factor when it comes to generating new cells in the brain.

While it's remarkable that the brain can regenerate, it can grow only a limited number of new cells. Yet a limited number of new cells can have a profound effect when you consider their connections to other neurons. Exercise has a direct effect at the cellular level throughout the brain: it promotes healthy new pathways between neurons and also rejuvenates existing mechanisms within neurons.

Producing Brain Growth Factors: Growth factors are proteins that stimulate existing cells, promote brain cell growth, and also maintain the health of mature neurons. Think of them as fertilizer for neurons. Aerobic activity has been shown to increase the synthesis of BDNF (brain-derived neurotrophic factor) in the brain: one study suggested that aerobic activity resulted in a threefold increase in BDNF. Other important factors that promote neuroplasticity (brain cell repair) and neurogenesis (new brain cell formation)—including superoxide dismutase (SOD), endothelial nitric oxide synthase (eNOS), insulin growth factor-1 (IGF-1), and vascular endothelial growth factor (VEGF)—also increase with aerobic activity.

Reducing Inflammation: In a systematic review and meta-analysis of forty-three studies published between 1995 and 2012 (which included over 3,500 subjects), researchers at Kent State University found that a structured exercise program significantly lowered inflammatory markers in the blood. These dramatic results were seen after only four weeks of exercise.

Increasing Klotho Levels: Klotho is a hormone associated with both longevity and protection against cognitive decline. Researchers at UCSF found that people who carry the klotho gene perform better on a number of cognitive tests. Other studies show that klotho levels can increase after only twenty minutes of intensive aerobic exercise in healthy adults.

Resistance Training

Though aerobic exercise has been studied most extensively, resistance training (the use of weights to build and preserve muscle) has also been shown to positively affect brain function. While our idea of "lifting weights" is often limited to teenagers and young adults trying to achieve the perfect physique, this form of exercise is so much more important when we're older given its impact on both the body and brain. Resistance training reduces bone loss, maintains muscle, increases balance, and decreases the risk of falling (a major concern for the elderly, especially those with cognitive decline and dementia). Research has shown that leg strength in particular is correlated with better cognitive function, likely because strong leg muscles help blood circulate up to the brain. You don't need to do barbell squats with fifty-pound weights to experience this benefit—just strengthening the legs with partial squats while holding on to a chair has a significant positive effect on the brain. Additionally, people who weight train are stronger and more flexible, which allows them to exercise later in life and avoid many of the limitations that prevent the elderly from exercising.

Scientific evidence of the positive effects of resistance training includes:

Improvement in White Matter: Researchers from the University of British Columbia found that twice-weekly resistance training for a period of fifty-two weeks resulted in a reduction of white matter lesions and improved attention in a group of elderly women.

Increased Growth Factors: Researchers at the University of Florida found that adults who participated in resistance training had a 98 percent increase in the level of BDNF in their blood after an exercise session.

Improved Frontal Lobe Function: In a study at the University of British Columbia, individuals who weight trained demonstrated better cognitive abilities than those who did stretching and toning routines. Resistance training seemed to affect reasoning and attention skills (in the frontal lobe) more than short-term and long-term memory (in the medial temporal lobe and hippocampus).

Better Vascular Health: Both short-term and long-term resistance training improve the health of arteries throughout the body, and the effects last long after the exercise is completed. Resistance training significantly reduces the formation of cholesterol plaques, therefore increasing the supply of essential nutrients to the brain.

Inflammation: Serum homocysteine, which leads to inflammation and subsequent damage to blood vessels, has been shown to decrease following six months of high- or low-intensity resistance exercise in older adults.

Recent studies on resistance training have given us further insight into how this form of exercise helps protect against cognitive decline. A study published in the *Journal of the American Geriatric Society* measured the effects of a resistance-training program (two to three times a week for six months) on a group of older adults with MCI. Researchers found nearly 47 percent of the participants achieved normal cognitive scores after the intervention, and that these results were maintained over a period of eighteen months. Greater leg strength was extremely effective at improving cognitive performance. Another new study in the *American Journal of Geriatric Psychiatry* found that a nine-week program combining strength training with aerobic exercise resulted in better brain function than an aerobic-only program.

———————

What all this research proves, and what we've consistently seen in our clinic, is that regular exercise is a tremendously powerful way to heal your brain on a cellular level, increase its strength and resilience, and all but guarantee a life free of Alzheimer's. If you or someone you love is suffering from cognitive impairment, an exercise program will yield immediate benefits and may even reverse cognitive symptoms. The personalized program that follows this chapter will give you all the information you need to incorporate exercise into your daily life.

Other Benefits of Exercise

The benefits of any kind of exercise increase when a given activity involves multiple cognitive modalities. This is a topic we cover at length in Chapter 7, "Optimize," but the main idea is that activating multiple brain systems challenges the brain in complex, multimodal ways, thereby creating stronger connections and more resilience. Consider the difference between walking on a treadmill and participating in a sport like basketball that strengthens your reflexes, balance, and hand-eye coordination, and requires you to memorize different plays. Simply throwing a ball uses visuospatial awareness, attention, and motor control. Yoga involves awareness of specific muscle groups and also challenges balance, breathing, and attention. Nintendo Wii and other similar devices offer a constantly changing interface that keeps the brain active and engaged and can be a great alternative for those who get bored with bikes and treadmills. Everything we know about the brain suggests that more complex activities provide more protection against cognitive decline. The ultimate goal is to find something that keeps you active, challenges your brain, and makes you happier in the process.

Exercise of any kind positively affects the brain in two other interesting ways. First, exercise is a very effective treatment for depression, a condition that is correlated with Alzheimer's, as you learned in Chapter 2 (more information on depression and dementia can be found in Chapter 5, "Unwind"), and negatively affects both the brain's attention centers and important neurotransmitters like serotonin and dopamine. Exercise increases endorphins, which significantly elevate mood. As a lifestyle factor, exercise has an amazing power to promote overall health and wellness: the more you exercise, the better your body feels. The better your body feels, the better your mind feels. And the better your mind feels, the more motivation you have to keep exercising and implement other healthy lifestyle practices like proper nutrition and restorative sleep. The inverse is also true—the longer you go without exercising, the harder it becomes to motivate yourself to start, and because you lack energy and endorphins, other lifestyle factors can feel like they're out of reach. Whenever possible, we begin comprehensive lifestyle plans with exercise because of its almost immediate effects on mood.

Exercise also creates discipline. Any repeated behavior that requires initiative and planning, stamina and inhibition of laziness (which comes naturally to us) strengthens the brain's pathways between the frontal lobe (planning and problem solving), limbic system (the seat of instinct and mood), and basal ganglia (responsible for motor control, learning, and habits). Research has shown that people who exercise create better connections in these crucial habit pathways. At the same time, people who are disciplined enough to exercise regularly are much less likely to abuse their bodies in other ways. Studies show that teenagers who exercise are much less likely to abuse drugs and alcohol—and the same is true for adults.

Exercising with Injuries and Physical Limitations

Exercise can be a challenge for people in their fifties, sixties, and beyond. How do you get your heart beating fast when you have bad knees, or sciatic disc problems, or pain in your hips, ankles, and shoulders? One out of three people over the age of sixty-five has some kind of ankle, knee, or hip problem, and almost everybody has had a complaint or two about their lower back. Maybe you can't lift a lot of weight or jog around the neighborhood, but there are exercise options available for everyone. Elliptical machines and recumbent bikes are wonderful for reducing pressure on the joints. If you have limitations with your legs because of osteoporosis or arthritis, you can concentrate on arm exercises. Foot pedal machines work just as well for the arms, and you can do this kind of exercise easily in your home while watching television. There are even self-moving pedal machines and bikes. These machines work well for elderly people without much mobility or strength, and can safely increase fitness over time.

Though there's a lot of evidence for the remarkable effects of aerobic exercise and resistance training on the brain, there are also studies that show the cognitive benefits of gentler activities like swimming, tai chi, dance, and yoga. A 2016 study from Thailand found that people with mild cognitive impairment who practiced tai chi three times a week had significantly better cognitive performance; another study from 2012 found that a forty-week tai chi program significantly increased brain volume. The meditative aspect of tai chi appears to be especially beneficial for cognitive health. Additionally, a 2016 study at St. Luke's Hospital in the Philippines tested the effects of ballroom dancing on a sample of elderly patients. Researchers found that after twelve months, the patients demonstrated better executive control, cognitive functioning, and general well-being.

Swimming is especially useful for those with injuries and physical limitations. The buoyancy of water relieves stress on the joints, allowing you to exercise without risking further injury. You can do kicks in the water, walk back and forth to strengthen the legs, or even use resistance paddles on the arms and legs to build muscle. Proximity and ease are essential for a long-lasting exercise program, so some of our patients invest in a small, six-by-eight-foot swimming pool that gives them ample space for both aerobic exercise (steps and kicks) and resistance training.

Exercise Myths

- **If you're not running, you're not exercising:** You can raise your heart rate just by stepping up and down on a small, stable stool in your living room, or taking the stairs at work.

- **If you can't use your legs, you're not getting a good workout:** The body is a closed system. If you exercise the upper body, your whole body will experience the benefits.

- **All you have to do is work out for twenty minutes and then you can relax for the rest of the day:** Extended periods of sedentary behavior negate the benefits of twenty to thirty minutes of exercise.

- **No pain, no gain:** Extreme pain and discomfort will discourage you from exercising, but a little pain is helpful because it serves as a reminder that you worked toward your goal. The expression should be: "A little pain = a long-term gain."

- **You can work through injuries:** Never push through injuries or they could become permanent. Instead, exercise other parts of your body while you heal.

- **You need to take protein powders and supplements to build muscle when you're working out:** We get more than enough protein from a regular diet—even a vegan diet.

- **If you didn't exercise when you were young, it's dangerous to start when you're older:** It's never too late to start. Everyone experiences the benefits—even the elderly. You just need to start slowly and proceed with caution, being mindful of any injuries or limitations you may have.

- **Working out at a gym is better than working out at home:** We believe that working out at home is better. Exercise programs need to be easy and convenient. What's easier than doing some aerobic exercise in your living room at night while you're watching the news? Or taking a brisk morning walk through your neighborhood? You may choose to join a gym or pursue other outside activities, but consider them an addition to exercise at home.

Jerry's Follow-Up

When Jerry returned for his follow-up, he bore little resemblance to the man in slow motion that Dean had met three months earlier. He seemed focused and energetic, and as Dean spoke with him, his cognitive lag was much less pronounced. Jerry proudly showed Dean his detailed daily exercise records, which included the workout time and intensity, and how he felt afterward. He'd gotten into a great routine: every day he'd come home from work, eat dinner, and then watch TV while using his recumbent bike. By week six he was doing fifteen-minute intervals of high-intensity biking. He said he felt incredible after exercising, and this feeling helped him continue to increase the aerobic aspect of his program. Now, at three months, he was doing intensive biking continuously for twenty-five minutes—and he did this workout five to six days a week.

When Jerry returned after another three months, his focus, attention, and thought processing had returned to normal. These kinds of results are truly astounding given the usual progression of cognitive decline. Our approach showed Jerry that instead of waiting for a magic pill, he had the power to save his own life. So many patients come to us in Jerry's state, when an Alzheimer's diagnosis seems not only inevitable, but certain to arrive soon. Yet by taking advantage of just one lifestyle factor, Jerry avoided a diagnosis and returned to a normal, happy, and, by his own account, much improved life. He not only avoided an Alzheimer's diagnosis but put himself at a much lower risk of cardiovascular disease, diabetes, and other chronic conditions that he likely would have developed in the future. Jerry told Dean he was now getting up early to bike around the neighborhood before work. He'd bought a new road bike, and sometimes he biked outdoors at night, too. Biking became his addiction, and from this positive change Dean was able to help him improve his diet and sleeping patterns as well.

After a year, Dean ordered another MRI. While the white matter damage was still present, it had visibly decreased—a profound change, and strong evidence for the impact of exercise on Jerry's brain. These kinds of changes on MRIs were unheard of just a few years ago, but we are now consistently seeing structural changes as a result of exercise and other lifestyle factors. A comprehensive neuropsychological test demonstrated improvement in executive function and speed of processing, which were the areas of Jerry's brain that had been most affected. His blood pressure was also lower. Jerry believed he was even better than what he would have considered "normal"—and Rose agreed. She was using the recumbent bike, too, and she'd cleaned up her diet along with Jerry. Little by little they found ways to be even more active. They bought some weights for the living room, took walks together. They said they'd never felt more energetic. "Exercise helped me get back to the moment," Jerry told Dean. "I was stuck in a parallel universe, but now I'm with everyone else."

Designed to Move:
The Truth About Sedentary Behavior

Michael had strong shoulders, a lean torso, and excellent aerobic fitness. He exercised at the gym for a half hour at least four nights a week, and his diet was relatively low in sugar and filled with fresh vegetables. But lately he'd been experiencing fatigue, dizziness, and lack of mental focus. Michael was an accountant, and during a typical day he sat at his desk for ten hours or more. His work was intensive—he rarely got up, almost never took a break. During the appointment, he insisted that he was still capable of rising to the challenges of his profession. Sure, he'd made some minor errors in his calculations, but he could remember events from forty years ago. "I just can't remember what I ate for breakfast," he told us. Unfortunately, this kind of short-term memory impairment often progresses to Alzheimer's. We knew we had to intervene as soon as possible.

Just as we saw with Jerry, any increase in daily exercise will positively affect the brain, but the latest research suggests that a quick thirty-minute workout after a day spent sitting isn't sufficient for promoting overall health, nor is it adequate for protecting the brain against cognitive impairment. We're now discovering that a sedentary lifestyle is a major risk factor for cancer, diabetes, and cognitive decline. Researchers in San Francisco measured the amount of time people watched television and tried to find a correlation with cognitive health. Not surprisingly, they found that those individuals who spent the most time watching television had an increased risk of developing Alzheimer's disease. Another study showed that sedentary behavior was associated with a decrease in gray matter volume, meaning that lack of physical activity can result in both impaired brain function and negative structural change.

We can't simply undo a whole day spent sitting with a few minutes of exercise. Never in our history as a species have we been less physically active than we are now. Only recently did we begin to spend so much time sitting, and only recently did we experience a dramatically increased risk of noncommunicable diseases like heart disease, diabetes, autoimmune disorders, and dementia. The problem is that people are focused on the number of hours (or minutes) of exercise per day. It's true that exercise is extremely important, but what's also important, and what likely has a greater impact on brain health according to new research, is the number of sedentary hours per day. Our patients are often shocked to hear this: the number of hours they sit per day is a much better predictor of future cognitive decline than their daily exercise regimen. We knew right away that Michael's sedentary hours were negating the exercise he was working so hard to incorporate into his schedule. We see this frequently in our patients because sedentary lives are so commonplace. How many hours per day do you sit at a desk without once getting up to take a short walk? How many hours a day do you sit in front of a television? Or in your car in traffic?

Research shows that four to five sedentary hours per day are more detrimental than a lifestyle that includes no formal exercise but regular movement. What the body—and brain—really needs is movement incorporated throughout the day in short bursts, ideally every hour. For example, slow biking coupled with a few intensive aerobic cycles each hour would be an almost perfect fitness regimen. This approach to exercise most accurately mimics the active lives humans have led for thousands of years—roaming in search of food, farming, chasing game. But how do we exercise in short bursts while we're stuck at the office? Most of us have desk-bound jobs. We're forced to sit in traffic. And with so much stress in our lives, watching television feels good at the end of the day.

It turns out that there are many creative solutions to this problem, and that the modern workplace is being transformed by what we now know about the consequences of sedentary behavior. Using a standing desk, for instance, is a great way to be more active while working. Standing burns far more calories than sitting, and it strengthens our leg muscles, which we know is important for both balance and vascular health. Some offices provide their employees with treadmill desks, which allow for constant movement throughout the day and also brief intervals of more intensive exercise that are so critical for cognitive health. There are also pedal exercisers for under your desk that cost roughly thirty dollars. Simply taking a brisk walk every few hours is a great way to get your heart pumping. Doing some squats sends blood to your brain after extended periods spent sitting.

We can apply this same movement-oriented philosophy at home. Basic weight training is easy to do in your living space, as are yoga, Pilates, and calisthenics. Time in front of the television should be time spent exercising. We often tell our patients that the world would be a very different place if televisions were attached to bicycles and you were forced to exercise while you watched your favorite shows. If you don't have an exercise bike, all you need is a staircase for aerobic exercise. And if you can't exercise on stairs because of injuries or arthritis, you can hold on to a chair and safely do fifty leg raises—again, easily in the comfort of your home.

After we taught Michael about the effects of sedentary behavior, he asked for a standing desk in his office. He also purchased a recumbent bike for his home so he could add more cardiovascular exercise at night. Michael was a very motivated, focused person who actually enjoyed exercise. We seized on his motivation and appealed to his detail-oriented nature by designing a daily exercise schedule: he committed to doing two, five-minute intervals of high-intensity exercise on the bike each night; he would also work at least two hours a day at his new standing desk.

We were confident that regular movement in Michael's day would improve his cognition and overall health because we'd seen this same transformation in our own bodies. We haven't always been in the best shape. The stress of medical school and raising young children took a toll on us. A few years ago, Ayesha would get winded on even a short staircase. She hated running. Dean was overweight, and he'd lost most of the strength he'd had when he used to play soccer. We knew we needed more exercise in our lives, so we set out to add movement to our daily routine.

We started with brisk walks outside at lunchtime that invigorated us for the second half of the day. Then we added frequent, short breaks in our office to do basic strengthening exercises like push-ups and sit-ups. We started small and increased our exercises by 2 percent every week, keeping careful track of how many repetitions we could do. We wanted to see our progress clearly—we knew we would need the motivation to stick with our program. Dean was shocked by how physically fit he became just through brief bouts of exercise in the office and at home. At age fifty, he can do 35 pull-ups, 120 push-ups, and 70 squats—way more than when he was an athlete. Ayesha gained a lot of strength in her shoulders and biceps, can do 50 squats without much effort, and even enjoys long-distance runs.

We've made a life where exercise is part of how we go about our day, how we work, and how we spend time together as a family. Now it's completely normal for both of us to take one minute out of every hour and knock out as many sit-ups as possible. We have standing desks in our office and a minielliptical machine that we use for 500 rotations throughout the day. We can do almost all our work at the standing desks, and the elliptical is great for listening to messages, replying to e-mails, and making audio recordings. As for exercising at home, even when we lived in an eight-hundred-square-foot apartment in West Hollywood, we had no problem working out as a family. We regularly do tae kwon do kicks in the living room to raise our heart rates. Squats help us build leg strength and balance. We always take the stairs. Of course, this lifestyle requires a strong commitment to family health, and it took us a few attempts to design the right system, but we're convinced that everyone can adopt similar programs without having to purchase a gym membership or hire a personal trainer.

When Michael came back for this three-month follow-up, he said he no longer felt peaks and valleys in his energy and attention throughout the day. In fact, his energy had increased. He couldn't believe that adding just two five-minute sessions could improve his focus and clarity so dramatically. He now had a habit of watching TV and biking every night, and he'd worked his way up to three sessions of high-intensity exercise for ten minutes each. He was also happier. His cognitive symptoms had been creating quite a bit of stress in his life, but now he felt relieved and better able to both work and relax.

Conclusion

Exercise is essential to cognitive health. It actively prevents dementia and Alzheimer's, repairs damage in important memory centers, and even grows new brain cells. We now have a body of research that's so compelling it can convince even the most reticent patient of the value of exercise—but starting an exercise program isn't easy. You need to identify your strengths and limitations and move step by step toward clear long-term goals. The best kind of exercise is whatever is easy, convenient, and sustainable for you. It's entirely possible to build your life around movement and experience dramatic improvement in cognition and mood. All you need is commitment and a well-designed exercise plan.

Your Personalized
EXERCISE
Program

A personalized, sustainable exercise program is crucial for long-term brain health. As you've now learned, aerobic exercise and resistance training are both incredibly effective at protecting the brain against age-related decline and even reversing the symptoms of early Alzheimer's. Sedentary behavior has been associated with many types of chronic disease, including cognitive impairment, so your goal should be to incorporate movement throughout your day. There is a form of exercise for virtually everyone—no matter the limitations or injuries—and the pages below offer many suggestions for tailoring a brain-healthy program to your unique needs. Keep in mind that we implement change most successfully when we experience immediate gains that are personally relevant, measurable, and visible. You'll find tools in this section for making your exercise program all three.

SELF-ASSESSMENT

Vision, Strengths, and Weaknesses: Assess your vision for an exercise plan, and identify factors that might help or hinder your efforts.

Vision: What is your ideal exercise plan for brain health? How often would you like to move throughout the day? How would the energy gained from exercise change other parts of your life? What symptoms could exercise improve? What kinds of exercise have you enjoyed in the past? Can you visualize yourself doing those activities now?

Strengths: What strengths and resources will help you achieve your vision?

Weaknesses: What are the obstacles to your vision?

1. How will you benefit from an exercise program?

Examples: I'll have more energy. I'll sleep better. I'll have greater focus and sharper thinking. I'll manage my glucose levels more efficiently. Complex tasks will be easier for me. I will have better balance, which will reduce my risk of falls. My digestion will improve (I'll have less constipation).

2. What are the most important areas for you to work on?

Examples: I want to develop an aerobic program that is fun, and one that I can do regularly. I want to exercise without aggravating my shoulder injury. I need an exercise program that's easy and convenient. My legs are weak—I need to build leg strength and improve my balance.

3. What obstacles might prevent you from exercising?

Examples: I don't have time. I've never liked exercise. I have knee pain. I don't have enough room in my apartment. I don't have money for equipment or a gym membership. I don't have the energy.

4. What might help you exercise? What are your resources?

Examples: There are exercise facilities at work that I could use at lunchtime, and as a backup I can do twenty minutes of foot pedal exercise at home while watching the news. I can walk with a friend during my lunch break. I have a bike that I haven't used for years. I have a whiteboard that I can hang in the living room to track my progress. I live on the fourth floor and can start taking the stairs at least three times a week. I can invest in a pair of weights or an exercise bike for my home. I could walk to work. I love dancing.

5. Who can help you and how?

Examples: I could ask a coworker who works out every day during lunch. My husband/wife wants to start exercising, too. My children can teach me how to use weights. I will organize a neighborhood walking club. I will take my dog out for walks twice a day. I will join a community center. I will join my church exercise group or start one. I will ask friends for old exercise equipment they may have.

6. When will you start?

Our Recommendation: You should start as soon as you have the time and resources. Beginning an exercise program without ease and efficiency will only lead to failure. At the same time, you don't want to put off exercising until you've developed the perfect program. Start with the first activity you want to focus on and pick an amount of time you can dedicate. Begin with the lowest intensity and then build fitness and the rest of your program around this initial activity.

BEFORE YOU START

A Disclaimer: Before starting any exercise program, it's very important to consult with your physician. Many people have medical conditions like heart disease or balance problems that can affect their ability to exercise. Anyone with a medical condition should only begin an exercise program under the supervision of a doctor.

On Exercising for Your Brain: Our goal is to help you build a better brain and avoid Alzheimer's disease. The following physical activity regimen isn't designed explicitly for weight loss or gaining muscle. You will lose weight and create stronger muscles as a result of this program, but our focus is on exercises that have been scientifically proven to help your brain age successfully and avoid future disease.

STEP 1: DESIGNING YOUR EXERCISE PROGRAM

Important Properties of a Successful Exercise Program

Convenience: Your program must be easy. If it's too difficult, you'll get discouraged.

Repeatability: A successful exercise program must be repeatable on a regular basis. Repeatable activities are easy, efficient, and ideally enjoyable.

Incremental Success: You have to see success in what you're doing. This could be as simple as being able to do nine squats instead of eight, or being able to pedal one minute longer than your baseline.

Measurable: You should be able to measure how much exercise you've done, and your progress should be visible at all times. You might use a whiteboard in your home, a notebook, or an app on your smartphone.

Three Insider Tips

Prioritize Exercise: It's easy to make excuses for not exercising. Commit to doing some form of movement every day: any exercise is better than none. If you really don't feel like exercising, vow to start and do it for at least five minutes.

Develop Daily Habits: Start with one activity you enjoy and focus on it until it becomes a habit (e.g., a brisk walk in the neighborhood every morning). If you don't enjoy any form of exercise, start with the activity that is most convenient and easy—and the one that you like the most or just dislike the least.

Beware of an Overambitious Exercise Plan: Start small and build from there. Always start at a pace and time that are slightly more than what you think you can do, and then increase by small increments each week. Keep notes detailing each increase. After you have some momentum—when you've achieved 50 percent of your goal—you can add in other exercises like stretching and strengthening.

Setting Up Your "Gym"

Although gym memberships are great for encouraging exercise, the home should be the base of your exercise program. At home you can work out whenever you want, and you're not forced to dress up, drive, and spend precious time and money just to get your daily exercise.

You can do an extensive workout at home without any equipment. Your task is simply to increase your heart rate and use resistance to build muscle (push-ups, sit-ups, planks, squats, bicep curls, and shoulder raises using any item in the room for a bit of weight). Pictures and explanations of the following exercises and more are available on our website at TeamSherzai.com. That said, equipment is helpful, especially for those who have less experience with exercise.

Recommended Items

- **Weights** (5- to 10-pound dumbbells; 1-, 2-, or 3-pound ankle weights) or a set of resistance bands

- **Mat** (if you don't have carpet)

- **Stationary bike** (optional, but strongly preferred; an excellent choice for those with balance issues; buying a comfortable seat will make biking more pleasant)

- **Foot pedal exerciser** (if there's no room for a bicycle; can be used with both legs and arms)

- **Stable chair** (to hold for balance exercises)

- **Treadmill** (optional, and only if you have no balance issues)

Injuries

Avoiding Injuries: Be sure to stretch properly before and after exercising. Please see the "Flexibility Training" section on page 172 for details.

Working Out with Injuries: For sprains and pulled muscles, use the RICE method (Rest, Ice, Compression, Elevation). Consult a doctor as soon as possible. Give the joint or muscle time to heal, and focus on exercising other parts of the body. For example, if you injure your knee, you can concentrate on strengthening your arms and shoulders while you recover.

If you suffer from a chronic condition that limits your activity and prohibits you from doing weight-bearing exercises, you can try a recumbent bike or exercising in a pool (resistance exercises or brisk walking in the shallow end), both of which reduce stress on the joints. You can also try less intensive exercises like yoga, tai chi, or even ballroom dancing. Keep in mind that there are different types of yoga and tai chi: some focus on gentle flexibility and movement (restorative yoga and slow-form tai chi); others focus on strength or aerobic fitness (power yoga and larger-frame tai chi). If you're attending live classes, you can call ahead and ask the instructor whether the style would be appropriate for someone of your fitness level and with your specific limitations. If you're searching for classes online, use keywords like "gentle" and "beginner's" to find the right style/level.

STEP 2: DAY-TO-DAY GOALS

Work Toward Increasing:

- Taking the stairs

- Moving while watching television

- Walking or riding your bike wherever possible

- Using a stepper while working

- Dancing, doing tai chi, or practicing yoga at home

- Squats or step-ups with a stool while at work or in the living room

- Wall push-ups whenever there is an opportunity

- Hamstring workouts with ankle weights in the kitchen/living room/bedroom

- Sit-ups in bed in the morning

Work Toward Eliminating:

- Long hours of sedentary behavior like sitting at an office desk or in your car

- Watching television without exercising

- Avoiding the stairs

- Days without any form of exercise

Types of Exercise

Now that you know the basics of exercising at home and in the office, here are some of the activities we recommend:

Aerobic Exercise

Choose one of these activities to do on a daily basis.

- Brisk walking

- Stationary bike, reclined or nonreclined

- Jumping jacks

- Stepper

- Stairs

- Dance

- Martial arts (tae kwon do, karate, kickboxing)

- Stepping up and down on a stable stool

While performing this exercise, you should be lightly sweating and have difficulty finishing the following sentence in one breath: "The train arrived at the train station in Boston one hour later than expected." If you have to stop in the middle of the sentence for a second breath, you have reached an appropriate intensity level. You can also be a bit more scientific about it. Below is a formula for calculating your maximum heart rate based on age (you can also find this formula on our website: TeamSherzai.com).

Maximum Heart Rate (MHR): Once your doctor has given you clearance to exercise, your goal should be achieving your specific MHR during periods of aerobic exercise.

$$207 - (Age \times 0.7) = MHR$$

For a person who is 70 years old, the calculation is as follows:

$$207 - (70 \times 0.7) = 207 - 49 = 158.$$

If achieving this heart rate is too difficult, then use the sentence referenced above as a guide.

Strength and Resistance Training

These exercises will help you build strength and stability. Choose one and do it every day. Feel free to switch exercises to create a more balanced workout. For videos of each exercise, please visit our website (TeamSherzai.com).

- Squats

- Lunges (forward, backward, side to side)

- Leg extensions

- Abdominal crunches

- Planks

- Bicep curls

- Tricep curls

- Shoulder raises

- Push-ups (regular and at the wall)

Balance Training

Below are exercises for balance. Choose one and do it every day. Have a chair next to you if you are just starting out or don't feel steady.

- **Heel-to-Toe Walk:** Place the heel of your foot in front of the toes of your other foot; both feet should be touching. Walk in a straight line while focusing on a point ahead of you. Do not stare at your feet.

- **Single Leg Balance:** Stand on one foot using a chair for support. Raise your leg, bringing the knee forward, and hold for 10–12 seconds. Lower your leg and repeat on the other side. For more of a challenge: do the leg raise without holding on to a chair.

- **Back Leg Raises:** Stand on one foot using a chair for support. Raise your leg, pushing the knee backward, and hold for 10–12 seconds. Lower your leg and repeat on the other side. For more of a challenge: do the leg raise without holding on to a chair.

- **Side Leg Raises:** Stand on one foot using a chair for support. Raise your leg, extending it sideways, and hold for 10–12 seconds. Bring your leg back to the midline and repeat on the other side. For more of a challenge: do the leg raise without holding on to a chair.

- **Yoga:** Tree pose is great for strengthening balance. To start, you can practice it with your back to the wall or the side of your body (standing leg) to the wall. As your balance improves, try stepping away from the wall. To further challenge the pose, you can try it with your arms reaching above your head or with your eyes closed. Chair and warrior 2 are other excellent poses for strengthening the leg muscles and core. Be sure to start slow and breathe.

- **Tai chi:** The Yang short form is best for beginners. Please visit TeamSherzai.com for a video.

Flexibility Training

Stretching or flexibility exercises are an important part of any physical activity program. They're designed to give you more flexibility in everyday activities and are especially helpful after aerobic exercise and resistance training. One of the main reasons people sustain minor injuries like ligament and tendon strains and tears is because they don't stretch properly. Those small injuries then become another impediment to regular exercise.

First, warm up with a few minutes of easy walking (stretching your muscles before they are warm may result in injury). Do each stretching exercise three to five times during each session. You should feel a little stretch or burn, but no pain. Slowly assume the desired position and hold the stretch for between ten and thirty seconds. Relax, breathe normally, and then repeat, trying to stretch farther.

Here are the nine main flexibility exercises that you should do regularly throughout the day:

- **Neck Stretch:** Tilt your head side to side and front to back. Follow with gentle neck circles.

- **Shoulder and Back Stretch:** Interlace your fingers and raise your arms above your head with your palms facing the ceiling. Extend your elbows and press your arms upward.

- **Shoulder Rotator Stretch:** Bend your right elbow and place your arm behind your back with your palm facing away from you. Holding a towel with your left hand, extend that arm overhead. Slowly bend your left elbow, bringing your left hand toward your right hand. Hold both ends of the towel firmly. As you breathe you may be able to bring the hands closer to each other, which increases the stretch.

- **Wrist Stretch:** Rotate the wrists in circles (both directions). Extend your arm and use your opposite hand to stretch your fingers both upward and downward.

- **Lower Back Stretch:** Sit on the ground with your back upright and legs extended in front of you. Slowly hinge at the waist and reach for your toes. Move slowly. Over time your abdomen will get closer to your thighs, and your head will get closer to your knees.

- **Hip Stretch:** Stand upright. Circle your hips in each direction. Then, with your hips stable, extend your torso to each side as you lengthen your waist.

- **Hamstring Stretch:** Stand upright. Fold at your waist, lengthening your torso over the fronts of your thighs. If your hamstrings are tight, bend your knees. Over time, as your muscles, ligaments, and tendons start to loosen, work toward straightening your legs.

- **Knee Stretch:** Circle your knees in each direction. Gently bend and straighten.

- **Ankle Stretch:** Rotate your ankles in each direction. While seated, use your hand to stretch your foot upward, downward, and to the left and right.

COMMON OBSTACLES

Physical Injuries: Rest the injured area. Seek help from your physician—ask for specific recommendations for how to heal the injury or prevent it from getting worse. Focus on exercising the uninjured areas. If you have a shoulder injury, for instance, focus on strengthening your legs.

Medical Conditions: Medical conditions such as heart disease, severe arthritis, and plantar fasciitis should be discussed with your physician to identify what exercises you can and cannot safely perform.

No Time: You can always modify your daily routine so that it includes some physical activity. You can take the stairs instead of the elevator or park farther away from your building. You can do a few push-ups and squats in your office during your lunch break, or bike to work when the weather permits. Our top choice is having a recumbent bike or foot pedaler in your living room so you can exercise while watching television or reading.

Bad Weather: Wear appropriate clothes, or exercise at home or indoors.

Disliking Exercise: You will dislike Alzheimer's disease and other diseases of the brain even more. Remind yourself why you're exercising. Think of the benefits to your brain and your overall health. Make exercise enjoyable by combining it with a satisfying mental activity. Many types of exercise don't require you to focus on what you're doing—you can put one foot in front of the other without conscious attention. Music, books on tape, podcasts, TV shows, and movies can all be enjoyed during exercise.

OUR PERSONAL APPROACH TO EXERCISE

- Our daily exercise routine happens in two locations: our living room and our office.

- In our living room we have a stationary bike, weights and resistance bands, a mat, a small step stool (for step-ups), and enough space for push-ups and sit-ups.

- In our office we have a stepper, minielliptical, dumbbells, and a mat for sit-ups. We also use standing desks.

- We like to exercise between meetings and seeing patients. We can also send e-mails and record audio files while using the stepper and minielliptical. We do a few minutes of high-intensity exercise regularly and are able to complete our program throughout the day without having to change our clothes or drive to the gym.

- We improve our stamina by taking the stairs, enjoying a brisk walk during lunchtime, and using the stationary bike in our living room while watching *The Big Bang Theory*.

- We do tae kwon do as a family three times a week.

- Our weekend relaxation always includes physical activities like swimming, playing tennis, biking along the beach in Santa Monica, and hiking in Topanga and Runyon Canyons.

- Our exercise goals appear on our Google Tasks list. We check them off every day and work together to ensure that everyone in our family succeeds with their exercise plan.

WEEKLY EXERCISE PLAN

Remember that an effective exercise plan needs to be convenient and easy. Do your best to minimize or eliminate long trips to the gym, overly complicated exercises, or exercises you find boring or uninspiring. We recommend that you start exercising in your living room or wherever you typically watch television and relax. Exercise either early in the morning, during your lunch break (in which case you can exercise in or around your office), or at home after work.

This one-week plan focuses on stretching, aerobic exercise, and strength training and is accessible to almost everyone (if adapted accordingly). You're welcome to choose other exercises from the previous lists or any physical activity that interests you.

Monday

STRETCHING: Begin by stretching for 5 to 10 minutes. Refer to the Flexibility Training exercises in this section as you stretch your neck, shoulders, hips, hamstrings, and ankles.

FOOT PEDAL EXERCISER: Find a comfortable chair. Turn on the news or your favorite television show and begin to pedal your foot pedal exerciser at roughly 1½ to 2 miles per hour. Increase your speed to 3 miles per hour during the first commercial break (slow down if you're unable to maintain this speed for the entire commercial break). At the end of the break, return to pedaling at 1½ to 2 miles per hour. Maintain a normal speed during the next commercial break. Continue with this pattern of low- to high-intensity aerobic exercise during every other commercial break, pedaling for 30 to 45 minutes total. It may take some time to build up to longer periods of intensity—consistency is most important when you're first starting an exercise program.

SQUATS: Separate your feet one and a half to two feet apart. Stand tall, and then bend your knees to roughly 90 degrees as you press your hips back. Pull your abdomen inward to support your lower back, and keep your knees in line with your feet to prevent knee pain. If balance is an issue for you, hold on to the back of a chair for additional support. You want to move slowly and with control. Start with 5 reps or as many as you can do without compromising your form. Increase the number of reps over time.

Tuesday

STRETCHING: Repeat yesterday's stretching routine. Be sure to challenge yourself with the flexibility exercises, but not to the point of pain.

FOOT PEDAL EXERCISER: Repeat yesterday's low- to high-intensity aerobic exercise routine for 30 to 45 minutes.

PUSH-UPS: Do 5 to 10 push-ups either at the wall or on the floor with your knees bent for extra support. If you're accustomed to doing regular push-ups, then do at least 10 with your abdomen firm and back straight.

Wednesday

REST

Thursday

STRETCHING: Repeat the stretching routine, but stretch more deeply this time if possible (though not to the point of pain).

FOOT PEDAL EXERCISER: Repeat the same low- to high-intensity aerobic exercise routine for 30 to 45 minutes. This time, try to increase your speed during each commercial break, and do your best to maintain your speed throughout the entire break.

SQUATS: Repeat the squats from Monday, but add at least one repetition while maintaining form and balance.

Friday

STRETCHING: Repeat the stretching routine and continue to challenge your flexibility.

FOOT PEDAL EXERCISER: Repeat yesterday's routine (increase your speed during each commercial break, and do your best to maintain your speed throughout the entire break).

PUSH-UPS: Repeat push-ups at the wall or on the floor with your knees bent. Add at least one repetition.

Saturday

REST

Sunday

REST

As you gain strength and confidence, your goal should be to exercise five or more days per week. Over time you can add extended periods of intense aerobic exercise, more repetitions for strength-training sets (adding one squat or push-up per week), and eventually two or more strength-training sets per session.

5.

Unwind

Colonel Thompson was a tough, no-nonsense Vietnam veteran in his early seventies. When we first met him and his wife, Clara, at the Veterans Affairs Hospital in Loma Linda, they seemed like they were enjoying retirement. They told us about their road trips along the California coast, and how they loved to visit their children and young grandchildren. But they'd come to see us because they were worried about the colonel's memory. He'd grown increasingly forgetful over the past year, and it was making him agitated.

"At first I thought he had selective amnesia," Clara told us, "but he's forgetting a lot more now. Sometimes he loses his train of thought before he can complete a sentence—and then he gets mad." She went on to say that when they'd met five years earlier, she suspected the colonel had some form of attention deficit disorder (ADD). He was an intelligent man with a quick moving mind that made it difficult for him to focus. The colonel agreed that he'd always had ADD, and that over the past few years it had gotten much worse. He admitted that his problems with attention were starting to affect complex daily activities like driving and managing their finances. Although he could still do these activities, they were increasingly difficult. He was also experiencing more anxiety than ever before. He kept pointing to his lack of concentration as the source of his problem. "My brain just doesn't work like it used to," he told us, "and that frustrates me." As the conversation continued, Colonel Thompson became more and more distressed. At times he was even tearful.

During his neuropsychological test, the colonel pushed back on some of the instructions, saying, "I know this. I don't need a test." The results showed that he was especially deficient in focus and recall. His MRI revealed some damaged blood vessels as well as shrinking of his entire brain. Because of these cognitive and physiological changes, we diagnosed him with MCI (mild cognitive impairment). During the physical examination, we also discovered that the colonel had an abnormally high resting heart rate of 96, and his blood pressure readings were 160/90 and 180/110 (elevated numbers had also been recorded during previous appointments). These high numbers were most likely the result of chronic stress and elevated adrenaline. Like so many of the patients we've worked with, he seemed to be caught in a vicious cycle: his inability to focus caused him stress, and this stress impaired his ability to focus.

Stress and the Brain

Stress comes in many forms. Conventional medicine focuses on two types of stress in the body: acute stress and chronic stress. Acute stress primes the body for action—giving a speech to a large group, for instance, or climbing a flight of stairs. This type of stress is time-bound. It comes in a short burst and then dissipates. But chronic stress lingers. It can be defined as our physical and mental response to a prolonged period of emotional pressure. This kind of stress can cause considerable damage to the body and especially the brain if not managed properly. The main difference between acute and chronic stress is the amount of time a person is exposed to it.

We prefer to look at stress a bit more comprehensively. Yes, the acute and chronic distinctions are useful, but they don't tell the whole story. Is all acute stress helpful? Is all chronic stress bad? That depends entirely on how you manage the stress. Acute stress sometimes overwhelms us, which can be unhealthy for many bodily systems. Studies have shown that acute bouts of stress can actually damage brain structures. On the other hand, chronic stress isn't always harmful. Pursuing long-term goals toward an important milestone (getting an academic degree, for example, or changing a lifelong habit) can seem overwhelming, but this kind of purposeful action actually creates significant cognitive reserve (a measure of the brain's resilience). The associated stress may in fact be chronic, but it fits your vision and purpose. The stress has both a direction and a time line: you set the goal, and you're in control. The two of us have experienced significant amounts of stress in medical school and as practicing physicians, and yet this stress is deeply connected to our goals as human beings. Pursuing these long-term dreams made us stronger and more resilient. Don't be afraid of this kind of stress: welcome it, as long as you're controlling it and are capable of managing it.

The type of stress we focus on when working with our patients is what we call uncontrolled stress—you don't own it and you didn't choose it. This kind of stress doesn't have a purpose or meaning, and there's no end in sight. Unrelenting, uncontrolled stress puts the body in autonomic overdrive and subsequently increases cortisol, a steroid stress hormone produced by the adrenal gland. The purpose of cortisol is to supply the body with energy in the midst of stress. Blood glucose levels spike in response. While higher blood glucose levels help us fight immediate threats, they also cause considerable long-term damage like anxiety and depression, digestive problems, disrupted sleep, and depressed immune function, which then makes us more vulnerable to infections and cancer. Chronic elevated cortisol may also lead to insulin resistance. The brain is especially susceptible to these physiological changes. Elevated cortisol has been shown in several studies to increase the risk of developing Alzheimer's disease. Cortisol has also been linked to shrinkage of the hippocampus. New evidence indicates that uncontrolled stress and high cortisol levels can even change how our genes are activated and deactivated.

The many negative effects of uncontrolled stress include:

Anxiety and Depression: Uncontrolled stress appears to inhibit the production of serotonin and other important neurotransmitters, and also impairs synaptic connections that help in coping with stressful situations. As a result, we experience increased anxiety and depression, both of which are significant risk factors for Alzheimer's.

Impaired Immune Function: Uncontrolled stress impairs the signaling of immune cells and also lowers the level of white blood cells. The body is then less able to defend itself against acute illnesses and also takes longer to heal. For the brain, this means that metabolic by-products build up and cause significant damage over time.

Impaired Attention: High levels of cortisol and epinephrine released during stress impair the growth of neurons in the frontal lobe, a brain region that controls concentration, attention, decision making, judgment, and memory formation.

Increased Inflammation: Uncontrolled stress can trigger a cascade of chemical reactions that disrupts cells and blood vessels and causes inflammation of the neural tissue.

Increased Oxidative By-Products: Reactive oxidative by-products created by uncontrolled stress can significantly damage brain cells and tissues.

Shrinking of the Brain: Stress literally shrinks the brain. Ongoing stress can interfere with the production of new cellular structures and destroy fully formed cells in the hippocampus, even after only a single stressful event. A study conducted by researchers at McGill University revealed that elderly subjects with increased cortisol levels had on average a 14 percent reduction in hippocampal volume and impaired hippocampus-dependent memory. When the hippocampus is damaged by cortisol, it struggles to regulate the body's stress system. This results in the secretion of even more cortisol, a vicious cycle that in turn damages more cells.

Increased Beta-Amyloid: There is some evidence that one specific stress-related chemical reaction—the release of corticotropin-releasing factor (CRF)—can contribute to the buildup of amyloid. One study found that elevated CRF in the brain appears to increase amyloid levels.

Gene Activation and Function: Uncontrolled stress alters our genes and their expression. Stress has been shown to decrease new cell growth and impair neuroplasticity (the ability of neural circuits to adapt and survive). One study found that changes in gene expression led to altered levels of BDNF (brain-derived neurotrophic factor): stress decreased the level of BDNF, thereby inhibiting the growth of new neurons and connections, while exercise, a stress-reducing activity, appeared to increase levels of BDNF.

Weight Gain: Uncontrolled stress has consistently been associated with weight gain, which we know is a risk factor for heart disease, cancer, and dementia.

Increased Heart Rate and Blood Pressure: The stress hormones cortisol and epinephrine cause increased heart rate and blood pressure, both of which are vascular risk factors that promote cognitive decline.

Disrupting Healthy Lifestyle Behaviors: When we experience significant stress, we're less able to process our emotions or access coping mechanisms. As a result, we quickly become exhausted, overwhelmed, and unable to sustain healthy behaviors: our sleep is disturbed, we tend to crave sugary, fatty foods, and fatigue keeps us from exercising.

A Plan for the Colonel

The key to reversing the colonel's cognitive symptoms and helping him avoid a further diagnosis was to decrease his stress and anxiety. Both were negatively affecting his memory and his quality of life. We'd learned a fair amount about the colonel during that first appointment. We knew that he was very resistant to pharmaceuticals, so an antianxiety medication was entirely out of the question. We could tell from his language and experiences—the way he spoke about his hobbies and his family—that he probably wasn't the kind of person to join an ashram, sit cross-legged, and repeat a mantra. That kind of meditation wouldn't work for him. But not all forms of meditation require sitting quietly. In the traditional Buddhist teachings of meditation, there are multiple ways of calming the mind: you can sit, walk, stand, or even lie down.

Because the colonel already spent most of the day sitting, we wanted to introduce a different kind of practice into his life. We suggested walking. Walking meditation has been studied in meditation centers and tested in various groups. People describe it as invigorating, and it can be a very helpful way of building concentration. For many of us it can even be more relaxing than sitting.

The colonel described his neighborhood as calm and walking-friendly, which was an excellent start. He would need a safe, mostly controlled environment in order to carry out a walking meditation. We told the colonel to choose a specific path, not wander aimlessly. Starting at one point and ending at another would create a sense of regimented activity—the groundwork for meditative thinking. When the body walks a familiar circuit, the problem-solving part of the mind can be put to rest, and we instantly feel more relaxed.

It was important that the colonel understood this was not an aerobic walk (though aerobic walking is very beneficial for brain health, as we showed in the "Exercise" chapter). We encouraged him to start walking more slowly than normal and to find a pace that gave him a sense of ease. His pace could vary depending on how he felt (sometimes walking fast can be calming when we're agitated). Once he found a pace that was easy for him to maintain, he would then let his attention settle. He could think of letting go of this body and allowing it to take him for a walk. We encouraged him to feel the ground beneath his feet, the tensing of his leg muscles, the easy swing of his arms.

To help the colonel stay present and focused, we suggested that he label his steps. He'd spent a lot of his life marching, and he had good memories of his time in the service, so we tried to make this exercise as regimented as possible. (We would never use associations with the military when working with a veteran suffering from PTSD, but this was not the case with the colonel.) We told him he could say, "One, Two" as he walked, but the colonel said he preferred, "Left, Right." The point of this labeling was feedback: if he looked down and saw that his feet weren't lining up with his verbal cues, he'd know that his attention had wandered. We told him it was normal to become distracted, that he shouldn't get upset with himself. If he saw something interesting or beautiful that captured his attention, he could look at it, but he should stop walking in that moment and tell himself that the meditation had stopped. Once he was ready, he could begin again.

To our surprise, this idea seemed to excite the colonel. He was grateful that we'd offered him an alternative to pharmaceuticals, and he agreed to start working on it right away.

Exploring Meditation

We used to get uncomfortable when someone mentioned the benefits of meditation. Our medical training hadn't taught us anything about it—there wasn't strong, evidence-based research supporting meditation for brain health or even overall health when we were medical students and residents. While we knew mindfulness activities could provide a sense of calm, we doubted that they had any therapeutic benefits for people with MCI or dementia. Then we moved to California. Almost all our patients here practice some form of meditation or yoga, and they constantly ask us about the benefits. We both decided we needed to investigate further.

First we looked at research that explored the brain waves involved in meditation. Brain waves are coordinated electrical impulses that result when neurons communicate with one another. We found many studies that showed how meditation induces theta waves, which confer a state of relaxed wakefulness. Almost all relaxing activities increase theta waves in different areas of the brain. Even when you're doing something that involves a complex motor routine, like playing the piano or skiing, you can find yourself "in the zone," a brain state in which you're simply experiencing the activity rather than thinking about it. This is sometimes called an optimal experience, or as Mihaly Csikszentmihalyi says, "flow." We knew that this type of mental state was critical to both focus and stress management.

We also knew that most of us spend our days in a very different kind of mental state. We live in a world of distraction. We're constantly interrupted by phone calls, e-mails, texts, and social media alerts. We've convinced ourselves that multitasking is the key to productivity, but what we're actually doing is rapid "task switching," which places enormous stress on the brain. A 2011 study in the *Proceedings of the National Academy of Sciences* showed that multitasking takes an especially big toll on working memory in older adults (ages sixty to eighty). Researchers asked the participants to watch a recorded scene and then interrupted it for several seconds with an image of a person's face. The participants were then asked to identify the person's gender and approximate age. Afterward, they were questioned about the original scene. The older individuals had a difficult time disengaging from the interruption and remembering the previous scene. A control group of younger adults (ages twenty to thirty) struggled far less with the same task. Researchers also looked at brain activity with functional MRIs and found distinct differences between older and younger brains: younger brains were easily able to return to the previous activity, whereas in older brains, the areas associated with the interruption remained stimulated. The study concluded that multitasking in older adults can lead to significant memory disruption.

We started to think of meditation as an antidote to modern distraction. If it could help us focus, it could also help us reduce stress, especially in the brain. Meditation isn't "doing nothing" with the mind. It's not a passive activity. Meditation is really the practice of cultivating concentration and focus—and these are the first cognitive domains (specialized brain regions) to be affected by dementia.

Now we have a collection of intriguing studies that demonstrate the effects of meditation on cognition and stress reduction. While none of these studies is perfect (we still need more research on how meditation actually works in the brain), research suggests that meditation is a powerful tool for cognitive health. A 2014 comprehensive review and meta-analysis from Johns Hopkins University investigated the effects of meditation programs on stress reduction. Researchers reviewed forty-seven trials that included a total of 3,515 participants and found that eight-week meditation programs, especially those in group settings, can reduce the negative effects of stress, anxiety, and depression. Beyond stress reduction, meditation has been shown in other studies either to increase the brain's volume or slow the rate at which the brain loses volume due to normal aging or disease. In a study conducted at Harvard Massachusetts General Hospital, functional

TYPES OF MEDITATION

There are hundreds of types of meditation. Some of the more popular styles, which themselves are often divided into different schools and practices, include:

Kirtan Kriya: a twelve-minute yoga meditation with chanting

Kundalini Yoga: focus on postures and breathing techniques to awaken energy

Metta Meditation: focus on loving-kindness toward self and others

Mindfulness-Based Stress Reduction (MBSR): focus on bodily sensations to increase relaxation; has been shown to reduce anxiety and depression

Qijong: focus on slow body movements and breathing techniques to release "life energy"

Transcendental Meditation (TM): use of repeated sound to focus attention

Vipassana Meditation: focus on breathing, thoughts, and sensations with the goal of cultivating insight

Zen Meditation: eyes open, focus on breathing and experiencing thoughts and sensations

---

MRI was used to measure cortical thickness in twenty individuals who were experienced in meditation. Brain regions associated with attention and sensory processing were thicker in meditators than in matched controls. These differences were most pronounced in older participants, suggesting that meditation might offset age-related changes in brain volume. Another study matched Zen practitioners with nonmeditators and found that meditation helps us maintain brain volume, especially in attention centers. Two other recent studies also found an association between meditation and brain volume: 1) A 2015 study at UCLA showed that meditation increased hippocampal volume; and 2) Researchers at the University of Pittsburgh showed that meditation resulted in increased volume in both the amygdala and caudate area, two brain regions involved in emotional management. Yet another study found that mindfulness-based training was associated with reduced hippocampal atrophy and improved connectivity between the hippocampus and other areas of the brain, both of which could enhance memory.

Which type of meditation is best for brain health? There is no one technique that has been proven to be superior, and people may respond differently to different styles. If you're just starting out, we recommend trying simple breathing exercises, like the ones we've included in the Unwind Personalized Program. People with more experience may be drawn to more advanced mindfulness techniques. The best technique for you is one that interests you and brings you a sense of calm.

Making Sure It Works

Dean once had a patient named Monika who was very passionate about meditation. She studied with gurus, went to international retreats, and had been practicing for over a decade. She was also a high-powered businesswoman with an extremely successful public relations agency. Distraction was what finally prompted her to see a neurologist. She was struggling quite a bit with memory and recall, and to Dean, she didn't seem all that relaxed.

Dean took Monika's medical history and completed a physical exam. During her neuropsychological test, Monika made mistakes on two measures of distractibility. She was even talking as Dean tested her—it was extremely difficult to get her to focus.

Afterward Dean told her that he respected her meditation practice, and that she should continue studying. But he also wanted her to try something else. Something really simple—no mantras, no mala beads, just a basic relaxation exercise. He asked Monika to close her eyes and then tense all the muscles in her body starting with her forehead and eyes, moving down to her neck, shoulders, and back, and eventually all the way down to her toes. After five seconds, Dean told her to release the tension and take some deep breaths. They did the exercise together several times, concentrating on the difference between tension and release.

"I actually feel relaxed," Monika said when she opened her eyes. And she looked it.

This exercise would be her daily assignment for the next month. When she returned for her follow-up, she reported positive changes in her attention and far less anxiety. Because Monika was overly enthusiastic about the process and ritual of meditation, she'd somehow lost sight of the desired outcome: relaxation. We're not saying meditation retreats aren't helpful— they're wonderful for many people. But make sure your chosen mindful activity actually makes you relaxed. If you don't feel a clear sense of ease or improved mental focus, ask questions to further refine your technique, and if that doesn't work, consider trying a different style.

Unwind Myths

- **Stress is most damaging to your heart:** Stress damages the entire body, but the brain is especially susceptible, even more so than the heart. Uncontrolled stress causes considerable damage in the temporal and frontal lobes, destroying both brain cells and the connections between them.

- **You have to sit cross-legged when you're meditating:** You can meditate while standing, lying down, or even walking. Walking meditation can be a great choice for elderly people who aren't comfortable sitting, or who find that sitting makes them tired.

- **You have to meditate for long periods of time to experience any benefits:** Any amount of meditation or mindfulness is helpful. Even a few three-minute sessions per day are likely to reduce stress and support your brain.

The Colonel's Transformation

Six months later, the colonel returned. As we entered the room, we saw a very happy couple waiting at the edge of their seats, eager to give us a full report. Before we could sit down, the colonel told us about how he'd been walking twice a day. It was a bit of challenge for him to focus at first, but now he loved his new routine, and Clara said his attention had improved considerably. After repeating the neuropsychological tests, we found that the colonel's attention and recall were much stronger. Even more remarkably, his anxiety and stress had all but disappeared. He also had better balance, stronger back and leg muscles, and had lost fifteen pounds. He stuck to his walking meditation and was able to manage his anxiety and stress long term without medication.

Alternatives to Meditation

Because meditation requires the cognitive ability to sustain attention and remember the goal of the practice, people with serious cognitive decline and dementia might not be able to meditate effectively. There are, however, many alternatives to meditation that afford similar benefits:

Walking: Just as we saw with Colonel Thompson, walking around your neighborhood can be a powerful meditative activity that allows the brain to rest and restore. Stick to the same route and work to minimize distractions and interruptions. Consider using the rhythmic cadence of walking as a form of mantra to help reduce stress.

Yoga: Though the research on yoga and cognition has been mixed, a few studies have uncovered some promising aspects of this meditative practice. A study conducted in India found that participants had significantly lower levels of cortisol after a three-month yoga program. A 2016 review also found that yoga has therapeutic benefits for those suffering from depression. Other studies have associated yoga with improvements in anxiety, depression, and overall sense of well-being. Though more research is needed, yoga certainly appears to be a powerful stress-relieving activity.

Listening to Music: Most of us know from personal experience that listening to our favorite songs can be a great way to combat stress. Research has shown that music has a direct effect on our cortisol levels. A study published in *Frontiers of Psychology* in 2011 found that people who listened to music during surgery had lower cortisol levels and also required less anesthesia.

Simplifying Your Physical Environment: Just like meditation and yoga help to organize thought processes in the brain, organizing your external environment can help you process new information more efficiently. We are products of our environment, and the environments we create reflect our mental and emotional health. When our homes or offices become disorderly, our physical and mental health can suffer. We're prone to distraction. Focusing is difficult. We experience more stress and anxiety. But a clean, orderly space makes it easier for us to focus on what's important and also encourages sustained quiet and self-reflection, both of which positively impact cognition. Simplifying your environment can also affect other aspects of healthy living. By getting rid of clutter in your living room, for instance, you could make room for a recumbent bike or a yoga mat or a set of dumbbells. Instead of surrounding yourself with things that cause you stress, you can surround yourself with tools that promote brain health.

Cultivating Healthy Relationships: Meaningful relationships have been shown to reduce cortisol levels and increase BDNF (the growth factor that creates new neurons and connections). Studies have also found that oxytocin, a hormone associated with decreased stress response, is released when a loved one hugs you or holds your hand. The Harvard Grant Study has shown over the course of seventy-five years that meaningful relationships keep us happier, healthier, less stressed, and less lonely.

Living a Purpose-Driven Life: Many studies have concluded that a sense of purpose is linked to a longer, healthier life as well as reduced disability and mortality. A sense of purpose keeps the mind active and therefore less susceptible to daily stressors. It also provides controlled stress that is driven by meaning and time, which can significantly increase cognitive reserve. The Blue Zones research consistently showed us that people age more successfully when they live with a sense of purpose and responsibility. A 2010 study at Rush University looked at American and Japanese elderly people and their sense of purpose as they aged. Americans experienced a significant drop in sense of purpose after the age of sixty-five, likely due to retirement. In Japan, however, people maintained a strong sense of purpose well into old age. If you're retired, consider volunteering or engaging in community service as a way to protect both your mental and physical health.

Conclusion

Stress management is a critical and often misunderstood aspect of a brain-healthy lifestyle. Healthy stress is controlled and useful for achieving long-term goals and navigating the challenges of modern living. Uncontrolled stress initiates a hormonal cascade that taxes the brain on many levels. It even changes the structure of the brain, destroying cells and decreasing its volume. When we include meditation in our daily routines, we can dramatically reduce the effects of uncontrolled stress and even expand important attention centers in the brain. Unwinding, just like all the lifestyle factors in this book, should be personalized to your own interests and strengths. Meditation can mean sitting, chanting, walking around your neighborhood, or living in a decluttered space that helps you unwind at the end of the day. Whatever method you choose should be simple, convenient, and most important, relaxing.

> # Your Personalized
> # **UNWIND**
> # Program

Though managing chronic stress can sometimes create even more stress, this lifestyle factor is essential to cognitive health. Stress affects each of us differently, but we're all vulnerable to uncontrolled stress, especially when it comes to the brain. Regardless of your stage of dementia or degree of risk, stress reduction is crucial to overall health and happiness. If meditation doesn't appeal to you, there are many other relaxing and enjoyable activities to help you stay calm. Please use the following assessment and exercises to build your personalized stress-relief program.

SELF-ASSESSMENT

Vision, Strengths, and Weaknesses: Assess your vision for a brain-healthy stress management program, and identify factors that might help or hinder your efforts.

Vision: What is your ideal stress-relief plan for brain health? What activities make you feel calm and relaxed? How often do you enjoy those activities and would it be possible to do them more often? What type of meditation from this chapter resonated with you the most? What are some of the uncontrolled stressors in your life that you'd like to manage?

Strengths: What strengths and resources will help you achieve your vision?

Weaknesses: What are the obstacles to your vision?

1. How will you benefit from reducing stress in your life?

Examples: I will have better focus and attention. I will experience less anxiety and depression. I will get better sleep. It will be easier for me to exercise and eat healthy foods. I will be able to enjoy life to its fullest.

2. What are the most important areas for you to work on?

Examples: I'll set aside twenty minutes a day to do something that I find relaxing. I'll explore different meditative activities. I'll go to a meditation workshop with my friend. I'll start a walking meditation either by myself or with a group.

3. What obstacles might prevent you from reducing your stress?

Examples: I have a very stressful job. I don't have much time to meditate. I've never tried mindfulness activities and don't know where to start. I've been stressed out all my life and don't know if I can change now. I don't have anywhere quiet to meditate.

4. What might help you manage your stress? What are your resources?

Examples: I can learn different relaxation techniques. I can set aside time every day to do something relaxing. I have a quiet and comfortable spot that I can use for meditation. I can visit TeamSherzai.com for more examples of relaxation techniques.

5. Who can help you and how?

Examples: My spouse can help remind me to take some time for myself. I can go to a yoga class with my friend. My family and I can reorganize the house so that it's less cluttered and more conducive to relaxation. My friend is a psychologist and can help me with relaxation techniques.

6. When will you start?

Our Recommendation: You should start once you've secured a quiet spot and some time that you can dedicate to stress management. You don't need to have all the resources in place right away (such as a friend or supportive group or time each day). Try to begin with three days per week, and then slowly increase to seven days a week. You can start with short, three-minute sessions with the intention of increasing to twenty- to thirty-minute sessions over time.

MEDITATION EXERCISES

To become acquainted with the practice of meditation, give these exercises a try.

Mindful Breathing

- Find a comfortable place where you won't be disturbed.

- Sit up straight. Consider using a wall to support your back.

- Close your eyes.

- Breathe slowly and deeply through your nose.

- When you've reached the natural point of exhale, breathe out slowly through your mouth.

- Once you've gotten into a rhythmic breathing pattern, typically after a minute or so, start to focus on the sounds around you. Don't analyze or memorize them. Just listen quietly and experience them.

- When other thoughts arise in your mind, don't engage them. Let them drift out of your mind and return your attention to what you can hear.

- Try this exercise for ten minutes each day. As you get more proficient, feel free to increase the time.

Variations on Mindful Breathing

- **Sensation:** Focus on different bodily sensations, like the floor beneath you, and the sensation of air entering your nose and exiting your mouth.

- **Progressive Muscle Relaxation:** Starting at the top of your body and moving downward, begin to tense all your muscles—your forehead, eyes, jaw, neck, shoulders, back, arms, hands, abdomen, buttocks, thighs, calves, and feet. Hold this tension for at least five seconds. Then take a big inhalation, and on your exhalation release everything. Take a few more deep breaths. Feel the difference between a tensed body and a relaxed body.

- **Visualization:** Imagine you're on a riverbank and that your thoughts are slowly riding a current that flows from left to right. When a thought arises, simply watch it float down the river and out of sight.

Alternatives to Traditional Meditation

These options are especially recommended for those individuals already struggling with cognitive decline.

Walking Meditation: Walk the same route every day. This will allow your brain to relax and focus on the pleasant sensations in your body. The goal isn't aerobic exercise (though aerobic exercise is very important for brain health). Instead, find a pace that feels natural and try to maintain it throughout your walk.

Yoga: There are many different types of yoga to suit your personality and your desired level of exercise and mental relaxation. Some classical yoga postures for stress relief include child's pose, spinal twists, gentle hip openers, cat/cow pose, legs-up-the-wall, and corpse pose. Please visit our website, TeamSherzai.com, for more information on these postures.

Simplifying Your Life: Live in a clean, uncluttered home. Approach your work in an organized, purpose-driven way.

Meaningful Relationships: Surround yourself with friends and loved ones. They naturally reduce your stress levels.

Listening to Music: This is one of the best ways to unwind. Try to fill your day with music as much as possible, and use it at night to relax before sleep.

Work Toward Increasing:

- Deep, cleansing breaths

- Time spent in nature

- Time spent in a clean, organized home

- Meditation

- Periods of quiet in your day, ideally without technology

Work Toward Eliminating:

- Situations that make you stressed out

- Relationships that make you stressed out

- Not giving yourself some time to relax each day

WEEKLY UNWIND PLAN

MONDAY: Find a quiet space for practicing mindful breathing. Assume a comfortable seated posture, but refrain from lying down, which might make you fall asleep. Close your eyes and sit quietly for 3 to 5 minutes. Your breathing should be deep but natural and comfortable. Do this once in the morning and once in the afternoon. If you have trouble focusing, consider using an app with a timer and calming background music or nature sounds to help you relax.

TUESDAY: Repeat mindful breathing for 3 to 5 minutes during both the morning and afternoon. Feel your body being cleansed with each exhalation.

WEDNESDAY: Begin with mindful breathing for 3 to 5 minutes. Then add progressive muscle relaxation, a variation of mindful breathing described earlier in this section. Feel each muscle as it relaxes, and how this physical relaxation encourages mental relaxation as well.

THURSDAY: Begin with a few minutes of mindful breathing and progressive muscle relaxation. Then add an element of visualization. Picture yourself sitting comfortably in a specific and calming location—on the beach, in the desert, or on top of a mountain. Imagine the temperature, wind, light, colors, and other sensory details. Relax deeply.

FRIDAY: Begin with a few minutes of mindful breathing with progressive muscle relaxation and visualization (try to use the same location you used yesterday; becoming familiar with a specific, calming location will help strengthen your meditation practice over time). Today you'll also add an element of focus. Choose a specific object that you see regularly—your favorite necklace or painting, for example—and imagine it in great detail. See all aspects of the object. Maintain your focus for at least three minutes.

SATURDAY: Today you're ready to combine mindful breathing and all the variations you've learned this week: progressive muscle relaxation, visualization, and focus. Challenge yourself to sit for at least 5 minutes both in the morning and afternoon.

SUNDAY: Practice the same elements of mindful breathing. If you feel comfortable, try sitting for 6 to 7 minutes.

Continue building your skills with the goal of increasing your daily meditation sessions to 15 to 20 minutes each.

- Constant distractions caused by cell phones, computers, and television

- A living space with nowhere quiet or calm to retreat to

COMMON OBSTACLES

Not Knowing How to Meditate: Try the exercises described in this program. They're simple, free, and highly effective. You can also find many free resources online, including instructional videos on YouTube.

Not Having a Quiet Space: You certainly don't need an ashram to start meditating. You could do a few minutes of mindful breathing in your bedroom when you wake up or before you go to sleep. You can even meditate on a park bench or while waiting for the subway. All that's required is focusing on your body and your breath.

Having a Stressful Life: Even a three-minute-per-day meditation practice can significantly relieve stress. Try not to think of mindful activities as a burden, but rather a solution to the stress you feel right now.

Not Having Anyone to Meditate With: While it can be relaxing to meditate on your own, and in your own space, you can also join a group or class at a community center, or find a meditation community online.

Being a Hyperactive Person Who Can't Easily Relax: Not everyone has to meditate the same way, or for long periods of time. Three-minute sessions are helpful for people who find it difficult to relax. Try several of these sessions per day, and gradually increase the time as you become more comfortable.

OUR PERSONAL APPROACH TO UNWINDING

- Our family uses Google Tasks to track our activities for the week and eliminate those that don't support our health. Though we're a very busy family of four, we try not to overschedule ourselves. If we have a particularly full day, we make sure to cancel meetings and events at night so we have enough time to decompress. If we have a research deadline, we focus on getting that one job done well. If we have a major trip out of town, we return at least a day before we go back to work. This way we have enough time to eat well, exercise, and sleep soundly as we jump back into our routine.

- We practice mindful breathing for five to ten minutes, four times per day.

- We spend our lunch hours walking the same path around the hospital. This is an opportunity for both exercise and relaxation.

- One of our favorite unwinding activities is listening to Beethoven's "Moonlight Sonata." We also enjoy listening to our daughter, Sophie, singing in the backseat of our van while we drive up the Pacific Coast Highway (Sophie is a classically trained opera singer and Alex, our son, plays classical piano). We often listen to classical music at a low volume throughout our home. Every hour or so, either Sophie or Alex plays a dance song. We have a rule that we all have to get up and dance, which is yet another form of stress relief.

6.

Restore

As neurology residents we were on call for the stroke team every three or four nights. We worked directly with patients for twenty-four hours straight, making critical decisions about their medical care. Sometimes we could sneak in a ten-minute nap, but not often. After our twenty-four-hour shifts, we'd then update patient files for another six to eight hours. Not sleeping became an art form in those years. We drank gallons of coffee and kept meticulous checklists to stay organized and avoid making mistakes. We thought this aspect of our medical training made us tougher, smarter, more resilient. We thought we were invincible.

And yet our research, creativity, and family relationships were all suffering. We were physically wrecked. Our minds felt like overloaded computers struggling to churn out a single coherent idea. At times the exhaustion was almost unbearable. After one twenty-four-hour shift, Ayesha was so tired she blacked out and couldn't remember where she was. Her professor quietly tapped her on the shoulder, took her patient notes, and sent her home. There was a special transportation service at the hospital for sleep-deprived residents who felt it was too dangerous to drive.

Resident hours became part of an ongoing public debate in 1984 when eighteen-year-old Libby Zion was admitted to New York Hospital with a fever and muscle spasms. She was seen by two overworked residents who were so busy with other patients that they didn't have time to check on her during the night. The next morning Libby's fever spiked and she went into cardiac arrest. She could not be revived. Her father was Sidney

Zion, a powerful journalist who had worked for the *New York Times* and the *Daily News*. When he found out his daughter had been evaluated by doctors-in-training who worked thirty-six-hour shifts with little to no sleep, he first sued the hospital and then fought to change the health-care system altogether. Because of his efforts, New York became the first state to limit resident hours in 1989, and by 2003 the Accreditation Council for Graduate Medical Education recommended that residents work no more than eighty hours a week, with a twenty-four-hour shift maximum. A follow-up study at Harvard showed that residents who worked eighty hours per week made 36 percent more mistakes, and 22 percent more serious medical errors, than those who worked sixty-three hours per week.

Our clinical experience has shown us again and again that restorative sleep is critical to cognitive function and overall quality of life. Put simply, good sleep leads to good health. Instead of juice cleanses or detoxes or any of the trendy wellness practices we see popping up all over Los Angeles, we should be doing the simplest, most important cleanse of all: beautiful, restorative sleep. Seven to eight hours of sleep do more to remove toxins, oxidative by-products, and amyloid—and even negative thoughts and memories—than any other cleanse you could find.

Sleep was designed especially for the brain. Our bodies are bound by an automatic daily cycle, shifting back and forth between wakefulness and passive rest, but the brain enters a completely different state during sleep. This energetic state promotes two important functions: 1) Detoxification of amyloid and oxidative by-products; and 2) Consolidation of memory and thought—short-term memories are converted into long-term memories, unneeded memories are eliminated, thought processes are organized, and new connections are built.

When you fail to get restorative sleep, your thinking and concentration suffer. The result is the "brain fog" that plagues so many of our patients with MCI and Alzheimer's. Lack of quality sleep impairs your ability to function during the day—your focus, processing speed, short-term memory—and also disrupts your circadian rhythm. It's easy to get into a pattern of poor sleep where you're always exhausted but still can't get good rest. This is an incredibly frustrating experience for anyone, especially for those struggling with cognitive decline. But as you'll learn in this chapter, there are many techniques for improving the quality of your sleep. The concept of "restore" goes well beyond a good night's rest to encompass healthy sleep patterns, prebedtime relaxation, managing light and noise in your environment, and making dietary choices that promote restorative sleep.

We've known for decades that sleep deprivation has dire physiological and neurological consequences, but new research has revealed that chronic poor sleep and lack of sleep (even if you feel good after sleeping only a few hours a night) both affect neural networks involving behavior, problem solving, and memory. Functional MRI scans of sleep-deprived individuals have shown decreased brain activation during both math and verbal tests. In the last decade, several studies have also connected sleep disorders to an increased risk of dementia. From a clinical perspective, sleep is a critical component of cognitive health, and oftentimes changes in sleep habits are an early sign of neurodegenerative disease. Somewhat surprisingly, there are no official sleep guidelines for patients with early memory and cognitive difficulties, MCI, dementia, or Alzheimer's, but we view sleep as an essential aspect of any brain-healthy lifestyle plan.

How Sleep Works

Sleep is a necessary biological function for almost every living organism. Pythons and opossums sleep for eighteen hours a day; dolphins get around ten hours, and horses just three. Even fish and fruit flies sleep. We've all heard the figure that humans spend roughly a third of our lives asleep, but few of us understand the purpose of sleep, the fact that each night the brain silently recovers from the previous day, cleaning, clearing, organizing, and consolidating. Though it's true that the brain is somewhat quieter at night, it is far from dormant.

Normal human sleep is characterized by two different types of sleep: NREM (nonrapid eye movement) and REM (rapid eye movement). NREM sleep is divided into three distinct phases:

Stage 1 (N1): Light sleep, which lasts between one and seven minutes. This is a transitional stage in which a person can be easily awoken with a soft noise.

Stage 2 (N2): During this stage of sleep, which lasts from ten to twenty-five minutes, it's more difficult to wake someone up, heart rate and body temperature fall, and memory begins to be consolidated from short term into long term.

Stage 3 (N3): The deepest stage during which we experience slow wave sleep (SWS) and are even less responsive to the external environment. Norepinephrine, serotonin, acetylcholine, and histamine all decrease, while growth hormone peaks. Memories from the previous day are processed, transmitted from cell to cell, and ultimately converted into long-term memories. Amyloid that has accumulated during the day is also cleared during this stage. PET scan studies have shown that when individuals learned the route to a destination in a virtual reality town, the same areas of the hippocampus that were activated during this memory task showed increased activation in SWS. The amount of activity in the hippocampus even correlated with performance the next day (more brain activity during sleep meant greater success with the virtual route). These findings have led scientists to conclude that the brain "replays" encoded information during SWS.

REM sleep, the second type of sleep, lasts between twenty and forty minutes each cycle. Our muscles are paralyzed and the brain's reticular activating system, which controls our level of consciousness, is inhibited. Researchers believe that REM sleep allows the brain to organize information and restructure itself by integrating memories into a larger neural network, a bit like defragging a hard drive. The rise of acetylcholine and cortisol during this phase has also been implicated in declarative memory processing.

The sleep cycle proceeds in the following order and lasts roughly ninety minutes:

Stage N1 → Stage N2 → Stage N3 → REM → Back to Stage N1

Each night we pass through an average of four to six cycles. Most sleep, about 75 to 80 percent, occurs during the NREM stages. REM sleep usually comprises 20 to 25 percent of total sleep. Slow wave sleep, in NREM

Stage 3, dominates the first half of the night, while the amount of REM is nearly doubled in the second half of the night.

The sleep cycle is an elegant and efficient process of restoring both the body and the mind—unless we tamper with it. Our sleep-wake cycle is strongly influenced by circadian rhythms, the body's innate twenty-four-hour biological processes. Though the circadian clock is a self-sustaining system, it is affected and adjusted by external factors like light and temperature. When we're exposed to daylight, the pineal gland, a pea-sized structure located just above the midbrain, goes to work producing melatonin, a hormone that makes us feel sleepy. When the sun goes down, the pineal gland then actively secretes melatonin and releases it into the blood at around 9:00 P.M. The levels remain high throughout the night, facilitating deep sleep. Roughly twelve hours later, at around 9:00 A.M., melatonin levels fall rapidly and we become alert for the day's activities.

Any disruption in light exposure negatively affects this natural rhythm. Studies have shown that long-term night-shift workers experience suppressed melatonin production at night due to continuous light exposure and are at an increased risk for cognitive impairment. A 2001 study in *Nature Neuroscience* examined the cognitive performance of transmeridian flight attendants. Researchers found that these individuals had smaller right temporal lobe volumes as well as impaired cognitive performance. Chronic disruption of circadian rhythms—over a period of four years in this study—seemed to have a cumulative negative effect on both cognitive function and cerebral structure. Other studies have found that TNF (a protein that increases at the time of usual sleep onset) is elevated in response to sleep disruption and deprivation. These abnormal TNF levels contribute to the exhaustion and confusion that characterizes jet lag.

Circadian rhythms are also affected by internal biochemical processes. We now have evidence that anxiety and depression both adversely affect circadian rhythms, and also that people with altered circadian rhythms tend to develop depression and anxiety more frequently. This strong relationship speaks to the power of neurotransmitters and hormones—like serotonin and cortisol—and their effects on the brain's limbic system, which controls anxiety and fear. Many people suffering from mood disorders may not realize there is such a direct, biochemical link to sleeping problems.

Disrupting the sleep cycle has significant consequences, but normalizing your schedule can have tremendous benefits. If you're experiencing short-term memory loss or other symptoms of cognitive decline, we recommend evaluating whether your work schedule or an undiagnosed mood disorder may be contributing factors. What's natural for the body is what's best for the brain—and when we go against the body's innate rhythms, the brain suffers the most.

How Much Is Enough?

How many hours do we need to sleep each night? That depends on how you sleep. The majority of people need at least seven hours per night, but more isn't necessarily better. People who sleep nine hours per night usually perform worse on cognitive tests (among the elderly, sleeping nine hours per night is also associated with cardiovascular disease). People who sleep six hours per night or less also perform poorly. Yet there are some people who sleep for six hours and experience no negative effects on their cognitive performance. Researchers have found that these individuals go through each sleep cycle and phase in a shorter amount of time, and still wake up fully rested. This is the case with many scientists we know—they sleep fewer hours a night but are energetic, successful people. World leaders also have a reputation for sleeping less than the general public. Margaret Thatcher famously claimed that she slept only four hours per night, but in her seventies she developed dementia. This is just observational evidence—we don't know whether her sleep was restorative or not—but chronic lack of sleep, irrespective of how you feel on daily basis, can still do considerable cognitive damage over time.

Studies have shown that while many people claim to sleep very few hours a night (three or less), they're actually sleeping closer to six. The fact is that people who sleep three hours or less per night are extremely rare, and we have little data on long-term effects. What we do have is overwhelming data that a minimum of six hours per night, and an average of seven hours per night, is extremely beneficial. For this reason we strongly recommend that you get no fewer than six hours of sleep per night. Ultimately, the quality of sleep is what matters most. It must be restorative, and you must feel refreshed. If you sleep less than seven hours a night but lead a fully energetic and active life, you are likely achieving the restful sleep you need. If you're skimping on sleep and using caffeine to mask your exhaustion, sleep is especially critical for you because long-term chronic exhaustion is strongly associated with cognitive decline.

Our own sleep requirements are highly individual. Ayesha loves—and needs—her sleep. She needs to get seven to eight hours of sleep every night, and if she doesn't sleep at least seven hours, the next day is going to be extremely difficult. Dean's current average is six and a half hours of sleep a night. If he sleeps just five and a half hours a couple nights per week, he doesn't experience any negative side effects. He learned from a sleep study (more on this later) that he does in fact achieve very deep sleep in five to six hours. If he sleeps eight to nine hours, on the other hand, he wakes up with a headache. It's critical that you know and respect your own personal requirements. Be willing to honestly evaluate how you feel when you wake up in the morning: Do you feel refreshed, or do you immediately rush to the coffeemaker? And do you have energy throughout the day, or do you often feel exhausted in the afternoon or evening?

The Many Benefits of Restorative Sleep

We now have a strong body of research that illuminates the connections between sleep and brain health. Studies have shown that BDNF (brain-derived neurotrophic factor) repairs the brain at night, and both neurons and their supporting glial cells appear to regenerate during sleep. In 2009, researchers at Washington University in St. Louis found that when people don't get regular sleep, they actually have more amyloid plaques in their brains, which puts them at a greater risk for developing Alzheimer's. Just four years later, researchers at Oregon Health & Science University found that the brain appears to clear out toxins during deep sleep, including those toxins that lead to amyloid buildup. Other large studies have shown that people who don't get enough sleep experience atrophy in important memory centers like the hippocampus and also have smaller brain volumes in general, suggesting that lack of sleep can negatively affect both the brain's structure and function.

There are many other scientifically proven ways in which restorative sleep (or lack thereof) influences our cognition and health:

Overall Health: People who sleep better spend less time at the doctor's office. One study found that individuals who sleep appropriately spend 11 percent less on health care. Those with sleep disorders (like sleep apnea, which we cover in greater detail later in this chapter) typically have many other medical problems—including heart disease, stroke, and diabetes—due to chronic lack of sleep. Getting quality sleep reduces your risk for all these diseases.

Immunity: Better sleep leads to fewer colds and immune-related disorders, and even a lower risk of cancer. Restorative sleep seems to have a particularly profound effect on the body's response to inflammation. C-reactive proteins and other inflammatory markers like homocysteine seem to be lower in those who sleep better. Lower inflammation decreases amyloid buildup in the brain, thereby decreasing the risk of developing Alzheimer's.

Mood: People who sleep appropriately are happier. There is a direct correlation between restorative sleep and both qualitative and quantitative measures of happiness. Many studies have indicated that quality sleep results in better mood, insight, social engagement, and overall quality of life. One study found that college students with healthy sleep patterns experienced better psychological and physical health and improved academic performance. A good night's sleep can also help us process emotions and therefore provide a buffer against negative feelings. Another study conducted by scientists at UC–Berkeley and Brown University demonstrated that poorer sleep quality can impair our ability to process and regulate negative emotions on a daily basis.

Focus and Attention: Focus and attention are the foundation of cognition—not just memory processing but all kinds of complex functions like visuospatial and motor skills. Both are disproportionately impaired by sleep disorders and significantly improve with proper sleep. A 2005 review in *Seminars in Neurology* found that executive attention is especially affected by sleep loss. Neuroimaging of participants revealed frequent cognitive lapses in the frontal and parietal lobes, showing how insufficient sleep affects the way in which we perceive and process information.

Learning: People who sleep well have better short-term and long-term memory, processing speed, recall, visuospatial skills, driving skills, and even athletic skills.

Coordination: Lack of sleep can blunt our responses to the environment, making us more likely to drop objects and struggle with intricate or even simple actions. In elderly patients, slight aberrations in sleep seem to negatively affect hand-eye coordination, which increases the risk of both car accidents and falls.

Decision Making: People who sleep regularly are less likely to make bad financial decisions. Sleep-deprived individuals tend to be biased toward inappropriate risks. It appears that sleeplessness inhibits the frontal lobe, causing you to favor immediate, visceral choices over more complex choices.

Alcohol and Drug Abuse: Better sleepers are less likely to abuse alcohol and other drugs (which again speaks to the frontal lobe's ability to inhibit inappropriate choices). This is true in adolescence, midlife, and even late life. Regardless of your age, restful sleep makes you much less likely to abuse substances that will negatively affect your cognition.

Diabetes: People who don't sleep enough are more likely to develop type 2 diabetes. Studies have shown a direct link between sleep and your body's ability to process insulin. Adults who slept seven to eight hours per night (compared to those who slept six hours) were 1.7 times less likely to develop diabetes; those who slept only five hours were

2.5 times more likely to develop diabetes. Prediabetes and diabetes have both been repeatedly linked to dementia and cognitive decline.

Stroke: Lack of quality sleep increases the risk of stroke. This is a strong relationship that has been reproduced in multiple studies, showing that sleep is critical to healthy vascular function.

Headaches: People who sleep better experience far fewer migraines and tension headaches. This benefit was illustrated in a study where forty-three women were trained to improve their sleep with sleep hygiene techniques. All participants except for one experienced fewer headaches, and most were headache free for long periods of time. We also know that lack of sleep, or too much sleep, can trigger migraine headaches.

Weight Regulation: In a thirteen-year study of 500 individuals, researchers found that those who regularly slept less than seven hours per night were 7.5 times more likely to be overweight, even after controlling for activity levels and family history. Sleep seems to have a significant effect on weight gain. There are many reasons for this: Sleep-deprived people experience inhibition of the frontal lobe, which makes them more vulnerable to cravings. Abnormal circadian rhythms also play a role in weight gain, as does the hypothalamus, which houses the brain's satiety and hunger centers. Being short on sleep causes cravings for high-fat foods and sweets and releases both leptin and ghrelin, two hormones that increase appetite. Restricted sleep also appears to increase snacking.

Libido: People who get more sleep have better libido and increased testosterone levels. The opposite is also true—less sleep results in lower testosterone. Low libido can cause depression and diminished quality of life, both of which affect cognition and memory. Studies have also linked low testosterone to Alzheimer's risk in people with endocrine disorders that lead to low testosterone, as well as individuals on testosterone-lowering medications.

Brain Atrophy: A new study from 2017 revealed that sleep deprivation can cause microglia (the brain's specialized waste clearance cells) to destroy healthy neurons and their connections. This innate detox system is essential for clearing harmful by-products, but when we're chronically sleep-deprived, the system turns on itself, pruning the very cells it would otherwise preserve. The damage sustained by this abnormal process appears to be cumulative over the long term, and may explain the brain shrinkage found in individuals who consistently fail to get enough sleep.

Chronically Sleep-Deprived, Chronically Sick

Despite the fact that sleep is critical to so many aspects of our health and well-being, studies show that many of us are failing to get enough rest. The Centers for Disease Control and Prevention (CDC) calls insufficient sleep a major public health concern and estimates that 30 percent of American adults are chronically sleep-deprived. That's 40.6 million people. Night-shift workers, particularly those in transportation and health care, are most at risk for not getting adequate sleep. Excessive sleep is a problem as well, partly because people who sleep too much have less time to activate their brains, which makes them more vulnerable to decline, but also because excessive sleep is often due to underlying medical problems like anemia, sleep disorders, cardiovascular disease, and many types of cognitive disease.

The elderly are particularly affected when it comes to disordered sleep. Stage 1 of NREM sleep—the beginning of the sleep cycle—changes the most as we age. Older people tend to stay in this initial stage longer, which means they spend less time in the deeper, more restorative sleep of Stages 3 and 4. This is likely because our ability to absorb daylight declines as we age. After we reach the age of sixty, as much as 40 percent of daylight fails to be absorbed by the retina into the brain's optic centers. One of these centers is the ventral lateral preoptic nucleus, which is essentially a sleep switch that sets the circadian clock of the brain. Many cells in this region appear to die off in midlife.

Somewhere between 50 and 70 percent of elderly people have at least some degree of sleep disorder. Night after night of lost or low-quality sleep often leads to perpetual daytime drowsiness. Research shows that daytime sleepiness over a three-year period is associated with an increased risk of cognitive decline and dementia in the elderly. A recent study reinforced this conclusion, finding that a reduction in sleep time was associated with a 75 percent increase in the risk for dementia and a 50 percent increase in the risk for Alzheimer's. Yet another study controlled for depression, age, gender, and vascular health and found the same association between lack of sleep and cognitive decline. Elderly people with MCI, dementia, or Alzheimer's are even more significantly affected by poor sleep. These patients often experience increased confusion later in the day, in part due to chronic exhaustion, a phenomenon known as "sundowning."

Restore Myths

Skipping an hour or two of sleep won't hurt me: Studies show that skipping sleep affects your memory, processing speed, and mood. Loss of sleep—even if it's only an hour or two—is especially detrimental long term.

Your brain rests when you sleep: The brain is incredibly active during sleep as it consolidates memories and clears away waste products (including amyloid) that accumulate during the day.

Snoring is common and nothing to worry about: For some people snoring can be harmless, but for others it can be an indication of sleep apnea. It's best to undergo a sleep study if you suspect you may have this common sleep disorder.

Older people don't need as much sleep: The elderly need just as much sleep as other adults (an average of seven to eight hours per night) but struggle to get adequate sleep due to biological changes in the brain that occur as we age.

I can sleep less during the week and make up for it over the weekends: You can sleep in and pay back some of the sleep you missed, but it's not the same as getting regular, quality sleep all week long, which is the best option for cognitive and overall health.

The Danger of Sleep Medications

Sleep medication is a common over-the-counter solution to disordered sleep for the general population and especially the elderly. Many people taking sleep medication assume their sleep is restorative. But research shows that while sleep medication may help you fall asleep after a day fueled by stress and caffeine, it also negatively affects your sleep cycles. We now know that many of these medications prevent you from entering Stages 3 and 4, where deeper, more restorative sleep occurs. This might be why many people who take sleep medication wake up after seven or eight hours and still feel groggy. Their cognitive symptoms continue, and the longer they take medication, the more they lose touch with what's really causing their sleep problems, with what in their routine and lifestyle they need to change in order to sleep well on their own.

We routinely see older patients taking high doses of medication in a desperate attempt to get quality rest. Over time they build up a tolerance to the medication and require more and more and more. One such patient in her late sixties, Catharina, came to see us after hearing one of our talks on Alzheimer's. She'd attended the talk for her husband, who had the disease, but he had since passed away from a heart attack. Catharina told Dean that her sleep problems had gotten much worse since the death of her husband. She'd gotten to the point where she was taking two different sleep medications every night—both at three times the normal dosage. Even though Catharina was sleeping more regularly, she felt like she was in a fog. She struggled in conversations, often losing her train of thought or forgetting the names of new acquaintances. She prided herself on her relationships, and not being able to function in social settings had given her great anxiety, especially now that her husband was gone. Catharina sensed that the medications weren't helping, but without them she couldn't sleep at all. She didn't know what to do.

All of Catharina's labs were normal. So was her MRI. It was clear that sleep medications were her main problem, and we knew we'd have to rehabilitate her sleep to slowly and methodically decrease her dosage. In talking with Catharina, we realized that her problems with sleep were deeply connected to the anguish of losing her husband. She had also been struggling with sleep for so long that even a conversation about what she did before bed caused her significant stress. Given her troubled relationship with sleep, we decided to refer Catharina to a specialist for an eight-week course of cognitive behavioral therapy (CBT) to decrease her anxiety. This was the best first step we could take in reforming her sleep habits. We offer you many of the techniques used in CBT in the Personalized Restore Program at the end of this chapter.

As part of this treatment, Catharina was asked to keep a detailed sleep diary, like the one you'll find on page 226. She recorded when she went to sleep and woke up each day, and how she felt in terms of energy and mental clarity. Catharina's afternoon naps seemed to be interfering with her ability to sleep at night, so she stopped napping and stayed up later. This process tired her out in the beginning, but after a few weeks she was sleeping through the night, something she hadn't done in nearly a decade.

Once Catharina felt more rested, we introduced sleep hygiene techniques to optimize her prebedtime routine and even her daily activities—all with the goal of facilitating regular, restorative sleep. Sleep hygiene techniques are simple practices you can use to transform your sleep, like getting sunshine early in the morning and decorating your bedroom with calming colors. Not eating before bed gives your brain more energy to repair itself during the night. Cutting out late-day caffeine can have profound effects on the quality of your sleep. So can exercise, meditation, and the right temperature and bedding. You'll find a complete list of sleep hygiene techniques in the Personalized Restore Program.

Most people benefit greatly from using just two or three of these techniques. For Catharina, this meant walking every morning (for both physical activity and exposure to daylight), drinking coffee no later than 2:00 P.M., and turning off all electronics thirty minutes before bed. Her sleep continued to improve, so we began to slowly reduce her medication. We cut her dosage by 25 percent for the first month. After we examined her to make sure she wasn't experiencing withdrawal, we reduced it by another 25 percent for the second month. Catharina had some difficulty adjusting to this dosage and called us a few times to discuss the problems she had getting to sleep. Together we agreed to let her acclimate for an additional month. At the end of month three, we reduced her medication by another 25 percent. She stayed at this dosage for several more months, which gave her body time to re-create a healthy sleeping pattern. A common mistake is to decrease sleep medication too quickly, which can cause headaches, anxiety, depression, and a number of other side effects. Rather than adhering to some prescribed regimen, we always consider the patient's resolve, medical history, and compliance to new lifestyle practices when designing an appropriate schedule. The whole process often takes several months to a year or more.

Our intervention successfully altered the course of Catharina's cognitive health. Though she still requires low levels of medication, she's seen clear improvements in her memory and processing speed. And as with so many of our patients, the more improvements Catharina experiences, the more motivated she is to change. Had she stuck with her regimen of sleep medication, poor-quality sleep, napping, and caffeine, she would have undoubtedly experienced further decline. But by methodically reforming her sleep, Catharina saw a full reversal of her symptoms and is now enjoying a healthier, happier life.

SLEEP APNEA: A MEDICAL EMERGENCY

Jim, an engineer in his midfifties, came to see us because he was having memory problems and difficulty concentrating. He said he regularly forgot where he parked his car. Once he had to look for nearly an hour. He told us he'd had a great memory when he was younger, but he could feel it getting worse by the day. He was especially worried because his grandmother had developed dementia in her sixties. He figured he was headed down the same road.

During the medical history Jim reported that though he slept through the night, he always woke up tired and was fatigued throughout the day. He said that he used to love to drive through the canyons and mountains of Los Angeles, but for the last few years, if the drive was more than half an hour, he started feeling sleepy. On a couple of occasions he'd nearly had an accident. He didn't even feel rested on the weekends when he slept in. We asked him whether he snored. Jim said that he'd gotten divorced six years ago and had felt too ➤

tired to have a serious relationship since. He wasn't sure whether he snored *every* night, though a few times his snoring had woken him up.

We did a complete workup and didn't find any metabolic abnormalities or abnormal imaging patterns on the MRI, but Jim's neuropsychological testing revealed he was struggling with attention and recall. He couldn't count a sequence of numbers forward and backward, nor could he keep track of a two- or three-step command. This pattern could have been suggestive of many different problems, some of them psychological, like depression, but there were no signs of that.

An overnight sleep study (or polysomnography) told us everything we needed to know. During this test, Jim's sleep stages were recorded with electrodes placed on his scalp, eyelids, and forehead, while additional electrodes on his chin and legs detected movement. His heart rhythm was monitored with an EKG machine, and we also tested the airflow at his nose and mouth, the effort he used to breathe, and the oxygen levels in his blood. The sleep study revealed that during the night Jim stopped breathing a total of forty-three times.

Sleep apnea is one of the most common sleep disorders. Experts believe that one in fifteen people (or 18 million Americans) have sleep apnea. Men are more at risk than women—20 percent will experience some form of sleep apnea in their lives, compared to 9 percent of women. Sleep apnea is tragically underdiagnosed, and because of its detrimental effects on the brain and how little people know about it, we believe sleep apnea is a veritable medical emergency.

Many people associate sleep apnea with obesity. While it's true that this condition is prevalent in those who are overweight, it's also pervasive in the general population. Obstructive sleep apnea is by far the most common form. The obstruction happens when the pharynx and the soft tissue in the back of the mouth block the flow of air. This is especially common when people lie down. Individuals who have large tongues, tonsils, or adenoids; short, thick necks; or a narrow cavity in the back of the mouth are at a much higher risk, regardless of their body weight.

Often the airway is obstructed for more than ten seconds, and this can happen as many as twenty to thirty times per hour. Each sleep cycle is disrupted, and the brain is literally starved of oxygen, which injures neurons and contributes to chronic exhaustion, headaches, and difficulty concentrating. Research suggests that the lack of oxygen and blood flow to the brain directly contribute to cognitive decline. The medial temporal lobe, a brain region heavily involved in memory, seems to be particularly sensitive to lower oxygen levels. In our own research, published in *Circulation* in 2015, we discovered a strong relationship between COPD—a pulmonary disease that deprives the brain of oxygen in a manner similar to sleep apnea—and subsequent diagnosis of Alzheimer's. When we looked at the prevalence of dementia in those diagnosed with sleep apnea as part of our nationwide study, we were able to detect a significantly greater increase in dementia rates for sleep apnea sufferers. We also found that once the disorder is diagnosed and treated, subjects were less likely to develop dementia, though further research is needed to better delineate this important finding. In a review and meta-analysis of seven studies published in 2015, which included more than 13,000 participants, scientists at the University of South Florida reported that sleep apnea increased the risk of Alzheimer's disease by 70 percent. This should be grounds for a national campaign to detect and treat sleep apnea.

We shared this research with Jim after giving him the diagnosis and insisted that he use a sleep apnea device called a CPAP (continuous positive airway pressure). The CPAP is a mask worn over the face and nose that ensures a steady supply of oxygen throughout the night. We were honest with Jim: the mask can be uncomfortable. We always remind our patients that there's nothing you can do in terms of lifestyle to overcome this serious lack of oxygen to the brain. The CPAP device is necessary, and though it takes some getting used to, it's possible to learn to sleep with it and experience dramatic cognitive improvement.

Jim came back after three months. He admitted that he'd had a difficult time getting used to the device, but he persevered and eventually learned to sleep through the night. Follow-up cognitive testing showed improvements in both memory and attention. Even more important, Jim felt a boost in his mood and energy, and he was much more confident at work. We've seen him several times since, and his cognitive test results continue to improve.

Conclusion

Chronic lack of sleep is a major contributor to cognitive decline. Sleep medications, sleep disorders, and our prebedtime routines all affect the quality of our rest. If you're struggling with memory or attention problems, or persistent, unexplained exhaustion, you should be tested for sleep apnea. And if you're relying on heavy medications to get to sleep, you're missing out on deeper sleep stages where the brain does its most important organizing and cleansing. Through the use of sleep hygiene techniques, you can rehabilitate your sleeping patterns and decrease your dependence on medications. Simple behavioral modifications can have a tremendous impact on sleep quality and cognitive health. As the newest research proves, whenever we think about optimizing the brain, we should carefully consider the quality of our sleep.

```
┌─────────────────────────────────────────┐
│                                         │
│          Your Personalized              │
│            RESTORE                      │
│             Program                     │
│                                         │
└─────────────────────────────────────────┘
```

Restorative sleep has emerged as a critical aspect of cognitive health and resiliency. Any brain-healthy lifestyle intervention must address the quality of your sleep, and as you've now learned, restorative sleep encompasses more than just getting six to eight hours of sleep per night. It also involves optimizing your prebedtime routine, using sleep hygiene techniques, and understanding the many ways in which quality sleep protects and strengthens the brain. The program below includes a self-assessment, a sleep diary, and techniques to help you optimize your sleep.

SELF-ASSESSMENT

Vision, Strengths, and Weaknesses: Assess your vision for a restorative sleep plan, and identify factors that might help or hinder your efforts.

Vision: What is the ideal restorative sleep plan for you? How many hours of sleep would you like to get each night? How do you feel in the morning? How do you feel throughout the day? What cognitive symptoms—like confusion or nighttime anxiety—do you hope to eliminate?

Strengths: What strengths and resources will help you achieve your vision?

Weaknesses: What are the obstacles to your vision?

1. How will you benefit from healthier sleep habits?

Examples: I will have more energy. I will work more efficiently. My mood will improve. I'll have much better focus. I'll be able to manage my weight. My memory will improve. I'll have a reduced risk of both heart disease and dementia.

2. What are the most important areas for you to work on?

Examples: I won't drink coffee after 2:00 p.m. I'll stick to a regular sleep schedule. I'll stop eating a few hours before I go to bed. I'll make sure I exercise in the mornings. I'll turn off the TV and all my electronic devices thirty minutes before bed. I'll make sure I get enough natural light during the day. I'll keep the lights in my bedroom dim at night. I'll practice meditation as a way of relaxing before sleep.

3. What obstacles might prevent you from getting restorative sleep?

Examples: I find it difficult to relax. I'm addicted to caffeine. My husband snores. I'm a shift worker and have to sleep during the day. There's too much light in my room. My mind races before sleep. I often wake up in the middle of the night.

4. What might help you get restful sleep? What are your resources?

Examples: I can remove the TV from my bedroom. I can eat dinner earlier. I can use incandescent light during the day to help set my circadian rhythm (more on this on page 223). I can commit to exercising each morning. I can learn different meditation techniques for relaxation. I can apply techniques I learn from cognitive behavioral therapy to get better sleep.

5. Who can help you and how?

Examples: I will see my doctor for a sleep evaluation. My spouse will help me keep a normal sleep schedule. If I still have trouble sleeping after trying several sleep hygiene techniques, I will see a sleep specialist. My family can help me manage my responsibilities at home so I can reduce my stress levels.

6. When will you start?

Our Recommendation: Start with two sleep hygiene techniques, like going to bed and waking up at the same time, and adjusting the light, temperature, or sound in your bedroom to promote better sleep. Use a sleep diary to identify the most important areas to work on first.

TECHNIQUES FOR A BETTER NIGHT'S SLEEP

1. **Normalize Your Sleep Schedule:** Go to bed at the same time each night and get up at the same time each morning. Keeping regular hours helps your brain know when to rest and when to be alert. We evolved to sleep with the fall and rise of the sun. An erratic sleeping schedule interferes with the daily hormonal processes that help facilitate restful sleep.

2. **Avoid Eating Late at Night:** When your gastrointestinal system is working to digest food, you don't sleep as deeply and are more likely to wake up. Dean had a long-standing habit of eating sugary cereal with almond milk a few hours before bed. It was his reward at the end of the long day. But he started to have difficulty sleeping after the age of forty. At first he couldn't figure out what the problem was, but one night after he ate his cereal he heard a low rumbling in his stomach. His digestive system seemed to be working very hard, and he wondered whether eating the cereal earlier would have any effect on his sleep. The sugar could have been keeping him up as well. The next night he ate his cereal three and a half hours before bed. He had no problems sleeping. Eventually he swapped the sugary cereal and almond milk for oats and berries and was able to relieve his digestive distress as well.

Conducting your own personal experiments like Dean did can help you figure out what's disrupting your sleep.

These foods can be especially disruptive to sleep:

- Sugary foods give your body quick energy that interferes with relaxation and sleep.

- High-fat foods can cause indigestion and acid reflux.

- Spicy foods can irritate the stomach and also cause acid reflux.

- Chocolate contains sugar and caffeine, both of which negatively affect sleep.

3. **Avoid Certain Drinks Too Close to Bedtime:** Caffeine can stay in your body for over eight hours. We recommend drinking coffee and other caffeinated drinks no later than 2 P.M. Ayesha loves coffee and used to drink her last cup at 5 P.M. When she cut out late-afternoon coffee her sleep improved significantly. Small actions like this can have major health consequences.

Other drinks to look out for:

- One or two glasses of wine can be relaxing, but more than this will disrupt sleep cycles and often cause you to wake up in the middle of the night to use the bathroom.

- Citrus juices can cause acid reflux and irritate the bladder.

4. **Avoid Exercising Before Sleep, But Be Sure to Exercise Earlier in the Day:** A brisk walk in the morning has wonderful effects on your sleep. Getting out into the light helps set your circadian cycles and wakes you up for the day, and exercise has been shown in many studies to increase the depth of sleep. Walking after dinner (ideally at dusk) is also a great option. Your brain reacts to the changing light and naturally prepares for sleep. Be sure to complete exercise—especially intensive aerobic exercise—at least three hours before bedtime.

5. **Low Light at Night, Bright Light During the Day:** Your brain needs bright, natural light during the day, and softer light at night. If you find it hard to get adequate natural light, light boxes are a great solution. They provide twenty to forty times more light than regular lamps and mimic natural light. Many studies have proposed light therapy as a treatment for seasonal affective disorder and depression, but it can also help with the sleep-wake cycle. Light boxes should always be used in the morning—otherwise they could interfere with your sleep. Use only soft lights in your bedroom at night, and turn off electronic devices that emit bright light.

6. **Avoid Playing Games, Watching Stimulating Movies, and Working on Your Tablet in Bed:** The idea is to calm the brain, not rev it up. Try reading instead—something enjoyable but not too engrossing. This allows the mind to relax and helps you avoid the blue light in electronic devices that has been shown to interfere with sleep. It's best to reserve the bedroom for sleep and sex only.

7. **Avoid Napping:** For most of us, napping during the day will interfere with our ability to fall asleep at night. We don't recommend daily naps unless you have a long-standing habit of napping. Even then you should set an alarm so that you sleep no longer than ten to thirty minutes. Anything beyond that can result in sleep inertia, a groggy feeling after awakening that can impair performance. If you're trying to establish a regular sleeping pattern, we recommend that you stay awake during the day (unless sleepiness could put you or others in danger). You'll be tired enough at night that you'll fall asleep earlier and faster, which will help you normalize your schedule.

8. **Use Meditation:** Meditation is a wonderful addition to your prebedtime routine. This powerful practice physiologically relaxes the body by slowing both breathing and heart rate and has also been proven to reduce stress.

9. **Sound- and Light-Proof Your Bedroom:** Both sound and light can wake you up and disrupt your sleep cycles, robbing you of the deep sleep your brain requires. Try using white noise or natural soft sounds. If

WEEKLY RESTORE PLAN

MONDAY
Work on reducing the amount of light and sound in your bedroom. Try thick curtains to block light and either earplugs or a simple fan to help you sleep through the night.

TUESDAY
Establish a regular sleep schedule. You should go to sleep at the same time every night and awake at the same time every day. Remember that almost all of us require seven to eight hours of a sleep per night. If you're tired during the day, avoid taking a nap as it might interfere with your sleep cycle.

WEDNESDAY
Stop eating at least three hours before going to sleep tonight. Stop drinking fluids at least two hours before going to sleep. Avoid caffeine, chocolate, and sugar in the afternoon and evening.

THURSDAY
Aim to get at least one to two hours of natural light during the day, perhaps by taking a walk at lunchtime or early in the morning. If you don't have time to walk outside, consider using a light box in the morning.

FRIDAY
Make sure you exercise today, ideally in the morning, as it significantly improves the quality of your sleep.

SATURDAY
Stop using electronic devices at least a half hour before sleep (an hour is even better). Lower the lights in your bedroom, and avoid stimulating movies and music before sleep.

SUNDAY
If anxiety is preventing you from getting restorative sleep, visualize a calming physical location, like the beach or a lush forest, to help you relax. If your anxiety persists, consider visiting our website (TeamSherzai.com) for more information on cognitive behavioral therapy or booking a session with a qualified therapist.

you have consistent loud noise, consider egg crating the room and insulating the windows and doors. Blackout curtains are great for keeping your room dark.

10. **Get Comfortable:** Do you prefer a warm blanket or cool sheets? There seems to be a difference in temperature preference between men and women. Women prefer a slightly higher temperature, men slightly cooler. This is certainly true with the two of us. We use dual blankets (one warmer and one cooler) so we can sleep together and also enjoy our preferred sleeping temperatures. There are also beds with dual temperature settings, and even pillows designed to maintain certain temperatures throughout the night. Because of hormonal fluctuations throughout the sleep cycle, the temperature pattern for the most restful sleep seems to be: 1) falling asleep at a temperature just slightly above body temperature; 2) the temperature slowly dropping throughout the night; and 3) a minor rise in temperature before waking up.

11. **Address Dependence on Medications:** Use these techniques under a doctor's supervision to slowly reduce your need for medication.

12. **Use Cognitive Behavioral Therapy (CBT) if Necessary:** Seek help from a qualified therapist if you are experiencing excessive anxiety or distorted sleep patterns. CBT is most effective for those who still experience anxiety after trying both the relaxation techniques in the "Unwind" chapter and the sleep hygiene techniques presented here. Anxiety that doesn't respond to any of these techniques may require an initial round of therapy.

13. **Look for Signs of Sleep Apnea:** If you suspect you might have this common sleep disorder, ask your doctor to order a sleep study (this is the only way to know for sure). Review the results and then discuss the best solution for improving your sleep.

SLEEP DIARY

Use the following chart to document your sleep, daily routine, and energy levels for a period of one to two weeks. This process is helpful for identifying what in your lifestyle and schedule you can change to achieve more restorative sleep.

	SAMPLE	MONDAY	TUESDAY
Time I went to bed last night:	12:00 midnight		
Time I woke up this morning:	8 a.m.		
Number of hours I slept last night:	8		
Number of awakenings and total time awake last night:	3 times 3 hours		
How long I took to fall asleep last night:	45 minutes		
Intensity of running thoughts. The thoughts kept me from sleep for: 1 = 15 minutes 2 = 30 minutes 3 = 1 hour 4 = 2 hours or more	3		
How awake did I feel when I got up this morning? 1 = Wide awake 2 = Awake but a little tired 3 = Sleepy	2		
Number of caffeinated drinks (coffee, tea, hot chocolate) and time I had them today:	2 drinks 6 p.m. and 6:30 p.m.		
Number of alcoholic drinks (beer, wine, liquor) and time I had them today:	3 drinks 10 p.m.		
Nap times and lengths today:	2:30 p.m. 20 minutes 5:30 p.m. 30 minutes		
Exercise times and lengths today:	9 p.m. 20 minutes		
Amount of sunlight I got today:	45 minutes		
How sleepy did I feel during the day today? 1 = So sleepy I struggled to stay awake during much of the day 2 = Somewhat tired 3 = Fairly alert 4 = Wide awake	2		

WEDNESDAY	THURSDAY	FRIDAY	SATURDAY	SUNDAY

PROGRESSIVE MUSCLE RELAXATION: AN EXERCISE YOU CAN DO IN BED

Try this exercise when you have trouble falling asleep.

- Take a deep breath. Hold it for five seconds, and then breathe out.

- Take another deep breath. This time contract all the muscles in your feet and hold for five seconds. Then breathe out and completely relax your body. Feel the contrast between tension and relaxation, the way your body releases deeply after holding tension.

- Move slowly upward, contracting and releasing your ankles, calves, thighs, hips, abdomen, lower back, upper back, fingers, forearms, upper arms, shoulders, neck, jaw, mouth, cheeks, nostrils, eyelids, temples, and forehead. Be sure to inhale deeply and exhale completely each time.

Work Toward Increasing:

- Relaxation before bedtime

- Time spent without electronics

- Enjoying a regular schedule

- Meditation

- Light during the day

- Exercise earlier in the day

Work Toward Eliminating:

- Bright light late at night

- Eating before bed

- Drinking coffee at night

- Noise that wakes you up at night

- Physical activity and exercise later in the evening

COMMON OBSTACLES

Undiagnosed Sleep Disorders: Have your doctor order a sleep study if you're experiencing unexplained chronic exhaustion.

A Snoring Spouse: Have your spouse evaluated for sleep disorders like sleep apnea. Doing so will help both of you get better quality rest.

Erratic Sleeping Schedules: Establish a nighttime routine and use an alarm to help you keep a normal schedule. It's especially important to adhere to this schedule on the weekends, when there's a tendency to stay up late and sleep in, thus disrupting the body's sleep patterns.

Waking Up in the Middle of the Night and Not Being Able to Get Back to Sleep: Try the progressive muscle relaxation exercise described on the previous page. If you still can't get to sleep, leave the bedroom, read something soothing for thirty minutes, and then try going back to sleep.

Too Much Light / Too Much Noise: Make sure your bedroom is free of light and unwanted noise. Buy blackout curtains. Invest in a white noise machine, or use one of the many white noise apps.

OUR PERSONAL APPROACH TO RESTORATIVE SLEEP

- Dean used to sleep at all different times of the night. Now he keeps a regular sleep schedule, even on the weekends.

- We put our computers away at least thirty minutes before sleep.

- We still enjoy coffee and tea, but only before 2:00 P.M. Ayesha experienced much deeper sleep after cutting out late-afternoon caffeine.

- We stop eating three hours before bedtime. This was especially helpful to Dean, whose digestive problems had been waking him up and causing chronic exhaustion.

- We exercise in the morning and throughout the day, but save our evenings for relaxation.

- We make sure to get enough light during the day to maintain a healthy circadian rhythm (walking during our lunch break is a great way to do this).

- In our home, we have created a special sleep therapy room that's free of light and sound. We got the idea after staying in a friend's basement and getting the best sleep we'd ever had. Just as we can create space in our living room for exercise, we can also design our home so that it facilitates restorative sleep.

7.

Optimize

Dean and a group of twelve residents entered Mrs. Collins's room to find her propped up in bed, staring blankly at the television. She was the fourth patient they'd seen that morning as they conducted rounds in the neurology ward at Loma Linda University Medical Center. The resident neurologist who was assigned to Mrs. Collins stepped forward to present her case.

"Eighty-four-year-old right-handed female with a past medical history of hypertension, hypercholesterolemia, and forty-year history of smoking," he began. "She was diagnosed with Alzheimer's eight years ago. Patient has been a resident of a local nursing home for the past six years and has been stable, alert, and oriented." After reviewing her entire medical history, he explained that she'd been admitted to the hospital because of a sudden decline in her cognition during a bout of pneumonia. Mrs. Collins did respond to noxious stimuli—like a pinch of her nail beds—but was otherwise globally aphasic, meaning that she didn't communicate or respond to any commands. According to hospital staff, she hadn't made eye contact with anyone in over a month. The family said that prior to her admission, Mrs. Collins was able to speak and make at least some connections. They were alarmed by her precipitous decline.

The resident said his plan was to treat the pneumonia further, send Mrs. Collins to rehabilitation, and eventually transfer her back to the nursing home.

"Tell me a little more about her," Dean said.

"Her electrolytes were normal, and her lumbar puncture came back negative. Her MRI revealed no new stroke or other lesions."

"I understand the labs, but tell me about *her*," Dean said. The resident fumbled for more detail.

"She lives in the area," he said. "Her daughter brought her in last month."

"Tell me about her life," Dean clarified. This was an unusual request for the young doctor, but he dutifully grabbed the chart and reviewed it with the other residents. Dean pointed to a summary of her personal history: Mrs. Collins had been a piano teacher for more than sixty years.

"Music is a huge part of her personality," Dean told the group. "It's her identity, her sense of self." He reminded the residents that even when patients are unresponsive, their identities are still intact. Their brains still hold a lifetime of rich experiences that are stored not as dots or slivers of information but as complex networks with many different points of entry. The mind has centers of specialization—Broca's and Wernicke's areas for understanding and producing language, the occipital lobe for visual processing, the frontal lobe for executive function, and the temporal lobe for short-term memory and speech recognition. These specialized areas process different types of sensory input (sound, sight, touch, etc.) and give rise to the fluid thoughts, memories, and emotions in our brains. When these thoughts, memories, and emotions connect to a significant set of life experiences, an integral aspect of our selfhood like a lifelong artistic pursuit, they form islands of consciousness, our anchors of personality, identity, and meaning. The more complex and meaningful the experience, the larger and more resilient the island. For Mrs. Collins, music was a way of understanding both herself and the world.

Dean stood in front of her, looked her in the eye, and called her name a few times. Mrs. Collins didn't respond. The residents watched skeptically. Some of them looked anxious, knowing they had many more patients to visit that morning.

"Mrs. Collins!" Dean said again, his eyes trying to connect with hers. Again, nothing. Then he asked, "Who was a better composer: Mozart or Beethoven?" As he said this, her eyes didn't exactly move, but Dean felt that he'd somehow gotten through to her. He leaned in and asked again.

After a long pause, she said in a soft voice, "What a stupid question." The residents gasped.

"There it is," Dean said. "Now we've connected."

Imagine what it took, cognitively, for Mrs. Collins to answer Dean's question. She had to take in the sound of his voice, understand it, filter it through the vast library of music in her mind, connect the music with specific composers, form an opinion, and then verbalize her response. It was an incredibly complex cognitive process, and she'd done it effortlessly. Music was a main island of consciousness for her, one so central to her cognition that it served as an anchor to awareness and alertness. It helped her reconnect with the world despite the damage caused by Alzheimer's.

Dean and the resident physician asked Mrs. Collins's daughter to bring music to the hospital, to play her mother's favorite songs, talk about her favorite composers, favorite students, and anything else they could think of to engage this important aspect of her consciousness. She had always loved Beethoven's "Für Elise." When her daughter played it a few days later, Mrs. Collins identified it immediately. "Ah, Für Elise," she said, closing her eyes and resting her head as she took in the sound. After a few weeks, these associations with music became even stronger, and Mrs. Collins was able to return to the life she lived before she'd come down with pneumonia. She still had moderate Alzheimer's, but she could speak coherently and once again recognized her family.

Islands of consciousness arise from the interplay between domains of cognition (specialized brain regions) and the brain's many complex networks. Each domain governs a specific type of thinking; each network processes information, gives it a name and meaning, and then integrates it into existing memories. Here are some of the brain's most important domains and networks:

- **Attention and Concentration:** Filtering sensory stimuli and focusing where appropriate

- **Emotions and Emotional Processing:** Motivation, mood, sustained interest

- **Executive Function:** Problem solving, critical reasoning, planning

- **Language Processing:** Communication, understanding language and forming a response

- **Motor Speed and Coordination:** Complex movement, awareness of how the body moves in space

- **Speed of Processing:** How quickly you receive and interpret information

- **Verbal Learning and Memory:** Understanding written and spoken words

- **Visual Learning and Memory:** Visual recognition, naming, and memorization

- **Visuospatial Processing:** Defining visual information and incorporating it into existing stories and islands of consciousness

Islands of consciousness use different aspects of each of these cognitive functions to generate awareness about an idea, a story, or an image of self. In the context of music, for example, executive function allows you to understand the intricacy of a Mozart concerto. Your temporal lobe stores memories of the violin lessons you took as a child. The occipital lobe gives you the image of the audience applauding after your very first performance. All these functions come together seamlessly to create a three-dimensional, highly personalized story of music in your life.

It takes a special kind of connectivity—and a lot of it—to coordinate communication among these functions and create such a nuanced conscious experience. We can think of these connections as the bridges and highways that link different islands together, fortifying and reinforcing them. The construction of this island infrastructure starts when we're just forty-two days old as newly formed neurons begin to travel throughout the brain to establish the beginnings of networks. These networks proliferate so rapidly that the brain's volume increases fourfold by the time we enter preschool. Many structural changes are also taking place, including the growth of gray and white matter compartments, and the myelination of millions of neurons in order to facilitate electrical communication. As networks are formed, they're also pruned, or refined, through the process of apoptosis (programmed cell death), leaving us with the brain structure we'll have for the rest of our lives. The measure of network connectivity generated during early childhood is known as brain reserve. You can think of brain reserve as a kind of scaffolding, the structure that remains after brain development is complete.

Cognitive reserve, on the other hand, is a measure of the connectivity we develop throughout life. This capacity is determined by how much we challenge our brains, how much information we take in, all the trauma, risk, adventure, joy, and knowledge we experience over a lifetime. It's a product of the quality and quantity of connections between cells, brain regions, and islands of consciousness. Cognitive reserve is essentially the integrity of the brain, and it's the result of how we live our lives. Brain reserve is determined early on, but cognitive reserve is within our control and can expand even late in life.

What does this have to do with Alzheimer's? Consider this remarkable fact: almost all people in midlife and late life have at least some of the brain pathology associated with Alzheimer's disease—brain atrophy, or amyloid—yet only a portion of people experience cognitive decline. Why is this? Because both types of reserve afford the brain tremendous protection in the form of redundancy and interconnectivity. Multidomain networks—the kinds that result from brain reserve and especially cognitive reserve—are connected tens of thousands of times over, which allows us access to the same memory, fact, or idea via many different bridges and highways. We need these redundant structures so we can cope with the pathology of normal aging: say one bridge to a childhood memory is destroyed by vascular trauma due to a diet high in saturated fat, another by an amyloid plaque, and a major highway is blocked by tau tangles. If your brain has sufficient reserve, you can endure all of this pathology and still access the memory because it's connected thousands of different ways. This kind of redundancy makes it nearly impossible for a connection to be severed, for the waves of aging to cause serious damage, for an island of consciousness to be lost.

Built for Complexity, Sustained by Complexity

So how do we build cognitive reserve? How do we promote the interconnectivity and redundancy that allow our brains to withstand both normal aging and neurodegenerative disease? In essence, how do we optimize our brains? The conventional answer to this question has been memory games and crossword puzzles like sudoku and tangram. It seems intuitive that engaging the mind through these activities must be good for cognition and brain health. And there is some evidence that brain games help. In a randomized longitudinal study conducted by the University of Florida, elderly people seventy-four years of age and older took part in speed-of-processing cognitive training (a simple computer game that involves quickly identifying objects flashed on the screen). There were two control groups: one that took memory and reasoning classes, and one that did not partake in any cognitive training. The first group, those who trained with the simple computer game, were found to have a 48 percent lower chance of developing Alzheimer's disease in the following ten years. This was the first time that cognitive training was shown to protect against Alzheimer's in a large population. What's especially intriguing is that it took only ten to fourteen hours of cognitive training during the ten-year study for these results to manifest. This study shows that even the most rudimentary games may boost our attention, executive function, and short-term memory skills.

The problem, however, is that memory games and puzzle books are mostly linear activities—but there's nothing linear about the brain. Much of the memory-enhancement industry seems to have overlooked this fact, which has led many patients to invest time and effort in activities that afford only minor benefits. Sudoku, for instance, challenges a mathematical center in the posterior parietal area of the brain. While you do need to read and process visual information to play this game, you're not actively challenging multiple areas of the brain, nor are you increasing the connections between them or engaging any personal or historical islands of consciousness. The same is true for crossword puzzles (which mainly challenge the language centers of the brain) and tangram (which challenges our visuospatial capacity). All these games engage the brain on only a simple level of thought processing. Simple memories and thoughts like these are encoded via small, local connections, resulting in small networks that are limited to a single region of the brain. They do provide some infrastructure and support for the brain's larger islands, but to a limited degree. Our comprehensive meta-analysis of all the studies to date on cognitive exercises for MCI supports this theory: some of these exercises do help with memory processing, though the effect is minimal.

But let's say you use more complicated brain games and memorization exercises. Moderately challenging activities—those that engage multiple cognitive domains at the same time—use the brain's associative power to create more complex connections. These networks are for the most part still local and impermanent, but they're stronger than simple networks and can also result in neuronal growth. Association and chunking are two such moderately complex mental processes. Association means connecting a new piece of information to something that already exists in the brain, a memory, image, or idea that is most proximal by some measure, be it structure, character, story, or meaning. Here's an example: When Dean visited Singapore for the first time, he discovered dozens of new tropical fruits, including durian, a sweet yellow fruit with a thorny husk. He saw it everywhere in Singapore. There was even a theater in the shape of a durian. The memory of this fruit is now categorized in his brain according to several different associations. There are similarly shaped objects with which it is associated, like a baseball, and the fruit's strange spikes are associated with an image of a porcupine. Durian is also connected to the memory of passion fruit and lychee, two other tropical fruits that Dean also found on this trip, as well as general memories of Singapore. While these associations aren't connected to any strong personal history that's essential to Dean's consciousness, they're more substantial than those arising from a simple memorization exercise.

Chunking involves reducing long strings or segments of information into shorter, more manageable chunks. Most of us can't memorize a long series. Instead, when we encounter a large data set, we use an intrinsic method of organizing facts into smaller parts, with each part integrated into a story that connects to an island. This process yields an incredible memorization tool.

Both association and chunking can be very useful for exercising the brain, strengthening its connections, and therefore contributing to its resiliency. These powerful techniques have been shown to improve memory in several different studies. One such study, published in *Neuron* in 2017, assessed the memorization skills of World Memory Championship experts and people with average memories. The experts had superior skills to start with, but when the normal participants learned a memory technique called the "method of loci," which uses a familiar scene—a favorite room, for instance—in order to help memorize long lists, they became nearly as adept as the experts. And they achieved these results in only six weeks. After four months, their new memory skills remained. You'll find a long list of these types of exercises in the Personalized Optimize Program as well as other suggestions for exercising your associative and chunking skills.

Simple and moderately difficult exercises do in fact contribute to cognitive reserve, as our meta-analysis showed, but this study also revealed that complex, personalized activities afford us even greater protection. These findings speak to the tremendous power of complexity when it comes to long-term brain health. Complex activities directly strengthen the bridges and highways that lead to central islands of consciousness. Thought processes at this level of cognition are permanent and resilient and highly personal. This kind of intentional connection to the major islands of self is extremely difficult to sever: main neural roads are constantly repaved and reinforced, and they result in complex, overlapping communication between all the brain's domains.

Music is a perfect example of a multidomain, multifunction activity. Playing the piano, as in the case of Mrs. Collins, requires the brain to coordinate its efforts across many modalities: motor skills (pressing the right keys), visuospatial skills (the body moving in space and reading notes), attention (the particular timing of the music), mood (the way in which you play or respond to the music), executive function (following multiple steps in a complex sequence), and language (how to transform notes on a page into sound). Building a model ship is another challenging, multimodal task. You're required to follow written instructions, stay focused and attentive, understand the spatial properties of the ship, and predict how one piece will fit with another. For those at risk of developing Alzheimer's, these complex, multidomain activities provide the best way of building significant reserve and protecting against decline.

As you've now learned, our brains are designed for complexity at an early age, and sustained by complexity in old age. Here are some of the remarkable studies that beautifully illustrate this principle of human cognition:

Navigation: A 2006 study at University College London identified differences in hippocampal gray matter volume in London taxi drivers and bus drivers. Researchers found that taxi drivers consistently had a larger hippocampus. They controlled for other factors such as stress and years of driving experience and concluded that the difference in brain volume was due to the complexity of daily activity: bus drivers followed the same predetermined routes, while taxi drivers constantly navigated to new locations. More complex navigation led to more complex spatial knowledge, which in turn led to a bigger, more resilient brain.

Second Languages: There is evidence that second languages (or early bilingualism) appear to confer similar benefits based on complexity. In 2014, researchers at Ghent University found that lifelong bilingualism could delay the onset of dementia by about four and a half years. On average, monolinguals were diagnosed with dementia at 72.5 years old, while bilinguals were diagnosed at 77.3 years old. A 2016 study conducted by the NIH found that bilingual elderly people who were diagnosed with mild Alzheimer's disease had stronger brain networks and maintained better cognitive reserve than monolingual people, suggesting that bilingualism could possibly delay the onset of Alzheimer's disease. Another study conducted in Spain in 2016 found that bilinguals had lower cerebrospinal fluid markers of Alzheimer's (tau protein) and scored better in tests of executive function compared to monolinguals.

Music: Researchers have found a similar phenomenon in musicians. Gray matter was shown to be highest in professional musicians and significantly lower in nonmusicians in a number of brain regions that support the complex behavior of playing music.

Dance: A study published in the *New England Journal of Medicine* in 2003 looked at the association between dementia risk and a number of physical activities, including dance. Dance is a complex activity involving coordination, motor control, memorization, mood, and an intricate understanding of music, and in this study it was associated with a lower risk of dementia.

Formal Education: We now have a significant amount of data showing that formal education is correlated with late life cognitive reserve and the avoidance of dementia. A study published in 2007 looked at a group of British individuals and found that formal education in early adulthood was associated with greater cognitive ability later in life, specifically in the areas of verbal ability and fluency. Many recent studies have confirmed these findings. And education doesn't have to take place early in life to be protective: in a 2011 study conducted in Brazil, researchers found that formal education undertaken after the age of sixty also improved cognitive performance.

Lack of access to formal education may be a contributing factor to the disproportionate number of women who develop Alzheimer's (two-thirds of patients are women). Most people in their sixties, seventies, and eighties who are now developing this disease grew up in a time when women weren't encouraged to pursue a formal education. Later in life, these women have less cognitive reserve and thus less protection against Alzheimer's.

Complex Professions: Research on different types of professions has also shown that complexity throughout life leads to cognitive resilience. New research from 2016 by scientists at the Wisconsin Alzheimer's Disease Research Center and the Wisconsin Alzheimer's Institute demonstrated that complex jobs protect against dementia. The 284 participants in this study had an average age of sixty and were at a greater risk for Alzheimer's based on family history. Researchers assessed the complexity of the participants' jobs and determined whether they worked mostly with people, data, or things. Occupations involving mentoring other people (social worker, physician, school counselor, psychologist, and pastor) were especially protective, as were more intellectually demanding jobs like doctor and engineer. People in these professions developed more cognitive reserve than those who worked as cashiers, grocery store stockers, and machine operators.

Interestingly, brain scans showed participants with complex jobs had better cognitive performance despite the presence of white matter lesions in their brains, which may be indicative of vascular disease and increased risk for dementia. This study is further proof of the protective power of cognitive reserve: a complex, mentally stimulating lifestyle can lessen the effects of the harmful structural changes associated with Alzheimer's.

Additional studies from 2016 found that lifestyles involving complex work with others can even undo the neurological damage caused by a poor diet.

Uncomfortable Challenges: Another new study at Massachusetts General Hospital looked at seventeen "superagers" in their sixties and seventies who not only avoided cognitive decline but had the memory and attention of healthy twenty-five-year-olds. Researchers identified a set of brain regions that were thicker for superagers and thinner for regular agers. In the superagers, these brain regions were virtually indistinguishable from those of people in their twenties. Most of these regions were associated with emotional function as well as language, stress, interpreting information from the five senses, and overall communication. What kind of behavior led to these multifunctional, interconnected superaging brains? Anything that provided a challenge. Researchers concluded that brain-boosting activities should be challenging enough that they cause some unpleasantness (though not considerable stress). It's pushing through these areas of discomfort in the face of challenge, and exerting more effort than you might want to, that leads to successful cognitive aging.

Virtual Reality: In a systematic review of virtual reality cognitive training for people with MCI and dementia, considerable improvement was seen in attention, executive function, and memory (visual and verbal). There were also significant reductions in depressive symptoms and anxiety, both of which increase the risk of cognitive decline. Several studies in this review suggested that these cognitive benefits could be maintained even after the training was completed.

ACTIVITIES THAT BUILD COGNITIVE RESERVE

All activities involve all aspects of the brain. In fact, we use 100 percent of our brains 100 percent of the time—even when we're sleeping. Some activities, however, present specific challenges to different brain functions. The most complex activities, like those listed below, challenge multiple functions and do so to a greater extent, thereby resulting in greater cognitive reserve.

1. **Learning a New Language.** Main functions involved: language processing (new words and expressions), memory centers (memorizing, calling upon old memories to understand new material), frontal lobe (understanding the language in context), problem solving (forming a written or verbal response).

2. **Learning a Musical Instrument.** Main functions involved: motor skills (the physicality of playing), basal ganglia and cerebellum (fine motor movements), memory centers (memorizing notes, tunes, scales), processing (learning a sequence of steps), mood (understanding the emotional subtleties of the music).

3. **Computer Programming.** Main functions involved: memory centers (memorizing new codes), processing (knowing how the codes work together), attention (selecting which codes to use), motor skills (typing).

4. **Writing a Book.** Main functions involved: attention and focus (typing passages), memory centers (recalling research, stories, and ideas), processing (organizing and structuring the material), mood (re-creating emotions on the page), motor skills (typing).

5. **Karaoke and Singing.** Main functions involved: language centers (reading and performing lyrics), mood (interpretation of the song), cerebellum (modulating your voice), memory centers (recalling a particular song).

6. **Performing Stand-Up Comedy.** Main functions involved: memory, mood, executive function, and language.

7. **Learning to Dance.** Main functions involved: motor skills (physical coordination), basal ganglia and cerebellum (fine motor movements), mood (responding to music), memory centers (memorizing choreography), processing (understanding different dance techniques).

8. **Chess Club or Group Card Games (bridge, gin rummy, poker, etc.).** Main functions involved: memory centers (remembering your cards and the rules for each game), processing (step-by-step strategy), attention and focus (concentrating on the game), problem solving (planning how you will win).

9. **Mentoring Others in Your Field.** Main functions involved: memory centers (remembering and drawing from your expertise), attention (focusing on the mentoring activity), mood (reading another person's emotions and motivations), problem solving (coming up with options and solutions).

10. **Volunteering to Teach Children Math, English, or Any Subject You Enjoy.** Main functions involved: memory centers (remembering the subject matter), attention (focusing on the teaching), mood (responding to the students' needs), processing (examining and explaining multistep solutions).

11. **Jewelry, Crafts, Models, or Art.** Main functions involved: visuospatial skills (understanding complex designs), memory centers (memorizing techniques and patterns), attention and focus (concentrating on the activity), motor skills (the physical act of assembly).

12. **Taking Community College Courses.** Main functions involved: Memory centers (memorizing new words and concepts), processing (understanding multistep thinking), problem solving (applying new theories to find solutions).

The future of the memory-enhancement industry seems to be in virtual reality games that engage the brain across multiple modalities and challenge individuals according to their specific deficits and difficulties. Sometime soon you'll be able to exercise your brain while discussing quantum theory with Einstein, or talking politics with Lincoln. We'll all have access to games that are challenging, adaptive, and highly personalized.

Music as Medicine

John's nickname was "The Horn." He was a short man with a deep voice who came to see us with his partner of forty years. John was sixty-eight at the time. He'd retired a decade earlier from his demanding job as a publisher and had since become much less active, especially in recent years. Both John and his partner spoke of his declining memory, which was now affecting his ability to do complex daily tasks. John needed his partner to remind him to take his medications, and over the last few months he had routinely forgotten to do chores like washing the dishes and walking their dog. Once he even left the water running in the kitchen. Part of their home had flooded.

We did our customary labs and brain scans, which revealed no metabolic or structural abnormalities. John's personal history told us that he had once been very active, both in his career and in his hobby of playing the French horn in a local band. Though he'd always loved music, he'd given it up when he retired.

We knew John's past experience with music presented an ideal means of challenging his brain, so we asked him whether he would consider playing again. He didn't seem that interested. When we pressed him further, he would simply say, "I don't feel like it," or "I just don't play anymore." This kind of psychological resistance is something we often see in our patients, especially those who have lost their confidence due to memory problems. In John's case, he had developed a conflicted relationship to music. It was at once a source of some of his happiest memories and an activity that now made him uncomfortable. Our job as doctors is to disentangle the emotions and discomfort and figure out why a patient is avoiding something they used to love.

One of the most common limitations that causes older people to withdraw from life is hearing loss. Loss of hearing creates dissonance in conversation. The person is always a step behind and as a result he or she disengages, either subconsciously or consciously. A 2013 study published in the *Journal of the American Medical Association Internal Medicine* found that hearing loss was associated with cognitive decline, especially in the areas of memory and executive function. Other studies have found that visual impairment has a similar negative effect on cognition. We tested John and found that he did in fact have some minor hearing loss. A hearing aid was a simple solution that allowed him to hear music more clearly and also increased his confidence in social situations.

Minor pains are another reason older people withdraw from the activities they love. When patients say they have small joint pain, we pay special attention. John had lost some dexterity in his fingers due to arthritis, and though most doctors would tell him this was a part of normal aging, we were eager to treat it. We always place the patient at the center of our approach, not the generalized expectations of the health-care system. John's cognitive activities depended on the dexterity of his fingers—to us, fixing this problem was the key to his mental engagement. Though pharmaceuticals aren't often our first inclination as physicians, in this case we decided to treat his arthritis with medication. We also prescribed a course of physical therapy for John, and he experienced significant improvement as a result of both of these treatments.

Because John had physical limitations, he needed to adjust his expectations. He'd lost proficiency and speed in his playing since he'd been away from music, and he was also experiencing some cognitive deficits. All this meant that he played at a level lower than he was accustomed to. We made sure John understood what to expect when he returned to music. If he expected to play like he did twenty years ago, he was bound to be disappointed. Instead, we recommended that he start with a simple song, one he loved when he first began playing the French horn. John could begin with that song, rehearse it, and play it well. Then, once he felt comfortable with the first song, he could add another. We reminded him that this process would involve some physical and emotional effort, but that he would see improvement over time. We always tell our patients that the secret to life is managing expectations, especially your own, and especially if you're learning a new skill in midlife.

John agreed to start slowly, and after just a few months, he'd regained his musical skills and confidence. He was now dedicated to his music like he'd once been dedicated to his career. He could play more and more complex songs, which became great motivation to practice every day. After a few more months, he called a few friends he used to play with and together they decided to start a band. Some of his friends had children who played instruments, so they joined as well. Even a grandchild became part of the group. They rehearsed just for fun at first, but they started to realize they were actually pretty good. Eventually they were hired to play at a local restaurant. It was a wonderful social outlet for all of them, and they felt good about donating the money they earned to charity.

John had met his limitations, committed to challenging himself physically and mentally, and learned how to harness the power of motivation. Now he had cognitive complexity, positive emotions, and social engagement in his life again. He'd found his way back to himself, back to one of his greatest loves and one of his most significant islands of consciousness. Of all the incredible things we've learned as neurologists, this is perhaps the most beautiful: your rescue is in your stories, in what made you who you are. No puzzle book could ever compete with an activity that connects you to deeply personal, emotional islands. It might take a little investigating to unearth or remember your passions, but everyone has them, and everyone can benefit from them.

After six months we found that John's blood pressure and cholesterol levels had dropped. He was much more awake, alert, and focused, and he had no complaints about his memory. His partner was astonished by what he'd seen, but we weren't all that surprised. A study conducted in the Netherlands in 2013 found that engaging in music had physiological effects similar to those of exercise. Another study from India, published in 2015, found that individuals who listened to music had lower blood pressure and experienced less stress than participants who engaged in diet, exercise, and other common lifestyle measures.

Optimizing John's cognition had been the only aspect of our initial treatment plan, but as we so often see, positive changes in memory and social interaction made him more aware of diet and physical activity. During the follow-up appointment he asked for guidance on other lifestyle factors, and we drew up a personalized plan with the same kinds of measurable and achievable goals. John continued to improve and even reported greater happiness and satisfaction. After a year, a follow-up MRI showed that his medial temporal lobe was slightly bigger in size. Music and all its associated benefits had increased the volume of his brain and afforded him a retirement he could truly enjoy.

Optimize Myths

Puzzle books are the best way to exercise my mind: Puzzle books are beneficial to a certain extent, but complex activities are far more beneficial because they strengthen many of the brain's domains as well as the connections between them. Complex activities with a social component are even more beneficial.

It's almost impossible for people struggling with memory problems to learn new things: Learning new things is entirely possible if you work slowly, manage your expectations, and seek the support of family and friends. Technology offers an additional source of support and community.

You naturally lose mental sharpness in old age: Many people never experience cognitive decline. Your outcome depends on your genetic risk, but even more so on your lifestyle and the extent to which you generate cognitive reserve.

I'm forty—I'm too young to worry about cognitive function: In fact, it's at around this time that there is a pivotal change in the population. One group maintains health, and some people in this group actually improve their health. The other group starts a downward spiral. Your goal should be to live a healthy life from birth to death, but it's especially critical to make healthy choices when you're in your forties and fifties.

Social Interaction:
Another Kind of Complex Cognition

Joanne barely made eye contact. Every time Ayesha asked her a question she looked to her daughter. Like many of our patients, she'd grown accustomed to having others speak on her behalf. Joanne had always been active in her church and also worked as an organizer at a senior center. These responsibilities brought her great joy and a sense of meaning postretirement, but when she learned she had entered the early stages of Alzheimer's, she gave up both positions.

Her daughter reported that Joanne often complained of minor pains, though she couldn't identify exactly where the pain was located. She was also distracted, especially while she ate. Though she spent a long time sitting in front of her dinner plate, she never completed a meal. It took her family a while to realize this, and by the time they did, Joanne had lost almost thirty pounds. This loss of appetite is common in dementia patients, often in preclinical stages before memory symptoms emerge.

To Ayesha, Joanne seemed resigned to the fact that she had Alzheimer's. She was frail, not responding much, and withdrawing from social interaction into her own experience, which was largely the perception of physical pain and discomfort. This is unfortunate but common among Alzheimer's patients: They can't follow what people are saying. They're embarrassed because they repeat themselves. They feel like they're disappearing. In Joanne's case, she knew her disease couldn't be cured, and she had given up hope on any improvement or slowing of her symptoms.

Human beings are designed for social interaction. All evidence suggests that isolation is bad for human health. Loneliness itself can be a killer: the mortality rate in recently bereaved people is much higher, presumably because of a mixture of grief, loneliness, and reduced social interaction. One study found that people who don't engage in social activity are at a 50 percent greater risk of dying, suggesting that social behavior is just as important as diet, exercise, and other major lifestyle risk factors.

Many fascinating research projects have shown the different ways in which healthy social behavior makes us healthier in turn:

- The Blue Zones all have a strong social dimension that contributes to health and longevity. Religious communities are common in the Blue Zones, as we observed in the strong faith- and service-based community in Loma Linda. Maintaining family relationships is also common among these groups: having lifelong partners, living near parents and grandparents, and staying close to children were all found to increase life span and lower the risk of disease. The Okinawans even have a "moai," a group of five friends who remain close and support one another at all stages of life.

- The renowned Grant Study at Harvard followed 286 men throughout their lives, searching for the traits and decisions that led to happiness and fulfillment. The data from this study has consistently shown that the quality of your relationships affects your happiness and health as you age. Men who had poor relationships with their mothers were found to have an increased risk of developing dementia in their later years, while those who were close to their mothers earned an average of $87,000 more per year. "Social aptitude," the ability to cultivate and maintain relationships with the people around you—parents, siblings, other family members, mentors—consistently led to better physical and mental health in old age.

- The immunologist Esther Sternberg has written about the connection between social interaction and the immune system. Quality relationships help us deal with stress and therefore have a direct effect on the health of our hormones, nerves, and immune function.

Research also shows that social engagement is associated with a reduced risk of dementia. One study published in *JAMA Psychiatry* found that people defined as "lonely" had double the risk of developing Alzheimer's. A 2013 study from the University of New South Wales in Australia found that being married was associated with a lower risk of late-life cognitive decline. People with more extensive social networks also have a reduced risk of cognitive decline. How social you are turns out to be one of the most reliable determinants of your cognitive health.

Social activities, just like cognitive activities, range from simple to moderate to complex. Simple cognitive activities involve going into public and being part of a social situation: interacting with a clerk at the grocery store, going to the movies, or going out to dinner. Moderate social activities usually involve networks of people. You might get together with a group of old friends, for instance, and share stories and experiences. This kind of social activity will create more cognitive reserve than basic activities, but you still may not be fully engaged—perhaps you listen to the conversation but are mostly quiet. Complex social activities, those that require you to be truly engaged and participatory, are the most protective for the brain. These activities are purpose driven and involve active conversation, complete attention, and often complex cognitive behavior as well. They define who we are. They create and connect islands of consciousness. They may take time and effort on the patient's part, but the rewards are exponentially greater.

Social behavior, especially complex social behavior, works on many levels to increase cognitive reserve:

- Social interaction requires complex communication skills that involve different brain functions: face recognition, memory, focus, attention, auditory skills, and language skills.

- Social interaction generates emotions that are important for motivation and finding meaning in one's life.

- Social interaction decreases depression and low mood states, which we know increase the risk of cognitive decline.

- Social interaction facilitates action. For example, a friend might encourage you to exercise when you would not otherwise do so.

- Social interaction helps facilitate the expression of emotions, which has been shown to be important to overall health as well as cognitive health.

Social interaction also adds a real-life dimension to any cognitive activity. Combining a challenging, multidomain cognitive activity with social interaction yields the most complex behavior available to us. Eating with others, for example, is more cognitively complex than eating on your own. The same goes for exercise and pretty much any activity you can think of. Imagine one woman with MCI doing sudoku alone in her house, while another woman with MCI plays bridge with a group of friends. The woman playing bridge is benefiting from an activity that uses many cognitive domains—not just focus, attention, memory, and problem solving involved in the bridge game, but also the sensory and emotional processing involved in the social setting. According to all the evidence we have so far, the woman playing bridge is engaged in a far more challenging and beneficial activity. She'll build stronger connections and therefore experience slower decline.

Given this convincing research on social interaction, Ayesha's first step was to address Joanne's withdrawal and help her reconnect to the outside world. To that end, she prescribed medications to treat Joanne's anxiety and depression. She also encouraged Joanne's family to help her focus on something other than her present state. They could do this by gently redirecting her attention to her favorite stories and experiences, and making sure the memories that brought her joy were part of her daily life. In talking to her more, Ayesha also realized that Joanne was suffering from hearing loss. It turned out that she had tried some badly fitting hearing aids a few years back, and because they didn't work, she thought nothing could be done. Ayesha explained to her that well-designed hearing aids might work much better, and that we now have sophisticated procedures like cochlear implants that can nearly reverse hearing loss. When Joanne was prescribed hearing aids that fit properly, she seemed much more alert and willing to participate in conversations.

After a few weeks, Joanne started to feel less inwardly focused and more drawn to what was happening around her. It was then time to reintroduce social activities. Together she and Ayesha explored the opportunities available to her: her church, the senior center (where she had previously worked as an organizer), and the local hospital. Joanne was hesitant, so they decided to start slowly. Joanne would attend church with her daughter and begin to volunteer a few hours a week in the health ministry. Ayesha also asked her to keep a brief weekly diary of her activities in which she reflected on her successes, failures, obstacles, and new interests. This would keep Joanne accountable and also allow her to see her progress.

Ayesha followed up with Joanne a month later. She'd gained a lot of confidence by talking to members of her church, and though she still had some difficulty with complex tasks, she compensated by taking notes in order to stay organized. To Ayesha's surprise, she had also arranged to begin volunteering at a local hospital. After a few months, Joanne was manning the hospital's front desk and helping patients and families find their

---

HOW TO BECOME MORE SOCIALLY ACTIVE WHEN YOU HAVE MCI OR EARLY ALZHEIMER'S

Social situations can be challenging for those with memory problems. Not being able to follow a conversation can create considerable anxiety. People become intimidated easily and often choose to withdraw so as not to embarrass themselves in public. Patients are sometimes told to be more social, but they aren't given any guidelines for how to navigate social settings when they're experiencing memory impairment. This traditional approach amounts to a tremendous opportunity lost and often results in patients either giving up or experiencing even more anxiety.

In working with thousands of patients, we've found that people who have withdrawn socially generally fall into three categories, each of which requires a different approach for encouraging social behavior:

Naturally Shy: This type of person has had a lifelong habit of isolation. They like keeping to themselves. They're introverts. It's a challenge to become more social in midlife, but it's definitely possible. People who fall into this category need to start slowly. They should have initial contact with the people who make them feel most comfortable—like family members and close friends—and who are aware that the person is struggling with some cognitive deficits. The family members and friends should make a concerted effort to support the person in social circles. Familiar settings will also make them more relaxed. Once they're more

way around. The irony was not lost on her: here she was struggling with her memory, yet she spent hours every day navigating what for many was a very intimidating building. When she first started, Joanne had promised herself that she would learn the hospital inside out. She began with one floor, one office, one department at a time. Whenever she was at the desk she studied a map, and sometimes she walked the floors just to strengthen her memory (she also took the stairs whenever possible, which increased her physical fitness). Within five months she knew her way around the

---

comfortable in social situations, they may want to venture into larger and less familiar settings.

Out of Practice: These patients have fallen out of the habit of socialization. They used to be social, but as they grew older they just didn't have enough time, or some of their closest friends passed away. If these people are not uncomfortable in social situations, they should push themselves to engage as much as possible. Family and friends provide wonderful sources of companionship, as do churches and other community centers. Joining a book club can also be a great way of meeting new people and exercising your brain.

Withdrawn: Withdrawn patients are those whose cognitive problems have forced them to disconnect. They have trouble navigating conversations because of their psychological and neurological deficits. They may also be withdrawing due to physical limitations like hearing loss. These people are most comfortable in familiar environments. They're best at discussing familiar topics. They gain confidence when accompanied by a spouse, child, or other close friend or family member who can look out for them in social settings.

entire hospital. This single act of volunteering had provided her a social outlet, mental challenges, an opportunity for exercise, and a greater sense of purpose.

A year later Joanne was tested again. Most patients diagnosed with early Alzheimer's experience significant deterioration within the first year. Ayesha wasn't expecting to see improvement, but she hoped that social engagement could slow the progress of Joanne's disease. Both the brain scans and neuropsychological tests showed no significant deterioration. Joanne kept volunteering, and when Ayesha tested her again after two and a half years, the results were the same.

Conclusion

Optimizing the brain requires complex activities that build connections and create significant cognitive reserve. The most challenging activities engage many of the brain's domains and functions. These activities are even more challenging—and protective against disease—if they also involve social interaction. Though puzzle books and memory games are readily available, passions are more important. The activities you love provide the most effective and rewarding way of optimizing your brain and finding a purpose in life, especially in your later years.

Your Personalized
OPTIMIZE
Program

Building a resilient, connected brain takes more than simple puzzles and memory exercises. The brain thrives on challenges, especially those that are personally relevant and involve multiple cognitive domains. While our patients are sometimes daunted by cognitive and social activities, there are options for everyone. As with the previous programs, start by taking the self-assessment below. Once you've identified what optimizing brain function means in your life, you'll then learn about memory-enhancing techniques and many activities that will boost your cognitive function and protect against decline.

SELF-ASSESSMENT

Vision, Strengths, and Weaknesses: Assess your vision for a plan to optimize your brain, and identify factors that might help or hinder your efforts.

Vision: What is your idea of a brain-optimizing lifestyle? What kinds of activities are you currently doing to stimulate your brain? Are there opportunities to expand on those activities or replace them with more cognitively challenging ones? What are you most passionate about, and how might you connect this passion with friends, family, and community?

Strengths: What strengths and resources will help you achieve your vision?

Weaknesses: What are the obstacles to your vision?

1. How will you benefit from optimizing your brain?

Examples: I will have more mental clarity. My memory will improve. I'll have an easier time concentrating and working efficiently. I'll be better at organizing my daily schedule. I'll spend more time with family and friends. I'll have a sense of purpose in my life.

2. What are the most important areas for you to work on?

Examples: I need to start a new hobby. I need to finally learn how to play the drums. I need to learn how to be less shy. I have to stop watching television alone. I could be more comfortable with challenging myself mentally and socially. I have to find a new group of friends that I can see regularly.

3. What obstacles might prevent you from optimizing your brain?

Examples: I'm intimidated in social situations. I've never played a musical instrument or learned a second language. I'm not an adventurous person who likes trying new things. I don't have a social circle. I'm too old to change my daily routine. I'm already having memory problems and find learning difficult if not impossible. I have a stressful job that doesn't leave me much time for challenging cognitive activities.

4. What might help you optimize your brain? What are your resources?

Examples: I can enroll in community college courses designed for senior citizens. I can join a local book club. I can learn a second language, take dance classes, or play a musical instrument. I've always been interested in writing a book. I can join some friends who get together once a week to play card games.

5. Who can help you and how?

Examples: My spouse can support me in social settings. My friends and I enjoy reading and discussing books. I have some coworkers I could socialize with after work. I can join a group at the senior center. I can talk to my pastor and see if the church has someone who can help me. My daughter and I could study Spanish together.

6. When will you start?

Our Recommendation: Take a few days to think about the kinds of activities you'd like to try. Be creative. Make a list of all possible activities, ranging from crossword puzzles and chess to playing cards with friends, joining a book club, volunteering, opening an antique shop, or writing the book you've been thinking about for years. Have at least fifteen to twenty items on your list. Next, see which activities you have access to, what resources you have, and what limitations you need to address. You might want to begin with easier activities and work your way up to more challenging activities in group settings. Complex activities with a social component should be your ultimate goal.

COGNITIVE EXERCISES

Set yourself up for success by starting with the exercises that are easiest for you. Try to practice for one to two hours at least five days per week. Over time you can work your way up to more difficult exercises. Remember that exerting effort means you're challenging your brain. That's a good thing, as long as you stay calm and focused.

Please use these exercises to jump-start your optimizing process, but also save some time for complex activities that will afford your brain even more protection (detailed in the next section).

The exercises we recommend focus on four main cognitive skills:

1. Memory

2. Problem solving

3. Visuospatial skills

4. Attention and focus

1. Memory

Long-Term Memory: You can challenge your long-term memory by recalling stories from your past and enhancing them with images and other sensory details. The idea is to make your memories as vivid as possible. These memories are islands from which you can build connections to other important memories.

Photo Albums: Go through old photo albums, try to remember the context of each picture, and write a few words about the event or memory. This activity can result in a fun family document, or even a book.

Personal Event: Sit down with another family member or a group of friends and discuss in detail a particular event from your personal history. Birthdays, vacations, and weddings work well for this exercise. See who can come up with the most details.

Short-Term Memory: Exercising short-term memory involves using emotional links, association, chunking, and repetition. The more senses that are involved, the better. Sight is especially powerful in making memories. For instance, if you were trying to recall the details of a vacation to Hawaii, having a photo would almost certainly enhance your memories. Stories are also integral to memory—they're the mind's currency—and linking them can be a powerful tool in building memory.

In order to build short-term memory, let's start with a list of objects. Below we explain two strategies you can use to memorize these items.

Fruits

Apples	Grapes
Bananas	Mangoes
Cantaloupes	Oranges

Office Supplies

Scotch tape	Sticky notes
Pencils	Stapler

Cleaning Supplies

Air freshener	Paper towel
Broom	Pine-Sol
Dish soap	Windex
OxiClean	

Kitchen Items

Cutting board	Salt
Olive oil	

Visualize a Room

This strategy uses a familiar room and its features to help you memorize a list of items. You could choose your bedroom, living room, childhood playroom—whatever you like. Let's say you choose your bedroom: as you enter the room, you see a bed with four pillows, a wooden table, a floor lamp, and a large window. When trying to remember a list, associate each item on the list with an item or specific location in your bedroom. For example: You enter the room to a strong scent of PINE-SOL. Your bed is in front of you, and suddenly you notice that your bedding is glaringly white because you used OXICLEAN to wash it. You look to the left of the bed and see the lamp, but it's actually a BROOM. The lampshade is made of a giant BANANA PEEL! Then you look at the window and see a STICKY NOTE tacked on with SCOTCH TAPE.

Chunking

We only have a limited capacity to memorize a certain number of items. Chunking items together, either by category or association, can increase this capacity.

Chunking by Category: You can chunk the list of twenty items into four categories: six fruits, four office supplies, seven cleaning supplies, and three kitchen supplies. This gives you a strategy for organizing items on a long list. You could also label these chunks as 6F, 4O, 7C, and 3K.

Chunking by Association: You can associate each item in the list with a story that involves familiar people and settings. For example, we can tell the story of the list of office supplies through a character named Mary:

Office Supplies

- **Scotch tape:** Mary is known for being incredibly organized. Imagine as you enter the room that she's taping a large To-Do list on the wall.

- **Pencils:** Mary grabs a pencil and adds another task to her already extensive list.

- **Sticky notes:** Mary writes on sticky notes and adds them to her list—she's almost run out of room.

- **Stapler:** Mary staples another page onto the original list and continues planning her day.

Additional Memorization Strategies

Mnemonics: These devices assist in memory formation.

Let's say you want to memorize the following number: 425-563-2359. As a brain-building exercise and also a fun tool, let's assign to each number a word with an equivalent number of letters:

The first number, 4, can be "John."

The second number, 2, can be "is."

The third number, 5, can be "happy."

The fourth number, another 5, can be "Jacky."

We'll continue as follows:

6 = "jumped"

3 = "out"

2 = "of"

3 = "the"

5 = "plane"

9 = "yesterday"

So the original number, 425-563-2359, becomes: "John is happy Jacky jumped out of the plane yesterday."

Ridiculous stories are often easier to memorize. At first glance, this mnemonic looks harder than memorizing the number, but the technique becomes quite useful with practice, and it's fun.

Association: The brain functions by building on bigger and bigger patterns of association. Games that link two or more concepts, ideas, or images can really expand your memory-building mechanisms. You might associate by category (apples and oranges are fruits), or by shape (round), or by taste (sweet).

An example: In college, Dean needed to memorize the word *gastrectomy,* which means removing the stomach. Here is Dean's silly association for this word: he imagined a gas truck with a huge stomach instead of a gas cylinder. It was such a striking image that he never forgot the meaning of the word!

Below is a list of similarly challenging terms. Try to come up with silly associations for each of them.

Arthroplasty: joint replacement

Costochondritis: pain and inflammation of the cartilage that connects the ribs to the breastbone at the center of the chest

Diglossia: the phenomenon in which different dialects of a language or different languages are spoken by a person in different social situations

Indolent: lazy

Proxemics: the study of personal distance and other culturally defined uses of space that affect communication

ACES: These exercises combine four different thought processes to enhance memorization:

A = Attention. Pay attention to the piece of information you're trying to remember.

C = Connect. Associate that information with other related information using a mnemonic device—something that will make the information distinctive.

E = Emotion. Create an emotional link to the information to consolidate it further.

S = Senses. Try to associate other senses with the information (images, smells, tastes, etc.).

Let's say you're trying to memorize a long list of words. The first two words are:

Apple

Peacock

Here's an example of how to use ACES to memorize these words:

Apple

> *Attention:* Visualize the apple
>
> *Connect:* Think of Sleeping Beauty biting the apple
>
> *Emotion:* Feel the dread as she takes a bite
>
> *Senses:* See the apple's color (a deep red), hear the crisp crunch, taste the sweetness, and say apple

Peacock

> *Attention:* Visualize the peacock
>
> *Connect:* Think of Sleeping Beauty surrounded by peacocks
>
> *Emotion:* Suddenly the peacocks start flying all around her
>
> *Senses:* See the peacocks' vibrant green feathers, touch their elaborate tails, hear them chirping, and say peacock

ACES help create memorable scenes for each item. The sillier and more emotional the better.

2. Problem Solving

Problem solving involves many parts of the brain and is especially challenging to the frontal lobe. Almost all tasks require some degree of problem solving, from crossword puzzles to building models, solving mathematical equations, sudoku, and interpreting a written passage. One of our patients liked to build intricate wooden games that required hours of planning for each piece. Another patient enjoyed summarizing books and articles and ended up making money from a few websites that published her work. Both of these were excellent problem-solving activities.

One mistake people make is not realizing that an activity that initially requires problem solving can become repetitive over time. Consider knitting, a hobby many of our patients ask us about. In most cases, knitting doesn't challenge problem-solving skills throughout the process. Once you've decided on a pattern, the problem solving ends. Knitting would continue to challenge your problem-solving skills if you kept changing the pattern—but that wouldn't make a very wearable sweater!

3. Visuospatial Skills

Many of the problem-solving examples above have a visuospatial aspect, but here are a few more: learning to play the piano with a small, light-up keyboard (which would also build motor skills and executive function), painting by numbers, designing jewelry, and jigsaw puzzles. There are also many entertaining games, like Legos and tangram, that improve visuospatial skills.

4. Attention and Focus

Attention and focus are critical to optimal memory and executive function and serve as the foundation of all other cognitive capacities. As we get older, our attention starts to deteriorate and we have more difficulty focusing. Be especially patient as you practice these exercises. They can initially be overwhelming. We recommend that you start slowly and build your skills over time.

- One simple way to work with focus and attention is to go back to the list on page 259 and see how many items you can visualize and recall after reading the list once. Expect not to remember many items at first. See if over time you can increase the list from three to five to ten and ultimately twenty.

- Another helpful technique is to enter a quiet room (preferably a room you've never been in, or one you're not very familiar with), sit down, close your eyes, and try to recall as many features of the room as possible. You might use an audio recorder to capture your thoughts. See if you can remember more visual features with practice.

- You can also build focus by doing mathematical calculations in your head. In this case, it's not about the complexity of the math but your ability to stay focused during the process. Try subtracting 3s from 1,000 all the way down to single digits. Then try subtracting 7s. If you have trouble, start with 100 instead.

- Reading also strengthens attention and focus. Read a long passage and then try to recall the number of "ands" in the article. This exercise challenges concentration because you're forced to pay attention to the article while keeping track of another element. You should still be able to understand the content of the article.

COMPLEX ACTIVITIES

As we explained in the "Optimize" chapter, complex activities dramatically increase cognitive reserve. They build connections in your brain that fortify it against both Alzheimer's and normal aging. If you had to pick only one exercise for optimizing your cognition, we would encourage you to choose from the following list, or find another activity that challenges many of the brain's functions:

- Learning a new language

- Learning a musical instrument

- Computer programming

- Writing an article or even a book

- Karaoke

- Stand-up comedy

- Learning to dance

- Joining a card game, backgammon, or chess club (or any other challenging games in a group setting)

- Mentoring others in your field

- Volunteering in your community (doing an activity that engages your mind)

- Making jewelry, crafts, and models

- Drawing, painting, and sculpting

- Taking community college courses

All these activities are even more beneficial if they involve social interaction. You might decide to write a book with your children, for instance, or take guitar lessons with a close friend.

It's most important to find something you truly love doing, an activity that can be a source of joy and meaning in your life. If you don't know what you love doing, take some time to reflect on the past. Everyone had an interest at some point.

1. Talk to friends and family members. They may be able to help you identify activities that you love or used to be curious about.

2. Write a list of activities you did in your teens and twenties.

3. Write a list of activities you never got to do but dreamed about.

4. If you're still not sure what you like, pick something and try it. If it's not the right fit, then try something else. If you end up not liking the second or third activity you try, this is still not grounds for quitting. It might take time to develop a passion and affinity for a new activity. Bring a friend along as extra motivation.

Managing your expectations is critical as well. Complex activities are challenging and require a learning process. Start at an easy level, be patient, and stick with it.

Work Toward Increasing:

- Time spent with friends and families

- Activities that you love

- Learning new, cognitively challenging activities
- Being a part of different social circles

Work Toward Eliminating:

- Time spent in front of a television
- Long periods of isolation
- Withdrawing from social activity because of anxiety
- Forcing yourself to do puzzle books when there are more complex activities that you actually enjoy

COMMON OBSTACLES

Memory Impairment: Start a new activity slowly and work step by step. You may have to exert more mental effort than you did in the past, but you will see improvement over time.

Being Shy: Have your spouse, partner, sibling, or child accompany you at social outings. Venture out with your closest friends. Find situations that you would be comfortable in, and try them out with friends and family.

No Social Circle: Book clubs, community centers, and faith communities are all excellent places to find people who may share your interests and values.

Lack of Interest: Everyone, at some point in time, was interested in something. Go back to your childhood passions. Look at old photographs. Ask your family members. Use your intuition to follow interests that you may have been discouraged from pursuing many years ago.

Physical Limitations: Don't be shy about using a cane or walker in public. The cognitive gains will far outweigh any social discomfort.

WEEKLY OPTIMIZE PLAN

Your first task is to make a list of 20 to 30 cognitive and social activities. Offering your brain different activities throughout the week will help you stay motivated and engaged.

MONDAY
Read a book chapter or magazine article. Once you've finished, write down as many details as you can remember. In a few sentences, summarize the author's intention and your own analysis of the chapter or article.

TUESDAY
Go online and find a local community for an activity you enjoy. You might be able to join an event and meet new people. You can also correspond with members of an online group who share your interests.

WEDNESDAY
Purchase a small keyboard and start learning how to play simple songs you know well. Most of the newer devices come with a selection of preprogrammed songs that you can learn with the help of light-up keys.

THURSDAY
Gather some friends and start a book club or hobby group. Or simply meet up and enjoy a good conversation. Card games are also a great occasion for getting together with friends.

FRIDAY
Download a memory game onto your phone, tablet, or laptop. There are many games designed to increase memory, problem solving, and processing speed. Tangram is great for building visuospatial skills. Electronic versions of card games and word games will also challenge your brain.

SATURDAY
Volunteer at a local shelter, nursing home, senior center, or hospital. Over the next few weeks, you may want to try volunteering at several different places so you can vary your activities and social environments.

SUNDAY
Try two cognitively challenging activities today—at least one of which has a social component. You might play your keyboard in the morning and have a cup of coffee with a friend in the afternoon. If you're not accustomed to social interaction, be sure to start slow and give yourself time to build confidence in social settings.

If prolonged pain is a limitation, address it aggressively with your primary-care doctor. Make sure it doesn't turn into a lingering, isolating problem. Vision and hearing problems should also be treated aggressively.

OUR PERSONAL APPROACH TO OPTIMIZING

- We actively use chunking and association techniques when memorizing phone numbers, addresses, birthdays, and passwords.

- When we go grocery shopping, we chunk our items by categories (fruits, vegetables, spices, grains, etc.), and then memorize the number of items for each category. This is an effective way of challenging our memory on a daily basis.

- Memorization techniques are also a part of how we approach our professional responsibilities. For example, Dean is able to categorize his current patients. He knows that among his 1,536 Alzheimer's patients, 836 are early stage, 318 are moderate, and 432 are late stage. He also uses chunking within each category (for instance, twenty-eight of the early stage patients have had a stroke). As we've both worked with these techniques over the years, they've become automatic and have helped us organize our thoughts more effectively.

- Music is central to our lives. Dean plays the guitar (poorly), and Ayesha plays the keyboard and sings (beautifully). We made sure our children grew up around music as well. We try to enjoy music together as often as possible, whether it's singing in the car or going to outdoor concerts.

- We've made a habit of inviting friends over for dinner and discussing current events, documentaries, and books. Our daughter, Sophie, calls these events "Meal Masters," and we've spent many wonderful evenings socializing with the people we love and discussing topics that interest all of us. Often we'll cook, play games, and enjoy music together. It's fun to see people who are normally shy break out into song because the environment is so relaxed and supportive. Our goal is to build bonds and brains. This is also a great way to try out new recipes!

Conclusion

Medicine progresses. We learn more about diseases like Alzheimer's every day, and we may in fact see a pharmacological treatment sometime in the future. But why wait for that moment, and why continue living a life that will force you to someday rely on medication? Lifestyle change is available right now, and as you've seen throughout this book, our patients have transformed their lives using simple, effective, personalized techniques. It's entirely within your power to do the same.

Personalized medicine, a model of medical care that customizes treatment based on individual differences in genes, proteins, and environment, has emerged as the new medical paradigm for chronic disease. There's a significant amount of funding for studies that use this approach—every field's medical specialists and scientists are trying to frame their research so that it fits some version of personalized medicine. The idea behind personalized medicine is that though humans are on the whole very similar, we are very different at the molecular level. Each of us has different combinations of genes, and those genes are turned on and off at different times. Each of us has different enzymes and levels of enzyme activity; we respond to environmental stimuli differently; we process nutrients, chemicals, and medications differently. Conventional medicine's approach has been to treat us as though we're all the same, to assume somehow that one nutrient, drug, or behavior fits all. One study says that a vitamin is good for you and we all decide to take it. A drug is found to decrease blood pressure and we're all given prescriptions. But now we know that our infinite differences profoundly impact the way medical treatments affect us, and also how effective they are. To date, personalized medicine has been used most successfully in the treatment of diabetes, obesity, and heart disease, where doctors look at the unique genetic and chemical constituents of an individual's disease, and, more importantly, implement lifestyle changes that take into consideration the individual's history, resources, limitations, and proclivities. This comprehensive approach is bringing to light what we discovered years ago: chronic disease, especially neurodegenerative disease, is highly complex and highly personal, and if given the right tools, people can change their lives.

The protocol we shared with you in *The Alzheimer's Solution* is personalized medicine for the brain. We know this disease is more than just amyloid and tau, and it's certainly not a one-size-fits-all condition. It's a multidimensional disease that at its core has glucose and lipid dysregulation, inflammation, oxidation, and degenerative components that are in turn affected by individual nutrient deficiencies, toxicities, and other immune, endocrine, and metabolic factors. We also know that Alzheimer's is deeply affected by the risks you accumulate throughout life, and that any lifestyle protocol designed to minimize these risks must take your unique situation into account. Each of these factors needs to be addressed on the level of the individual: a complex disease like Alzheimer's requires personalization at every step.

Bringing about lasting change in people's lives also demands this level of personalization. Compliance to medication varies, as does compliance to lifestyle changes, all based on our individual strengths and weaknesses, and the habits we've created over our lifetimes. Accounting for all these elements is the only way to fight a complex chronic disease like Alzheimer's, and when we do, we can transform not only our own health, but the health of entire communities.

This book showed you the future of neurology. Within these pages we've described a groundbreaking model for how to understand, prevent, and treat Alzheimer's on a personalized level. The next step is to bring our powerful approach to families, schools, churches, and cities. We're doing everything we can to spread this message, to challenge assumptions about Alzheimer's disease, and pave the way for a comprehensive cure.

A Note About Our Research

The research that forms the basis of *The Alzheimer's Solution,* our comprehensive clinical program, and our life's work, is the culmination of three varied scientific approaches: fifteen years of seeing patients who suffered from every stage of dementia and cognitive decline, one of the largest observational studies ever conducted on cognitive health and lifestyle, and scrutinizing twenty years' worth of published research from around the globe on dementia, Alzheimer's disease, Parkinson's disease, and stroke. In total, our research proves convincingly that Alzheimer's, dementia, and overall brain health are directly linked to lifestyle factors and can be influenced—and more importantly, prevented—by the choices we make every day.

We now lead the Brain Health and Alzheimer's Prevention Program at Loma Linda University, where we've had the unique experience of treating two drastically different patient populations. The Seventh-day Adventists of Loma Linda have a remarkably healthy lifestyle that protects them against Alzheimer's—in fact, during a six-year period, looking at more than twenty-five hundred patients in our clinic, and at the relationship between nutrition, physical activity, and education, we found that less than 1 percent of our dementia patients practiced healthy lifestyles (plant-based diets, regular exercise, stress management, community involvement, and higher levels of cognitive activity, which create resiliency in the brain). The more strongly individuals adhered to these tenets of healthy living, the more protected they were against cognitive decline. The residents of nearby San Bernardino, by contrast, live a typical modern life—standard American diets, lack of exercise, chronic stress, poor sleep—and suffer disproportionately from lifestyle diseases including high blood pressure, high cholesterol, diabetes, cardiovascular disease, and Alzheimer's. After observing and quantifying healthy lifestyle behaviors for over a decade, we began to apply them to patients who were suffering from cognitive decline. We found that each incremental step—a reduction of refined sugar in the diet, for instance, or the introduction of just fifteen minutes of exercise per day—resulted in profound changes in cognitive health. In our patients showing the early signs of dementia, we are consistently able to stop the disease in its tracks and reverse debilitating cognitive symptoms.

As researchers at Loma Linda University (considered the only "Blue Zone" in the United States due to the Adventists' plant-based diet and active lifestyle), we were given access to a segment of the Adventist Health Studies database, one of the largest and longest-running epidemiological studies in the world, and a database that has produced some of the most incredible scientific results in the world of epidemiology and chronic disease to date. Using this incredible data, we examined the associations between diet (plant-based vs. other diets) and cognitive health outcomes. We concluded that a plant-based diet is strongly correlated with greater cognitive function.

We have since performed three comprehensive reviews that investigate the associations between diet and stroke, diet and Parkinson's disease, and diet and dementia. Each review showed a strong relationship between a plant-based diet and lower prevalence of the given neurological disease. We also searched a nationwide database for relationships between insulin resistance and cognitive decline, finding a strong correlation between insulin resistance and lower memory scores; in a second paper, we concluded that among individuals with diabetes, the incidence of dementia was increased by 10 percent.

Using a different nationwide database, we also found that in general there was a greater prevalence of dementia in people who suffered from sleep apnea. When we looked at leisure-time behavior in a multi-ethnic population, we saw that regular physical activity dramatically reduced the incidence of vascular dementia—by 21 percent. Our most recent research project was a comprehensive meta-analysis of the efficacy of cognitive exercises in people diagnosed with mild cognitive impairment. The studies we examined revealed a positive relationship between cognitive training and a lower risk for progression to Alzheimer's disease, and this relationship was stronger if the cognitive exercise was more complex and targeted the person's specific weaknesses.

Our clinical experience, research, and lifestyle interventions are supported by a wealth of research from around the world. The claims and the program in *The Alzheimer's Solution* are based on many groundbreaking studies on lifestyle and brain health. Below are a few of the foundational studies that appear in the book:

- The Finnish Geriatric Intervention Study to Prevent Cognitive Impairment and Disability (FINGER), published in 2015, examined the effects of a two-year, comprehensive lifestyle intervention in 1,260 adults between the ages of sixty and seventy-seven. The participants were divided into two groups. The first group received the following interventions: a healthy, plant-based diet high in omega-3 fatty acids, a regular aerobic exercise and resistance training program, computer programs that challenged cognitive activity, and intensive management of metabolic and vascular risk factors including diabetes, high blood pressure, and high cholesterol. The second group received standard-of-care health advice (they were simply told to eat healthy and exercise). At the end of the two-year period, the intervention group had a significantly higher score in overall cognitive performance than the standard-of-care group. This is the first large clinical trial to prove that it is possible to prevent cognitive decline using a multidomain intervention among at-risk individuals, and was published in the esteemed journal *Lancet*.

- In a new study from 2017, researchers at Columbia University found that participants who ate a plant-based diet had a lower risk of cognitive decline over a span of six years compared with those who ate a standard American diet.

- In a recent study published in 2014, three dietary patterns— the DASH (Dietary Approach to Stop Hypertension), the

Mediterranean diet, and a hybrid of the two, the MIND diet—were tested in 923 subjects to assess how these diets affected the risk of developing Alzheimer's disease. After four and a half years, a total of 144 people developed Alzheimer's disease. Those who adhered to the MIND diet at the maximum level cut their risk of developing Alzheimer's by more than half (53 percent). Researchers found that the risk of developing Alzheimer's was reduced even among those who only moderately adhered to the diet (these subjects cut their risk by one-third or 35 percent). This important study showed that every incremental step toward a brain-healthy dietary pattern results in a decreased risk of cognitive decline.

- The Framingham Longitudinal Study, a famous longitudinal study of the residents of Framingham, Massachusetts, found that daily brisk walks resulted in a 40 percent lower risk of developing Alzheimer's later in life.

- In a 2011 randomized controlled trial of 120 older adults, researchers at the University of Pittsburgh showed that rigorous aerobic exercise increased the size of the hippocampus, the brain region responsible for memory storage and processing, leading to improvements in memory. Exercise training increased levels of BDNF, a chemical that promotes both new neurons and the connections between them, and also led to a 2 percent increase in hippocampal volume, effectively reversing the normal volume loss due to aging.

- In a 2010 meta-analysis of fifteen studies that collectively assessed more than 33,000 participants, researchers in Italy found that participants who performed a high level of physical activity lowered their risk of cognitive decline by 38 percent. Even those participants who engaged in low- to moderate-level exercise were found to have a 35 percent lower risk.

- In 2014, researchers at Washington University in St. Louis found that sleep-deprived individuals had greater amyloid plaque deposition in their brains (amyloid plaques are considered the hallmark pathology of Alzheimer's disease), and that improvement in sleep led to a reduction in amyloid deposition.

- In a ten-year study of older adults conducted at Johns Hopkins University, lifelong cognitive activity was shown to improve brain efficiency and prevent Alzheimer's pathology even in those subjects with a strong genetic risk.

We are now conducting the most comprehensive and conclusive research to date that explores lifestyle risk factors and the development of neurodegenerative diseases. Our lifestyle program at Loma Linda University is one of the most sophisticated in the world—we have the most advanced imaging techniques, the latest biomarker and neuropsychological tests, and a behavioral intervention protocol more thorough and personalized than anything ever developed. The results are staggering and support the conclusions of the book, and we hope they will revolutionize the way we understand and treat Alzheimer's disease.

Recipes

Bean and Butternut Squash Enchiladas

We love the bold flavors of Mexican dishes, and this enchilada is a favorite in our household. Packed with plant protein and fiber, this recipe is a divine combination of sweet butternut squash, meaty black beans, and smoky adobo sauce. The synergy of the monounsaturated fats, vitamin E, and B vitamins, along with the antioxidant power of the polyphenols, will boost your brain and your entire body.

Serves 4 to 6

For the filling
- 2 cups butternut squash, cubed
- 1 tablespoon grapeseed oil or EVOO
- Salt and pepper
- 1 15-ounce can black beans, slightly drained
- 2 garlic cloves, minced
- ½ teaspoon cumin
- A pack of corn tortillas

For the enchilada sauce (makes about 2¾ cups)
- 2 cups low-sodium vegetable broth
- ½ cup low-sodium tomato paste
- 2½ tablespoons chili powder

2 teaspoons ground cumin

2 teaspoons dried oregano

3 garlic cloves, minced

1 teaspoon tamari or low-sodium soy sauce

1½ tablespoons lime juice, plus more to taste

Toppings

Avocado, sliced

Fresh cilantro, chopped

Lime juice

Pumpkin seeds

Red onions, diced

Tomato, diced

Preheat oven to 400°F. In a bowl combine cubed butternut squash, oil, and a pinch of salt and pepper. Stir together and spread onto a baking sheet. Bake for 20 minutes or until tender and slightly golden on the edges. Remove from oven and set aside. Lower the oven temperature to 350°F.

While the squash is baking, make the enchilada sauce by combining the vegetable broth, tomato paste, spices, minced garlic, and tamari or soy sauce in a medium-size skillet and placing over medium heat. Bring to a simmer while mixing with a wooden spoon or whisk, making sure the tomato paste blends well. Let mixture simmer for 15 minutes, until the sauce thickens. Remove from heat and add the lime juice. Try the sauce and adjust salt and pepper to taste. Pour the sauce in a separate bowl and set aside. Using the same skillet, add the slightly drained black beans, garlic, and cumin. Stir and warm until the beans start bubbling. Then add the roasted butternut squash. Remove from heat and add 2 to 3 tablespoons of enchilada sauce. Stir well. Add lime and pepper to taste.

Now prepare the enchiladas. Cover the bottom of a 9 × 13-inch baking dish with 1 cup of enchilada sauce. Warm the tortillas in the microwave for 30 seconds or place them on the middle oven rack for about a minute to soften them. Place one corn tortilla in the baking dish. Add a couple generous spoonfuls of filling, roll up the tortilla, and set it seam side down at one end of the dish. Continue until you run out of space—there should be room for 8 to 9 enchiladas. Pour the remaining sauce over the top of the enchiladas. Cover the dish with foil and bake for 20 minutes at 350°F. Add toppings and serve warm.

Chickpea Sandwich

This sandwich is a breeze to make and is one of the best meals for days when you just don't want to go near your stove. It's a great brain-healthy meal when you're on the run, but also exciting enough to take to a potluck or picnic. Don't underestimate this easy-to-prepare dish: it's bursting with flavor and filled with powerful nutrients for your brain.

Serves 2

Lemon Tahini Dressing (included in the Buddha Brain Bowl recipe, page 298)

1 15-ounce can chickpeas, rinsed and drained

¼ cup roasted unsalted sunflower seeds

3 tablespoons tahini

½ teaspoon Dijon or spicy mustard

¼ cup finely chopped red onion

2 tablespoons finely chopped fresh dill

¼ teaspoon turmeric powder

½ tablespoon lemon juice (or the juice of half a lemon)

Pinch each of salt and pepper

4 pieces rustic bread

Sliced avocado, onion, cucumbers, tomato, and lettuce for serving

Prepare the Lemon Tahini Dressing and set aside.

Add chickpeas to a mixing bowl and lightly mash with a fork. Then add sunflower seeds, tahini, mustard, red onion, dill, turmeric, lemon juice, and salt and pepper, and mix with a spoon. Taste and adjust seasonings as needed. Lightly toast bread and prepare any other sandwich toppings you desire (tomato, onion, lettuce, avocado). Scoop a generous amount of filling onto two of the pieces of bread, add desired toppings and dressing, and top with the other two slices of bread and serve.

Bean and Lentil Chili

Chili is the ultimate comfort food that soothes and warms from the inside out. Many chili recipes call for meat, but here, plant proteins create a perfect brain- and heart-healthy meal.

Serves 3 to 4

2 tablespoons EVOO

1 large yellow onion, diced

1 green, red, or yellow bell pepper, diced

1 jalapeño pepper, diced with seeds

½ teaspoon each sea salt and black pepper, divided, plus more to taste

4 garlic cloves, minced

3 tablespoons chili powder, divided

1 tablespoon dried oregano

2 teaspoons ground cumin, divided

1 teaspoon smoked paprika

⅛ teaspoon nutmeg

3 tablespoons tomato paste

1 28-ounce can low-sodium crushed tomatoes

1¾ cup water, plus more as needed

¾ cup dry red lentils, rinsed in water and drained

1 15-ounce can kidney beans, slightly drained

1 15-ounce can black beans, slightly drained

2 tablespoons lime juice

Toppings

Red onions, chopped

Avocado slices and/or guacamole

Cilantro

Place a large pot over medium heat. Add the oil, onion, bell pepper, jalapeño, and a pinch of salt and pepper. Sauté, stirring frequently for 5 minutes. Add the garlic and stir for about 30 seconds, until fragrant. Then add

2 tablespoons chili powder, oregano, 1 teaspoon cumin, paprika, nutmeg, tomato paste, crushed tomatoes, and water, and stir to combine. Once the mixture starts boiling, add the red lentils and cover the pot. Allow to boil for about 15 minutes, stirring every 4 to 5 minutes. Then reduce the heat to medium-low and simmer. Cook for another 20 minutes, or until lentils are mostly tender. During the process, you may need to add more water if the mixture looks too dry or if the lentils aren't fully submerged.

Then add the kidney and black beans, ¼ teaspoon each salt and pepper, and stir in the remaining 1 tablespoon chili powder and 1 teaspoon cumin. Simmer over medium heat, and once the mixture starts bubbling, cover the pot, reduce heat to low and cook for 20 minutes. Stir occasionally. More water may be needed if the chili boils down too much (about ½ cup to 1 cup).

Remove from heat and add the lime juice. Adjust seasoning as needed.

Serve as is or garnish with cilantro, red onions, and avocado slices or guacamole.

Oatmeal Amaranth Porridge

Breakfast is the most important meal of the day because it sets your metabolic pattern, which affects mood, energy, and motivation. Why not start today with a hearty whole-grain porridge? Amaranth may look like bird food, but it has more protein and iron than almost any other grain. Amaranth also contains lysine, an important amino acid found in only a few grains, as well as calcium and manganese. Boost your anti-inflammatory intake by adding nuts and berries as toppings.

Serves 2 to 3

½ cup rolled oats
½ cup amaranth
2 tablespoons chia seeds
3 cups water

1 cup unsweetened almond milk

Pinch of salt

1 teaspoon cinnamon

Stevia for sweetness (optional)

Toppings

Blueberries or raspberries

Bananas, sliced

Walnuts, almonds, or hazelnuts

1 teaspoon almond butter

In a medium saucepan, add the whole grains, chia seeds, water, almond milk, and salt. Mix together and place over medium heat. Cook the mixture, uncovered, for about 20 minutes, stirring frequently and reducing heat if necessary, until the oats are softened and the mixture thickens. (If you plan to make this recipe the night before, combine the ingredients in a bowl and place in the refrigerator. Transfer the mixture to a saucepan in the morning, and simply heat and serve). Remove from heat and stir in cinnamon and stevia to taste. Serve with your chosen toppings.

The MIND Smoothie

This smoothie is inspired by the MIND diet, a dietary pattern that numerous studies have proven to be the most effective at preventing Alzheimer's disease. All of the ingredients top the dietary scoring chart for cognitive health. Here's a recipe based on the latest research and specifically designed for your brain—now that's public health at its best.

Serves 2

1 cup blueberries, frozen

1 cup mango, frozen

1 banana, frozen

¾ cup of fresh spinach leaves

1 tablespoon ground flaxseeds (also called flax meal)

¼ cup walnuts

¾ cup water

Combine all the ingredients in a blender and blend until smooth and creamy (duration depends on how strong the blender is). Add additional water if needed.

Stuffed Bell Peppers

This wonderfully colorful dish is worlds apart from the beige, brown, and neon of processed Western foods. The yellow, green, and red peppers, mint green avocado sauce, white cauliflower rice, dusty pink pinto beans, and deep purple onion are the result of powerful phytochemicals like anthocyanins, lycopene, chlorophyll, lutein, and carotenoids, all of which fight inflammation in the brain and help grow connections among neurons. The cauliflower rice provides a low-glycemic alternative to white rice.

Serves 4 to 6

For the peppers

4 large red, yellow, or orange bell peppers, or one of each

halved lengthwise, and seeds removed

For the cauliflower rice

1 head cauliflower

½ tablespoon EVOO

1 cup red, white, yellow, or green onion, diced

3 cloves garlic, minced (optional)

¼ teaspoon each sea salt and black pepper,

plus more to taste

1 15-ounce can pinto beans, rinsed and drained

⅔ cup salsa, plus more for serving (see recipe page 287, or

buy a ready-made chunky salsa)

2 teaspoons cumin powder

2 teaspoons chili powder

2 to 3 tablespoons lime juice

Optional toppings

Avocado Dressing (see recipe page 287)

Cilantro, chopped

Red onion, diced

Lime juice, fresh

Hot sauce

Preheat oven to 375°F and set out a 9 × 13-inch baking dish or rimmed baking sheet. Lightly brush halved peppers with EVOO or grapeseed oil. Set aside.

Prepare cauliflower rice. Wash a large head of cauliflower and remove its greens. Then shred the cauliflower. If using a box grater, cut the cauliflower head into four pieces and use the larger grating side (the side commonly used for cheese) to grate the cauliflower into the size of rice. Do not grate the stem. This can also be done in a food processor with the grater attachment.

Then heat a large rimmed skillet over medium heat and add EVOO, onions, garlic (optional), and a pinch of salt and pepper. Sauté for 1 minute, stirring frequently to prevent browning. Then add cauliflower "rice" and sauté for 2 to 3 minutes. Next add the pinto beans, salsa, cumin, chili powder, lime, salt, and pepper. Adjust the seasoning as desired. Stir thoroughly and then cover, steaming the rice for 1 minute. Remove from heat. Transfer the mixture to a bowl and set aside.

Take the halved peppers and place about ½ cup of the mixture into each, or until the peppers are stuffed to the rim. Place the pepper boats in the baking dish and cover tightly with foil. Bake for 30 minutes, then remove foil, increase heat to 400°F, and bake for another 15 minutes, or until peppers are soft and the edges are slightly golden brown. If you're using soft peppers, bake them 5 to 10 minutes more. Serve with Avocado Dressing, cilantro, onions, lime juice, and hot sauce.

Avocado Dressing

2 small ripe avocados

2 cups chopped cilantro

1 teaspoon apple cider vinegar

1 small garlic clove

5 small limes, juiced

½ teaspoon sea salt

½ teaspoon cumin, optional

¼ cup water, to thin

To prepare dressing, add all ingredients except for water to a blender or food processor and mix thoroughly. Add only enough water to encourage blending. Taste and adjust seasonings as needed, adding more lime, salt, and/or cumin.

Salsa

1 pound or about 2 cups chopped tomatoes

½ white onion or about ½ cup, chopped

2 to 3 garlic gloves, minced

1 jalapeño pepper, seeded and diced

Juice of one lime

½ cup cilantro, chopped

½ teaspoon salt

Mix everything in a bowl and let sit for about 20 to 30 minutes for maximum flavor. Optional: Pulse all the ingredients two to three times in a food processor for a smoother consistency.

Tofu Turmeric Scramble

Tofu can be intimidating, but this versatile plant protein takes on whatever flavor you give it. With every bite of this savory scramble, you'll feel your arteries opening and your brain detoxing. This filling breakfast will also help manage your blood sugar levels.

Serves 2 to 3

  1 8-ounce block firm or extra-firm tofu
  1 tablespoon EVOO
  ¼ red onion, chopped
  1 green or red bell pepper, chopped
  ½ teaspoon each salt and pepper
  ½ cup button mushrooms, sliced
  1 teaspoon garlic powder
  ½ tablespoon turmeric
  ¼ cup nutritional yeast
  2 cups fresh spinach, loosely chopped

Drain the tofu and squeeze gently to remove extra water. Crumble tofu into a bowl by hand—the smaller the pieces, the better. Prep vegetables and place a large skillet over medium heat. Add EVOO, onions, and bell peppers. Stir in a pinch of salt and pepper and cook for about 5 minutes to soften the vegetables. Then add mushrooms and sauté for 2 minutes. Then add the tofu. Sauté for about 3 minutes, a little more if the tofu is watery. Then add the rest of the salt and pepper, garlic, turmeric, and nutritional yeast and mix with a spatula, making sure the spices blend well. Cook for another 5 to 8 minutes until tofu is slightly browned. At the end, add the spinach and cover the pan to steam for 2 minutes. Serve immediately with sides of your choice. This tofu scramble makes a delicious breakfast burrito on a whole-wheat tortilla. We enjoy it with slices of avocado and hot sauce, but you could also try it with baked russet potatoes, black beans, and/or cilantro.

Spelt Pancakes with Chia Berry Sauce

In Greek mythology, spelt was a gift from Demeter (goddess of the harvest and fertility), and when you taste this delicious pancake, you'll understand its divine roots. What's more, the combination of flax, grapeseed oil, almond milk, cinnamon, and chopped nuts will help your brain perform at its best.

Serves 2 to 3

For the pancakes

1 flax egg (1 tablespoon flaxseed meal + 2½ tablespoons water)

1 tablespoon EVOO or grapeseed oil

1 teaspoon aluminum-free baking powder

½ teaspoon baking soda

Pinch of sea salt

½ teaspoon ground cinnamon

1 cup plus 1 tablespoon unsweetened plain almond milk, plus more as needed

¼ cup 100% whole-wheat pastry flour

¾ cup spelt flour

2 tablespoons chopped nuts (walnuts or almonds)

For the chia berry sauce

2 cups fresh blueberries, washed

2 cups raspberries, washed

1 cup water

2 tablespoons chia seed

1 cup water

1 teaspoon vanilla extract

1 teaspoon lemon juice

Pinch of salt

2 tablespoons of erythritol or 3 packets of stevia

Begin with the pancakes. In a large mixing bowl, add flaxseed and water and let sit for a minute or two. Then add EVOO, baking powder, baking soda, salt, and cinnamon, and whisk to combine. Add almond milk and whisk again until well combined. Then add whole-wheat flour, spelt flour, and nuts, and stir until just combined. Do not overmix. If the batter seems too thick, add 2 to 3 tablespoons of almond milk to thin. Let batter rest for 10 minutes while you preheat your cooking surface.

Preheat a large skillet to medium heat on the stove top, or an electric griddle to medium heat (or about 325°F). Lightly grease your skillet or griddle with a few drops of oil, or preferably, with a light spray of cooking oil. Pour about-⅓-cup scoops of the batter on the surface and wait for tiny bubbles to appear in the middle. At this point the edges should be dry. Flip pancake to cook the other side.

Then make the chia berry sauce. In a medium saucepan, combine all ingredients except for erythritol or stevia. Bring to a light boil over medium heat, then turn down heat and simmer for 15 minutes. Turn off heat and add the erythritol or stevia. Transfer to a glass container or jar. Serve with the pancakes while warm.

These pancakes can be frozen for up to two weeks and reheated in a toaster or an oven at 350°F.

Black Bean Burger Lettuce Wraps with Chipotle Sauce

A recent study looked at five different populations around the world and concluded that legumes (beans being the healthiest food in this group) may be the most important contributor to longevity. Researchers found an 8 percent reduction in the risk of mortality for every 20 gram increase in legume consumption. This may be the first time a doctor has told you to eat a burger for your health.

Serves 2 to 3

1 tablespoon EVOO
½ large yellow onion, finely diced

2 garlic cloves, smashed and diced

¼ teaspoon each salt and pepper

1 15-ounce can black beans, rinsed and well drained

¾ cup cooked brown rice (substitute cooked quinoa or
     farro for a chewy texture)

1 cup raw beet, shredded

2½ teaspoons ground cumin

1 teaspoon smoked paprika

½ cup walnuts, finely chopped into a meal

1 head iceberg, green leaf, or butter lettuce

Chipotle Sauce (recipe on page 292)

Heat a large skillet over medium-low heat and add some nonstick spray or a bit of EVOO. Then add the onion and garlic and sauté for 10 minutes until soft and fragrant. Season with a pinch each of salt and pepper. Then add black beans and roughly mash with a fork or a potato masher, leaving some texture. Remove from heat and transfer to a bowl. Add the brown rice, beets, spices, walnuts, and stir together. Adjust the taste by adding more paprika or cumin. Allow to cool for 15 minutes before making patties.

Next, preheat the oven to 375°F and grease a baking sheet with some EVOO or a nonstick spray. Make patties from the mixture, either roughly measuring about 2 tablespoons in your hand and shaping into a patty, or using a jar lid lined with plastic wrap for a consistent shape. Make sure the patties are not too thick, as they will take longer to cook, but also not too thin, as they will become very dry. Bake for a total of 30 to 45 minutes, gently flipping at the halfway mark.

To assemble, cut each lettuce leaf at the base and carefully peel away so that it stays as intact as possible. Use 2 or 3 leaves per burger patty. Drizzle Chipotle Sauce and add other toppings of your choice like avocados and onions. Wrap the lettuce around each patty as tightly as possible. Slice in half and serve.

Chipotle Sauce

- 1 cup water
- ½ cup raw almonds
- 1 chipotle pepper in adobo sauce
- 2 tablespoons lemon juice, fresh
- 3 tablespoons nutritional yeast
- 2 garlic cloves

Place all ingredients in a high-powdered blender (like a Vitamix). Slowly blend for one minute. Then blend on high for another 1 to 2 minutes or until smooth and creamy. Store in the refrigerator. Separation of sauce is normal—simply stir before serving.

Brain-Healthy Chocolate Chip Cookies

We use almonds and dark chocolate as the base of this recipe to boost brain health. After all the reading you've been doing, you deserve a cookie!

Serves 24

- 1¼ cups almond meal (ground from raw almonds)
- 1 tablespoon ground flaxseeds
- ¼ cup dairy- and sugar-free dark chocolate (bar or chips), chopped (such as Lily's Dark Chocolate)
- ½ cup finely shredded (desiccated) unsweetened coconut
- ½ teaspoon aluminum-free baking powder
- ¼ teaspoon sea salt
- ¾ cup pitted dates
- ¼ cup aquafaba (liquid in a can of chickpeas, low-sodium or no-salt version)
- 2 tablespoons safflower oil
- 2 tablespoons applesauce
- ½ teaspoon vanilla extract

In a large mixing bowl, stir together almond meal, ground flaxseeds, dark chocolate chips, coconut, baking powder, and salt. Place the dates in hot water, enough to completely submerge them, and soak for 15 minutes. Then drain and place in a small food processor and blend until pureed. In a separate bowl, beat aquafaba (using a handheld mixer or whisking vigorously) until light and fluffy with loose peaks. To the aquafaba, add the oil, pureed dates, applesauce, and vanilla, and beat or whisk to combine. Then add to dry ingredients and mix until just combined. You should now have a firm, semitacky dough. Loosely cover and chill in the refrigerator for at least 30 minutes or overnight. Preheat oven to 375°F. Scoop out 1 to 2 tablespoons of dough or use a small melon scoop to form balls. Press into discs on a parchment-lined baking sheet with 1-inch distance between each cookie to allow for spreading. Bake for 13 to 15 minutes or until edges are golden brown. Be careful not to overcook or burn the bottom. Remove from oven and let cool for 5 to 10 minutes. Transfer to plate with spatula and let cool at room temperature.

Cauliflower Steaks

Let's get one thing straight: these cauliflower steaks are not trying to be real steaks, but only their genuine, flavorful selves. Add the Sweet Potato Mash and Cremini Mushroom Gravy (recipes follow) and this healthy—and delicious—meal will both unclog your arteries and energize your brain cells.

Serves 2

1 head cauliflower

2 tablespoons EVOO, divided

3 garlic cloves, minced

½ teaspoon each salt and pepper

1 sprig fresh thyme, stemmed and chopped

3 sage leaves, chopped

1 teaspoon fresh rosemary, chopped

Fresh ground black pepper

Preheat oven to 400°F. Remove leaves from stem end of cauliflower, leaving the core intact. Place cauliflower core side down on a cutting board. Using a large knife, slice cauliflower into four steaks. Each steak should be approximately a half-inch thick. Place parchment paper on a baking sheet and grease the surface with a teaspoon of EVOO. Arrange the cauliflower steaks on the baking sheet along with any of the broken florets.

In a separate bowl, combine the rest of the EVOO, minced garlic, salt, pepper, and all the herbs. Brush the cauliflower slices generously on both sides with this mixture, making sure the oil and herbs cover all the crevices. Then roast in the oven for 20 minutes. Flip the cauliflower and bake for another 10 minutes until golden brown and cooked through. When the cauliflower steaks are done, remove from oven and transfer onto individual serving plates. Season again with a generous amount of fresh ground black pepper. Serve with mashed Sweet Potato Mash and Cremini Mushroom Gravy.

Sweet Potato Mash

It may be called a sweet potato, but this root vegetable has a very low glycemic index, which means it won't spike your blood sugar levels. Sweet potatoes are the ultimate source of healthy carbohydrates, and when coupled with the monounsaturated fat in extra-virgin olive oil, they make the perfect brain-healthy dish.

Serves 2 to 3

  1 pound or 2 large sweet potatoes, peeled and diced
  ⅓ cup unsweetened almond milk
  ¼ teaspoon sea salt
  1 teaspoon EVOO
  Fresh ground black pepper, to taste
  Fresh thyme sprigs

Fill a medium-size pot with about 2 inches of water and set a steamer basket over the top. Place potato pieces in the basket and bring water to a boil. Cover, reduce heat to medium, and steam until fork tender, about 15 minutes. Optionally, place the sweet potatoes directly in the pot with 1 inch of water, cover, and cook for about 10 to 15 minutes, stirring occasionally to prevent burning. Add more water if potatoes are not fork tender. Once done, turn off the heat, remove water, and transfer the potatoes back into the pot. With a potato masher, mash the sweet potatoes with almond milk, oil, thyme, salt, and pepper. Once mashed and smooth, they're ready to be served.

Cremini Mushroom Gravy

Mushrooms have been part of our diet for thousands of years. Cremini mushrooms are a great source of protein, selenium, antioxidants, copper, and potassium, and are rich in vitamin B12, one of the most important nutrients for the brain.

Makes about 2½ cups

- ¼ cup whole-wheat flour
- 2 cups vegetable broth, preferably Better Than Bullion brand, divided
- 1 tablespoon EVOO
- ½ medium yellow onion, diced small
- 8 ounces or 2½ cups cremini mushrooms, thinly sliced and chopped
- 2 garlic cloves, minced
- 1 teaspoon dried thyme
- 1 teaspoon dried sage
- ¼ teaspoon salt
- Several dashes fresh black pepper
- ¼ cup dry white wine (preferably chardonnay)
- 1 tablespoon nutritional yeast

In a medium-size bowl, whisk the flour with 1 cup of vegetable broth until well dissolved. Then add the remaining 1 cup of broth and mix. Set aside.

Preheat a medium saucepan over medium heat. Add the EVOO and onions, and sauté for about 5 minutes until soft and translucent. Then add the mushrooms, garlic, herbs, salt and pepper, and sauté for about 5 to 7 minutes. Then add the wine and turn up heat to bring to a boil. After 3 minutes of letting the wine reduce, add the broth and flour mixture and the nutritional yeast. Whisk for a minute to prevent lumps from forming. Lower the heat to low-medium and let cook for another 10 to 15 minutes, stirring frequently. Add salt and pepper to taste, and add more nutritional yeast for a savory kick.

Brain-Boosting Caesar Salad with Roasted Chickpea Croutons and Nut Parmesan "Cheese"

We love the briny taste of Caesar salad, but with all the chicken, saturated fat–laden dressing, nutrient-deficient white bread croutons, and artery-clogging cheese, it became off-limits for brain health. But not anymore! This neuron-loving recipe provides greens, beans, nuts, seeds, and poly-unsaturated fats without sacrificing an ounce of flavor.

Serves 6 to 8

For the nut parmesan "cheese"
⅓ cup raw cashews
2 tablespoons sesame seeds
1 tablespoon nutritional yeast
½ teaspoon garlic powder
Fine-grain sea salt, to taste

For the roasted chickpea croutons
1 15-ounce can chickpeas (or 1½ cups cooked), drained and rinsed
1 teaspoon EVOO
½ teaspoon fine-grain sea salt
½ teaspoon garlic powder
⅛ to ¼ teaspoon cayenne pepper (optional)

For the Caesar dressing (makes ¾ to 1 cup)

½ cup raw cashews, soaked overnight

¼ cup water

2 tablespoons EVOO

1 tablespoon lemon juice, plus more to taste

½ tablespoon Dijon mustard

½ teaspoon garlic powder

1 to 2 small garlic cloves (you can add another if you like it superpotent)

½ tablespoon Worcestershire sauce (use a gluten-free brand)

2 teaspoons capers

½ teaspoon each sea salt and pepper, or to taste

For the lettuce

2 heads romaine lettuce, chopped into bite-size pieces,
about 10 cups

1 small bunch of lacinato kale

First, soak the cashews for at least 4 hours, or better yet, overnight. If you're in a rush, pour boiling water over them, cover the container with a lid or plate, and let soak for at least 30 minutes to an hour. Proceed to make the chickpea croutons.

Preheat oven to 400°F. Drain and rinse chickpeas. Transfer them to a bowl and dab with a paper towel to dry. Add the oil, salt, garlic powder, and cayenne, and toss to mix. Transfer them to a baking sheet lined with parchment paper. Roast for 20 minutes, then gently roll the chickpeas around on the baking sheet. Roast for another 10 minutes, until lightly golden. Remove from oven and set aside.

Make the Caesar dressing. Add the cashews and all other dressing ingredients (except salt) into a high-speed blender, and blend on high until very smooth. If the dressing is too thick, add a tablespoon of water to thin. Add salt and lemon to taste.

Make the nut parmesan "cheese." Add the raw cashews to a mini food processor and process until finely chopped. Then add the rest of the ingredients and pulse until the mixture is combined. Salt to taste.

Rinse the romaine lettuce and dry in a salad spinner. Transfer to a large salad bowl. Then wash and destem the kale, and cut into thin ribbons. This is a very important step, as the kale will be chewy if not cut properly. Place into bowl along with romaine.

To assemble the salad, pour the dressing on the lettuce and toss to fully coat. Add the chickpea croutons and the nut parmesan "cheese" on top, along with a dash of black pepper. Serve immediately.

Buddha Brain Bowl with Lemon Tahini Dressing

A buddha bowl is a meal packed with minimally processed foods that are both nutritious and filling. There are numerous variations, but here we've designed a version specifically for nourishing the brain. Feel free to include any other vegetables or grains.

Serves 2 to 3

> 4 large carrots, peeled and cut into 1-inch slices, or lengthwise
>   into 2-inch sticks, depending on the size
> 1½ tablespoons safflower oil, divided into three
> ½ teaspoon each sea salt and pepper
> 1 teaspoon fresh or dried thyme leaves
> 1 large head broccoli, stemmed and florets separated
> 1 15-ounce can cannellini beans
> ¾ teaspoon garlic powder
> ¼ teaspoon each salt and pepper
> ¼ teaspoon turmeric
> ½ teaspoon paprika
> 1 bunch Swiss chard, rough stems discarded,
>   leaves cut into 1-inch strips
> 2 tablespoons water
> 1 tablespoon lemon juice

For the quinoa

1 cup white quinoa, well rinsed and drained

1¾ cups water

Pinch of sea salt

For the lemon tahini dressing

¼ cup tahini

½ lemon, juiced

1 teaspoon erythritol

Pinch of salt

2 to 4 tablespoons hot water to thin

Toppings

¼ cup pumpkin seeds

Preheat the oven to 400°F. Grease a baking sheet large enough to fit all the carrots in a single layer. Place the carrots in a large bowl, and toss with a half tablespoon of safflower oil, salt, pepper, and thyme. Spread in an even layer on the prepared sheet. Cover with foil, and place in the oven for 30 minutes. Place the broccoli in the same bowl you used for the carrots and toss with a half tablespoon of oil, salt and pepper to taste. After 30 minutes, uncover the pan, turn the heat down to 375°F, push the carrots to one half of the sheet, and add the broccoli to the other half of the sheet. Return to the oven uncovered for 10 to 15 more minutes until the vegetables are roasted and tender.

While the carrots are roasting, cook the quinoa. Heat a saucepan over medium-high heat. Once hot, add rinsed quinoa and lightly sauté for 2 minutes before adding water. Then add water and a pinch of salt. Bring to a low boil over medium-high heat. Then reduce heat to a simmer and cover. Cook for 20 minutes or until liquid is absorbed and quinoa is fluffy. Then open lid and fluff the quinoa with a fork. Remove from the heat and set aside.

Heat a large skillet over medium heat and add the cannellini beans and toss with seasonings and spices. Sauté for 5 minutes and remove. Then add the remaining half tablespoon of safflower oil and Swiss chard. Sauté on high heat for a minute, add the water and cover the pan to steam. After

2 minutes, remove the lid and season with a dash of salt and freshly ground pepper. Turn off the heat and remove from stove. Drizzle the lemon juice and toss. Set aside.

Prepare lemon tahini dressing by adding tahini, lemon juice, erythritol, and salt to a mixing bowl and whisking to combine. Add hot water until a pourable sauce is formed. Set aside.

To assemble, choose a bistro bowl or any wide-rimmed bowl. Divide the quinoa, carrots, broccoli, beans, and Swiss chard between the serving bowls. Pour a generous serving of tahini dressing over everything. Top with pumpkin seeds and serve.

Portobello Steaks with Argentinian Chimichurri Sauce

Portobello mushroom is a great source of protein, B vitamins, and minerals, and is famous for its wonderfully chewy texture and savory umami flavor. The accompanying chimichurri sauce is packed with greens and monounsaturated fats, some of the top-rated foods for maintaining cognitive health.

Serves 4

For the portobello mushroom steaks
2 tablespoons EVOO

¼ cup balsamic vinegar

¼ teaspoon smoked paprika

½ teaspoon black pepper

4 garlic cloves, minced

4 large portobello mushroom caps, wiped clean, stems removed

For the chimichurri sauce
1 ripe avocado

2 cups packed fresh flat leaf parsley, washed and dried, finely chopped

4 medium garlic cloves, peeled

2 tablespoons fresh oregano leaves

2 tablespoons EVOO

3 tablespoons lemon juice, or juice of a large lemon

½ teaspoon sea salt

½ teaspoon black pepper and more dashes of freshly ground pepper for serving

¼ teaspoon red pepper flakes (optional)

In a mixing bowl, add the EVOO, balsamic vinegar, paprika, pepper, and the minced garlic cloves and whisk vigorously to mix. Adjust to taste as desired (do not add salt, as it makes the mushrooms soggy). Place the mushrooms in a deep dish stem side (bottom) up and pour the marinade over them. Use a pastry brush to make sure the marinade covers them completely. Marinate for 10 minutes, turning the mushrooms over halfway through.

While the mushrooms are marinating, prepare the chimichurri sauce. Dice the avocado, place in a mixing bowl, and roughly mash with a fork, making sure that some of the pieces are still intact. Place the parsley, garlic, oregano, EVOO, lemon juice, sea salt, pepper, and red pepper flakes in a food processor. Pulse until finely chopped. Alternatively, finely chop the parsley, garlic, and oregano and mix with the other ingredients in a bowl. Add the mixture to the avocado and combine. Set aside at room temperature.

Now prepare the steaks. Heat a large skillet over medium-high heat. Cook mushrooms on each side for about 3 minutes, or until fragrant and a chocolate brown color. During the process, keep brushing the mushroom with any remaining marinade. When done, place on a serving plate, stem side down, and pour the chimichurri sauce on top. As an option, cut the mushrooms into four to five slices and arrange on a plate with room for the chimichurri sauce in the middle. Serve immediately. Try pairing with the Sweet Potato Mash (page 294), or serve the chimichurri sauce with Cauliflower Steaks (page 293).

Mindful Mac and Cheese

Sometimes you just want to chill out with a bowl of mac and cheese. But traditional mac and cheese isn't very healthy, so we took it upon ourselves to reform this favorite dish with brain health in mind. You can prepare this tasty recipe in thirty minutes using basic pantry items. We use cashews for the sauce, which create a dreamy creaminess without an ounce of cream, butter, or milk. Sauerkraut adds the tangy taste of aged cheese, and cannellini beans provide a healthy plant-based protein.

This dish tastes incredible on its own, but you can boost its brain health score by adding sides like steamed broccoli, roasted brussels sprouts, or steamed green beans. We like to add two cups of fresh spinach directly into the pot when we mix the macaroni and sauce.

Serves 3 to 4

1½ cups raw cashews, soaked for 4 hours or overnight

1 pound small pasta made of brown rice, quinoa, or spelt
  (elbow macaroni, shells, or chiocciole)

3½ cups broth, divided (use No Chicken Base, Better Than Bouillon brand)

2 tablespoons EVOO, divided

1 small onion, diced

4 garlic cloves, minced

½ teaspoon salt, plus a pinch

½ teaspoon turmeric

Dash of black pepper

1 cup canned cannellini beans

1 cup canned sauerkraut, well drained

2 tablespoons nutritional yeast (optional)

1 tablespoon lemon juice, fresh

First, soak the cashews for at least 4 hours, or better yet, overnight. If you're in a rush, place them in boiling water, cover the container with a lid or plate, and let soak for at least 30 minutes to an hour. Next, in a large pot, boil water and add a teaspoon of salt. Cook the pasta according to package instructions and drain. While the pasta is cooking, prepare the sauce.

Place the soaked cashews and 2 cups of the vegetable broth in a food processor or a high-speed blender (Vitamix or Blendtec) and blend for 2 to 3 minutes until smooth, scraping the sides of the food processor with a spatula occasionally to make sure everything is properly mixed. Set aside.

In the meantime, preheat a large deep pan or a 6-quart pot over medium heat (you will mix the sauce and pasta in this pot). In a half teaspoon of the oil, sauté the onions, garlic, and a pinch of salt with half a tablespoon of the oil, until onions are softened. Now add the turmeric, salt, black pepper, beans, and sauerkraut for one minute. Once the mixture is heated well, turn off the heat and carefully transfer to the blender with a large spoon or a spatula. Puree the content until smooth and silky. Make sure the texture is not gritty.

Transfer the sauce back into the pan and place over low-medium heat to warm through, stirring regularly. The mixture will thicken a bit. Add the lemon juice, pepper, and nutritional yeast to taste. Add the cooked pasta to the sauce and mix together. Serve immediately.

Blueberry Kamut Salad

Kamut is a high-energy, high-nutrient ancient grain that promotes vascular health. It's easy to digest, and is a great staple for salads and other meals. What's exceptional about this salad is that both blueberries and kamut are high in anti-inflammatory properties.

Serves 2 to 3

For the salad
- ½ cup kamut
- 2 cups water
- 5 ounces mixed salad greens
- ½ cup blueberries
- ½ cup roasted unsalted hazelnuts

For the dressing
  1 tablespoon EVOO
  2 shallots, minced
  ⅓ cup balsamic vinegar
  2 teaspoons erythritol
  ⅓ cup blueberries
  Pinch each of salt and pepper

Prepare kamut by rinsing thoroughly with cool water in a fine mesh strainer. Add to a small saucepan with water and bring to a boil over high heat. Then reduce heat to low and cook for 45 minutes or until soft and chewy. Drain excess water when ready. In the meantime, prepare dressing by heating a small skillet over medium heat. Once hot, add EVOO and shallots, and sauté until tender and slightly caramelized, about 5 minutes, stirring often. Remove from heat to cool. Add sautéed shallots to a food processor or blender with balsamic vinegar, erythritol, blueberries, and a pinch each of salt and pepper. Blend until pureed, scraping down sides as needed. Adjust seasonings to taste.

To plate, top the mixed greens with slightly cooled kamut, blueberries, and hazelnuts. Serve with dressing.

Blueberry Crisp

This scrumptious dessert is completely guilt-free. We all know about the incredible antioxidant properties of blueberries, and the crust is made of nuts high in omega-3s. These powerful ingredients combine to offer you not only a delightful dessert but also nature's best medicine for a healthy brain.

Serves 6 to 8

  5 cups fresh blueberries, or mixed berries (raspberries, blueberries, blackberries, and strawberries; if using strawberries, chop them)
  1 cup rolled oats

½ cup almond meal

½ cup walnuts, finely chopped into almost meal

½ cup dates, soaked in hot water and blended into a puree

½ cup erythritol

½ cup pecans, roughly chopped

¼ teaspoon sea salt

1 teaspoon ground cinnamon

½ cup unsalted almond butter

Preheat oven to 350°F. Place the washed berries in a deep 9 × 13 (or similar size) baking dish. In a bowl, add all topping ingredients. Stir to combine, then use fingers to break apart any clumps. Pour over berries in an even layer. Bake for 45 to 50 minutes (uncovered), or until the filling is bubbly and the topping is deep golden brown. Let rest at least 30 minutes before serving. This dessert tastes best when fresh but can be frozen for up to two weeks. Reheat at 350°F until warmed through.

Wholesome Blueberry Muffins

If you eat just one of these blueberry muffins per day, you'll have your daily recommended intake of fiber, omega fats, and antioxidants.

Serves 12 (makes 12 large muffins)

1 cup unsweetened almond milk

1 tablespoon ground flaxseeds

1 tablespoon apple cider vinegar

2 cups whole-wheat pastry flour

1½ cups wheat bran

2 teaspoons baking powder

¼ teaspoon baking soda

¼ teaspoon salt

½ cup dates, soaked in hot water and blended into a puree

2 tablespoons erythritol or 2 packets stevia

¾ cup unsweetened applesauce

1 teaspoon pure vanilla extract

1 cup blueberries, fresh or frozen

Preheat the oven to 350°F. Line a 12-cup muffin pan with silicone liners or use a nonstick or silicone muffin pan.

In a large measuring cup, use a fork to vigorously mix together the almond milk, flaxseeds, and vinegar. Mix for about a minute, until foamy and curdled. Set aside.

In a medium mixing bowl, sift together the flour, bran, baking powder, baking soda, and salt. Make a well in the center and pour in the milk mixture. Add the dates, erythritol, applesauce, and vanilla to the well and stir together. Incorporate the dry ingredients into the wet ingredients until mixture is just moistened (do not overmix). Fold in the berries.

Fill each muffin cup three-quarters full and bake for 25 minutes, or until a knife inserted through the center of a muffin comes out clean. Let the muffins cool completely, about 20 minutes, then carefully run a knife around the edges of each muffin to remove from the pan.

Chocolate Chia Pudding

In South America, chia seeds were considered so valuable for their nourishing and medicinal qualities that in certain regions they were used as currency. Mayan warriors knew that chia seeds were a fantastic source of energy. In fact, in the Mayan language chia means "strength." Chia seeds offer a rich supply of omega-3s, which provide healthy fat for the brain, as well as copper and zinc, two minerals required for proper functioning of the brain's enzymes. And chocolate? There is so much to say about the cognitive benefits of chocolate that we included it in our top 20 power foods for the brain.

Serves 2 to 3

1½ cups unsweetened almond milk

⅓ cup chia seeds

¼ cup unsweetened cocoa powder or cacao

½ teaspoon ground cinnamon or vanilla extract

¼ teaspoon sea salt

4 dates soaked in hot water and blended into puree, or

    2 to 3 tablespoons of erythritol

Add all ingredients except sweetener to a mixing bowl and whisk vigorously to combine. Then add sweetener to desired taste. Alternatively, you can blend the ingredients for a smooth consistency. Transfer into glass bowls and cover. Place in fridge overnight or for at least 3 to 5 hours. Leftovers keep covered in the fridge for two to three days, though this pudding is best when fresh. Serve chilled and topped with raspberries.

Tomato Bisque

There really is nothing more comforting than a warm cup of creamy tomato soup. The creaminess in this recipe comes from cashews full of brain-fortifying unsaturated fats, vitamin E (a powerful antioxidant), and zinc and copper (minerals needed for many enzymatic reactions in the brain). The other ingredients further boost the power of this soup: onions, carrots, tomatoes, and thyme are great sources of iron, copper, magnesium, and vitamins A and C.

Serves 4

½ cup cashews, soaked for at least 4 hours or overnight

1 tablespoon EVOO

1 medium onion, chopped

1 celery stalk, chopped

1 medium carrot, chopped

4 garlic cloves, chopped or smashed

⅛ teaspoon sea salt

5 cups low-sodium vegetable broth

1 15-ounce can fire-roasted tomatoes

1 15-ounce can diced tomatoes

2 to 3 sprigs of thyme

1 bay leaf

Juice of half a lemon, about 2 teaspoons

Finely chopped parsley for garnish

Soak cashews at least 4 hours before you plan to make the dish, or if short on time, pour boiling water on the cashews and cover the container with a lid for 30 minutes. The longer the cashews are soaked, the creamier they will be.

Place a stockpot over low-medium heat. Add the EVOO and heat for a minute. Add onions, celery, carrots, garlic, and sea salt, and cook for 15 minutes while stirring frequently to prevent burning. Add the broth and cook for 10 minutes, until the mixture starts boiling. Add tomatoes, thyme, and bay leaf. Raise the heat to bring soup to a boil and then reduce heat and simmer for 40 minutes.

Remove the bay leaf and thyme sprigs. Working in batches, transfer the soup into a blender with the soaked cashews (use small batches for a regular blender, covering the lid with a towel to prevent hot liquid from spilling out), and blend on high for 2 to 3 minutes (to make it very smooth). Pour the soup back into the pot and warm. Add the lemon juice and adjust salt and pepper to taste. Ladle into soup bowl. Garnish with parsley.

Roasted Spaghetti Squash with Pasta Sauce and Nut Parmesan "Cheese"

This healthy take on spaghetti uses squash in place of pasta and nut parmesan in place of cheese, resulting in a clot-busting anti-inflammatory meal your whole family will love.

Serves 2 to 3

1 spaghetti squash
1 teaspoon EVOO
Sea salt and pepper, freshly ground
Pasta sauce of choice

Toppings
Parsley
Pumpkin seeds
Nut parmesan "cheese" (page 296)

Preheat the oven to 375°F. If your squash is quite large, start by slicing off the stem. This makes it easier to slice through and also gives you a flat base to work with. You can do this on a cutting board or an old tea towel. Place squash flat end down. With a chef's knife, slice down the middle lengthwise. With a metal ice cream scoop or spoon, scoop out the seeds and guts. Brush halves with a small amount of olive oil (½ teaspoon oil on each). Sprinkle with sea salt and freshly ground black pepper. Place on a baking sheet lined with parchment paper, cut side down. Roast for around 35 to 45 minutes. The outer yellow skin will deepen in color. Remove from oven and flip each half. Use a fork to see if the strands easily come off. When ready, cool for about 5 to 10 minutes and then use the fork to scrape the squash so that if forms spaghetti-like strands. Serve immediately with pasta sauce of your choice. Garnish with parsley, pumpkin seeds, and nut parmesan "cheese."

Roasted Butternut Squash and Brussels Sprouts Salad

Butternut squash is a satisfying sweet vegetable that's rich in fiber, minerals, and vitamins A and C. Here we combine it with extra-virgin olive oil and avocado, two of the healthiest fats for the brain.

Serves 6 to 8

For the roasted butternut squash and brussels sprouts

1 large butternut squash (about 2 to 3 pounds) peeled, seeded, and
   diced (½-inch cubes, 8 to 9 cups chopped)
2 tablespoons EVOO, divided
1 teaspoon each sea salt and pepper, divided into two
2 cups brussels sprouts, washed and sliced in halves

For the salad

1 cup uncooked quinoa
1 large avocado, pitted and chopped
2 tablespoons EVOO, divided
1 tablespoon lemon juice, plus more to taste
1 teaspoon each fine sea salt and freshly ground black pepper, divided
5 cups of mixed salad greens or baby spinach
½ cup walnuts, chopped
¾ cup pomegranate seeds

Preheat the oven to 400°F and line two large baking sheets with parchment paper. Place the chopped squash in a bowl and add 1 tablespoon EVOO and ½ teaspoon each salt and pepper. Toss until well coated and then transfer onto one of the baking sheets. Repeat the process for the brussels sprouts by adding EVOO, salt, and pepper, and transferring onto the other baking sheet. Roast the vegetables until the bottoms are just starting to brown, about 45 to 50 minutes.

Prepare the quinoa. Rinse the quinoa in a fine mesh sieve and transfer to a medium pot. Add 1¾ cups water and bring to a simmer over medium-high heat. Reduce heat to medium, cover with a tight-fitting lid, and cook for 13 to 16 minutes, until the water is absorbed and the quinoa is tender and fluffy. Once cooked, remove from heat. Before serving, fluff quinoa with a fork and season to taste with a generous amount of salt and pepper. Let cool for about 10 minutes before serving.

Chop and slightly mash the avocado in a bowl. In another small bowl, whisk the EVOO, lemon juice, and remaining half teaspoon each of salt and pepper, and set aside.

Assemble the salad by adding the greens to a large bowl. Add the remaining EVOO and lemon dressing. Toss to coat the salad. Then add the avocados and mix. Spoon the quinoa onto the salad greens. Top with roasted squash and brussels sprouts. Garnish with walnuts and pomegranates. Adjust to taste with lemon juice and a few dashes of black pepper. Serve warm.

Zucchini Pasta with Red Lentil Bolognese

Inspired by the traditional meat-based Bolognese of Italy, this plant-based version features red lentils, which are high in protein and an excellent source of fiber (known to reduce the risk of vascular disease in the brain).

Serves 2 to 3

½ tablespoon EVOO

½ small onion, finely chopped

3 to 4 garlic cloves, minced

2 to 3 carrots, finely shredded

⅛ teaspoon sea salt, plus more to taste

1 15-ounce can tomato sauce

1 tablespoon tomato paste

Pinch of red pepper flakes

1 teaspoon dried oregano

1 teaspoon dried basil

½ cup water

¾ cup red lentils, rinsed and drained

2 medium zucchini, rinsed, with ends removed

3 to 5 large basil leaves, cut into thin ribbons

Nut parmesan "cheese" (page 296)

Heat a large, deep, rimmed skillet over medium heat. Add EVOO, onion, and garlic, and sauté for 5 minutes until the onions are soft and translucent. Then add the shredded carrots and salt. Cook for 5 minutes. Add tomato sauce, tomato paste, red pepper flakes, basil, oregano, water, and lentils. Increase heat slightly and bring mixture to a simmer, then reduce heat to low and continue cooking for 20 minutes until lentils are tender. Stir every 3 to 5 minutes to prevent scorching. Add a bit more water if mixture gets too thick.

Once lentils are cooked, taste and adjust seasonings as needed, adding more salt to taste, red pepper flakes for heat, or herbs for flavor balance.

While the sauce is cooking, spiralize your zucchini into noodles using a spiralizer, mandolin, or vegetable peeler. The goal is to make thin strands of zucchini. Place zucchini strands in a pasta bowl with tongs, and ladle generously with the red lentil Bolognese. Garnish with ribbons of basil and nut parmesan "cheese." Serve immediately. Zucchini pasta is very delicate and disintegrates if stored.

Roasted Vegetable Lasagna

Who says lasagna is bad for you? This delicious, gluten-free lasagna is a piece of plant-based art. With the white béchamel sauce, the green pesto, and the red tomato sauce, it evokes an Italian flag and the country's famous flavors, minus the heavy pasta and saturated fats from cheese and cream-based sauce. We roast the vegetables to bring out their full flavor and richness, reduce their natural moisture, and deliver the texture of a typical lasagna. Feel free to use different vegetables like squash, carrots, onions, or bell peppers.

Serves 9

For the tofu ricotta filling

12 ounces extra-firm tofu, drained and pressed dry

Juice of one large lemon

½ teaspoon salt

4 tablespoons nutritional yeast

¾ cup basil leaves

For the pesto

2 cups basil leaves

1 cup raw walnuts

¼ cup nutritional yeast

2 or 3 garlic cloves

¼ cup EVOO

1 teaspoon salt

For the cashew béchamel sauce

1½ cup raw cashews, soaked overnight

¼ cup nutritional yeast

2 garlic cloves

½ teaspoon salt

For the nut parmesan

½ cup macadamia nuts or cashews

3 tablespoons nutritional yeast

⅛ teaspoon salt

¼ teaspoon garlic powder

2 large sweet potatoes (organic if possible), peeled and thinly sliced
    (about ⅛ inch; bendable but not paper-thin)

2 large zucchinis, thinly sliced

2 eggplants, thinly sliced

2 large portobello mushrooms, thinly sliced

EVOO, to taste

Salt and pepper, to taste

Basic tomato sauce, either from a jar or homemade

The day before you prepare this lasagna, cover the cashews for the béchamel sauce with water and soak overnight in a covered bowl in the refrigerator.

For the tofu ricotta filling, add tofu, lemon juice, salt, nutritional yeast, and basil to a food processor or blender and pulse to combine, scraping down sides as needed. You want a semi-pureed mixture with bits of basil still intact. Taste and adjust seasonings as needed.

For the pesto, add basil, walnuts, nutritional yeast, garlic, olive oil, and salt to a food processor and pulse to combine into a semi-pureed mixture with bits of walnuts and basil still intact. Taste and adjust seasonings. We like the intense taste of garlic, but you can pick the flavors you like best. Add 2 to 3 tablespoons of water to thin pesto, if needed.

To make the béchamel sauce, drain the soaked cashews, setting aside the liquid. Add the cashews along with the nutritional yeast, garlic, and salt to a blender or food processor, along with ¼ cup soaking liquid. Puree, adding more soaking liquid a tablespoon at a time until you have a smooth sauce about the consistency of custard (not runny, but thick and spreadable).

To make the nut parmesan, add nuts, nutritional yeast, salt, and garlic powder to a food processor and mix/pulse into a fine meal.

Preheat the oven to 400°F.

Toss the sliced vegetables with the olive oil, salt, and pepper to coat evenly. Spread the coated vegetables onto baking sheets in a single layer (you'll probably need four sheets). Roast the vegetables until they're cooked through and just starting to brown (10 to 15 minutes). Take the baking sheets out of the oven and lower the temperature to 350°F.

To assemble the lasagna, divide the vegetables, tomato sauce, and pesto into four parts each, and divide the tofu ricotta into three parts.

Cover the bottom of a 10-inch dish with a layer of tomato sauce and then place a quarter of the vegetables in a single layer on top of the sauce, overlapping them slightly. Top with a third of the tofu ricotta, spreading with a spatula, and then drizzle a quarter of the pesto over that. Repeat this again with layers of tomato sauce, vegetables, tofu ricotta, and pesto for four total layers. Leave a quarter of the pesto for garnish at the end. The top layer should be vegetables. Spread the béchamel sauce over this top layer, cover with foil, and bake for 30 minutes. After 30 minutes, remove the foil and bake uncovered for another 5 minutes to brown slightly.

Let lasagna cool slightly before serving. Top the entire lasagna with the remaining pesto.

You can adjust the seasonings as needed, adding nutritional yeast for more cheesiness and lemon juice for more brightness.

This lasagna can be frozen for up to three weeks.

Mediterranean Brain Bowl with Roasted Sweet Potatoes and Chickpeas, Turmeric-Infused Quinoa, and Lemon Tahini Herb Sauce

This recipe sounds fancy but is deceptively simple. It's our go-to dish after a long day when the whole family craves an effortless brain-healthy meal.

Serves 2 to 3

1 large sweet potato or two small ones, skinned and
   chopped into 1-inch cubes
1 tablespoon EVOO, divided
1 can chickpeas, drained and rinsed
1 teaspoon turmeric
1 teaspoon coriander
1 teaspoon cumin
½ teaspoon smoked paprika
½ teaspoon garlic powder
½ teaspoon cayenne (optional)
1 cup uncooked quinoa, well rinsed and drained
1¾ cups water
¼ teaspoon turmeric powder
⅛ teaspoon salt
3 cups kale, sliced thinly, seasoned with a teaspoon of
   lemon juice and a pinch of salt

4–6 tablespoons Lemon Tahini Herb Sauce, divided (recipe follows)

2 tablespoons sunflower seeds

Dill leaves, stemmed, for garnish

Preheat oven to 375°F. Line a large baking sheet with parchment paper.

Spread the sweet potato cubes on one half of the baking sheet. Drizzle ½ tablespoon olive oil over the potatoes and toss until coated.

Place the drained and rinsed chickpeas in a bowl, drizzle with ½ tablespoon oil, and sprinkle with smoked paprika, turmeric, coriander, cumin, garlic powder, and cayenne. Toss gently to combine. Transfer to the other half of the baking sheet, spreading the chickpeas in one layer.

Place the sweet potatoes and chickpeas in the preheated oven. Bake for 15 minutes, then remove and gently flip the sweet potatoes and roll the chickpeas (for even cooking). Place back in the oven for another 10 minutes. Roast until the chickpeas are golden and the sweet potatoes are lightly browned and fork tender.

While the potatoes and chickpeas are roasting, cook the quinoa. Thoroughly rinse the quinoa with water in a fine mesh sieve. Heat a saucepan over medium-high heat. Once hot, add the rinsed quinoa and lightly sauté it for about 3 minutes, stirring frequently; this removes excess moisture and brings out the quinoa's nutty flavor. Then add the water, turmeric powder, and salt to the quinoa and bring to a simmer over medium-high heat. Reduce heat to medium, cover with a tight-fitting lid, and cook for 18 to 22 minutes until the water is absorbed and the quinoa is tender and fluffy. Once cooked, remove from heat and fluff the quinoa with a fork.

Place the seasoned kale in a large shallow bowl. Drizzle with 2 to 3 tablespoons Lemon Tahini Herb Sauce. Add a scoop of quinoa and a generous serving of sweet potatoes, and then sprinkle chickpeas on top. Drizzle with another 2 to 3 tablespoons of Lemon Tahini Herb Sauce. Garnish with sunflower seeds and stemmed dill leaves.

Lemon Tahini Herb Sauce

Makes ¾ cup

¼ cup tahini

1 garlic clove, minced

½ lemon, juiced

¼ cup almond milk

2 tablespoons chopped dill

⅛ teaspoon salt, or to taste

Combine all ingredients and serve. The sauce can be stored in the fridge for up to 3 days.

Creamy Sweet Pea Soup

This soup is the ultimate comfort food. The naturally sweet peas and creamy cashews are so satisfying you'll never miss the cream. We like to enjoy it with 100% whole-wheat bread.

Serves 4

½ cup raw cashews, soaked for at least 4 hours (or overnight)

1 tablespoon EVOO

1 medium onion, chopped

1 celery stalk, chopped

1 medium carrot, chopped

4 garlic cloves, chopped or smashed

⅛ teaspoon sea salt

5 cups low-salt vegetable broth

2 cups shelled peas, fresh or frozen

2 or 3 sprigs thyme

1 bay leaf

Juice of half a lemon, about 2 teaspoons

Parsley or chives for garnish, finely chopped

Soak cashews before you make the dish, or if short on time, pour boiling water on the cashews and cover the container with a lid for 30 minutes. The longer the cashews are soaked, the creamier they'll be.

Place a stockpot over low-medium heat. Add the olive oil and heat for 1 minute. Add the onion, celery, carrots, garlic, and sea salt and cook for 15 minutes, stirring frequently to ensure that the vegetables don't burn. Add the vegetable broth, peas, thyme, and bay leaf. Raise the heat and bring soup to a boil; then reduce heat to simmer for 30 to 35 minutes.

Remove the bay leaf and thyme sprigs. Working in batches, transfer the soup to a blender, add soaked cashews, and blend on high for 2 to 3 minutes (to make it very smooth). As you blend, cover the lid with a towel to prevent hot liquid from spilling out. Pour the soup back into the pot and heat through. Add the lemon juice, taste the soup, and adjust salt and pepper as needed. Ladle into soup bowls, and garnish with either parsley or chives.

Turmeric Milk

Also known as golden milk, this is a soothing, nutrient-rich beverage for brain health. It's packed with turmeric, cinnamon, and ginger, all of which repair and rejuvenate the brain, and the erythritol adds a lovely sugar-free sweetness.

Serves 1

    1 cup sugar-free almond milk
    ½ teaspoon turmeric powder
    1 teaspoon cinnamon
    ¼ teaspoon ginger powder
    1 teaspoon erythritol

Heat almond milk in a small saucepan or in a microwave. Stir in turmeric, cinnamon, ginger, and erythritol. Enjoy hot or cold.

Acknowledgments

We are indebted to our grandfathers, whose dedication to public health and education has shaped who we are as physicians and citizens. Both of these remarkable men faced many battles, but none greater than the battle they faced at the end of their lives. Witnessing their courageous fight with dementia was what brought the two of us together and ultimately led us to preventive neurology and community service. In every patient we've seen, in every attempt to understand the origins and causes of this devastating disease, we've glimpsed the struggles of these two great men. They inspired us to write this book. We hope it will make a difference in the lives of many grandfathers, grandmothers, fathers, and mothers.

We thank the many mentors who taught us the art of research and clinical practice, and the wonderful communities in Loma Linda and San Bernardino, most especially our patients, who allowed us to pursue our passion for prevention and made the experience less like a job and more a joyous journey of discovery.

We are extremely grateful for the guidance of Douglas Abrams, our agent and dear friend. His empathic approach and wisdom in every conversation has helped us not only bring this book to life, but has made us better people in the process.

We would like to thank the talented team at HarperOne—especially Gideon Weil and Sydney Rogers—for their steadfast support. A special thanks to the creative TriVision team for their incredible talent in bringing our message to life.

We also want to show our great appreciation for Howard Rankin, who listened to our ideas and helped us shape the framework of this book, and our chief editor, Amy Schleunes, whose amazing ability to hear our voices, see our experiences, and help us tell our story was second to none.

Last but not least we would like to thank our mothers, for providing all of the love and support we needed on this journey, and our children, Alex and Sophie, who endured many nights of writing, whiteboard sessions, and passionate discussions while listening and giving their own feedback.

Notes

You can find a comprehensive list of references on our website at TeamSherzai.com.

INTRODUCTION

Page 2, *In 2016, Alzheimer's disease was the sixth-leading cause of death in the United States*: Alzheimer's Association. (2017). 2017 Alzheimer's disease facts and figures. *Alzheimer's & Dementia, 13*(4), 325–373.

Page 3, *In 2015 alone, caregivers provided an estimated eighteen billion hours of unpaid care*: Wol, J.L., Spillman, B.C., Freedman, V.A., and Kasper, J.D. A national profile of family and unpaid caregivers who assist older adults with health care activities. (2016). *JAMA Internal Medicine, 176*(3), 372–379.

SECTION ONE

Page 9, *In November of 1901, a young German physician*: Cipriani, G., Dolciotti, C., Picchi, L., and Bonuccelli, U. (2011). Alzheimer and his disease: A brief history. *Neurological Sciences, 32*(2), 275–279.

CHAPTER 1. MYTHS AND MISUNDERSTANDINGS

Page 12, *A gene responsible for production of the protein apolipoprotein E*: Liu, C.C., Kanekiyo, T., Xu, H., and Bu, G. (2013). Apolipoprotein E and Alzheimer disease: Risk, mechanisms and therapy. *Nature Reviews Neurology, 9*(2), 106–118.

Page 15, *If you were to look at the brains of people with Alzheimer's*: Heneka, M.T., Carson, M.J., El Khoury, J., Landreth, G.E., Brosseron, F., Feinstein, D.L., Jacobs, A.H., Wyss-Coray, T., Vitorica, J., Ransohoff, R.M., and Herrup, K. (2015). Neuroinflammation in Alzheimer's disease. *The Lancet Neurology, 14*(4), 388–405; Ferreira, S.T., Clarke, J.R., Bomfim, T.R., and De Felice, F.G. (2014). Inflammation, defective insulin signaling, and neuronal dysfunction in Alzheimer's disease. *Alzheimer's & Dementia, 10*(1), S76–S83.

Page 15, *Because the brain works harder than any other organ in the body*: Raichle, M.E., and Gusnard, D.A. (2002). Appraising the brain's energy budget. *Proceedings of the National Academy of Sciences, 99*(16), 10237–10239.

Page 15, *Though the brain has special cells and molecules*: Good, P.F., Werner, P., Hsu, A., Olanow, C.W., and Perl, D.P. (1996). Evidence of neuronal oxidative damage in Alzheimer's disease. *The American Journal of Pathology, 149*(1), 21–28; Scheff, S.W., Ansari, M.A., and Mufson, E.J. (2016). Oxidative stress and hippocampal synaptic protein levels in elderly cognitively intact individuals with Alzheimer's disease pathology. *Neurobiology of Aging, 42*, 1–12; Wang, X., Wang, W., Li, L., Perry, G., Lee, H.G., and Zhu, X. (2014). Oxidative stress and mitochondrial dysfunction in Alzheimer's disease. *Biochimica et Biophysica Acta (BBA)-Molecular Basis of Disease, 1842*(8), 1240–1247.

Page 16, *One dangerous consequence of glucose dysregulation*: Talbot, K., Wang, H.Y., Kazi, H., Han, L.Y., Bakshi, K.P., Stucky, A., Fuino, R.L., Kawaguchi, K.R., Samoyedny, A.J., Wilson, R.S., and Arvanitakis, Z. (2012). Demonstrated brain insulin resistance in Alzheimer's disease patients is associated with IGF-1 resistance, IRS-1 dysregulation, and cognitive decline. *The Journal of Clinical Investigation, 122*(4), 1316–1338; Willette, A.A., Bendlin, B.B., Starks, E.J., Birdsill, A.C., Johnson, S.C., Christian, B.T., Okonkwo, O.C., La Rue, A., Hermann, B.P., Koscik, R.L., and Jonaitis, E.M. (2015). Association of insulin resistance with cerebral glucose uptake in late middle–aged adults at risk for Alzheimer disease. *JAMA Neurology, 72*(9), 1013–1020; Mosconi, L. (2005). Brain glucose metabolism in the early and specific diagnosis of Alzheimer's disease. *European Journal of Nuclear Medicine and Molecular Imaging, 32*(4), 486–510.

Page 16, *Studies have shown that individuals with diabetes*: Barbagallo, M., and Dominguez, L.J. (2014). Type 2 diabetes mellitus and Alzheimer's disease. *World Journal of Diabetes, 5*(6), 889–893.

Page 16, *Lipid dysregulation is the fourth biological process*: Sato, N., and Morishita, R. (2015). The roles of lipid and glucose metabolism in modulation of β-amyloid, tau, and neurodegeneration in the pathogenesis of Alzheimer disease. *Frontiers in Aging Neuroscience, 7*, 199.

Page 17, *APOE4, the most researched gene connected to Alzheimer's*: Huang, Y., and Mahley, R.W. (2014). Apolipoprotein E: structure and function in lipid metabolism, neurobiology, and Alzheimer's diseases. *Neurobiology of Disease, 72*, 3–12; Cutler, R.G., Kelly, J., Storie, K., Pedersen, W.A., Tammara, A., Hatanpaa, K., Troncoso, J.C. and Mattson, M.P. (2004). Involvement of oxidative stress-induced abnormalities in ceramide and cholesterol metabolism in brain aging and Alzheimer's disease. *Proceedings of the National Academy of Sciences, 101*(7), 2070–2075.

Page 21, *To date, more than twenty different genes have been implicated in Alzheimer's*: Karch, C.M., and Goate, A.M. (2015). Alzheimer's disease risk genes and mechanisms of disease pathogenesis. *Biological Psychiatry, 77*(1), 43–51.

Page 21, *APOE4, the most-researched Alzheimer's gene, is responsible*: Michaelson, D.M. (2014). APOE ε4: The most prevalent yet understudied risk factor for Alzheimer's disease. *Alzheimer's & Dementia, 10*(6), 861–868.

Page 22, *For the other 10 percent, those with genes like presenilin 1, presenilin 2*: Bertram, L., Lill, C.M., and Tanzi, R.E. (2010). The genetics of Alzheimer disease: back to the future. *Neuron, 68*(2), 270–281; Robinson, M., Lee, B.Y., and Hane, F.T. (2017). Recent progress in Alzheimer's disease research, Part 2: Genetics and epidemiology. *Journal of Alzheimer's Disease 57*(2), 317–330.

Page 22, *Consider individuals with Down syndrome*: Head, E., Powell, D., Gold, B.T., and Schmitt, F.A. (2012). Alzheimer's disease in Down syndrome. *European Journal of Neurodegenerative Disease, 1*(3), 353–364; Thiel, R., and Fowkes, S.W. (2005). Can cognitive deterioration associated with Down syndrome be reduced? *Medical Hypotheses, 64*(3), 524–532; Zana, M., Janka, Z., and Kálmán, J. (2007). Oxidative stress: A bridge between Down's syndrome and Alzheimer's disease. *Neurobiology of Aging, 28*(5), 648–676.

Page 23, *Researchers at King's College London*: Steves, C.J., Mehta, M.M., Jackson, S.H., and Spector, T.D. (2016). Kicking back cognitive ageing: Leg power predicts cognitive ageing after ten years in older female twins. *Gerontology, 62*(2), 138–149.

Page 24, *Two-thirds of people with Alzheimer's are women*: Mielke, M.M., Vemuri, P., and Rocca, W.A. (2014). Clinical epidemiology of Alzheimer's disease: assessing sex and gender differences. *Journal of Clinical Epidemiology, 6*, 37–48.

Page 24, *This relatively new scientific concept is at the heart of epigenetics*: Chouliaras, L., Rutten, B.P., Kenis, G., Peerbooms, O., Visser, P.J., Verhey, F., van Os, J., Steinbusch, H.W., and van den Hove, D.L. (2010). Epigenetic regulation in the pathophysiology of Alzheimer's disease. *Progress in Neurobiology, 90*(4), 498–510.

Page 25, *Research has shown that our genome actually changes over time*: Nicolia, V., Lucarelli, M., and Fuso, A. (2015). Environment, epigenetics and neurodegeneration: Focus on nutrition in Alzheimer's disease. *Experimental Gerontology, 68*, 8–12; Maloney, B., Sambamurti, K., Zawia, N., and Lahiri, D.K. (2012). Applying epigenetics to Alzheimer's disease via the Latent Early–life Associated Regulation (LEARn) Model. *Current Alzheimer Research, 9*(5), 589–599; Migliore, L., and Coppedè, F. (2009). Genetics, environmental factors and the emerging role of epigenetics in neurodegenerative diseases. *Mutation Research/Fundamental and Molecular Mechanisms of Mutagenesis, 667*(1), 82–97.

Page 26, *The Honolulu-Asian Aging Study found that Japanese people*: White, L., Petrovitch, H., Ross, G.W., Masaki, K.H., Abbott, R.D., Teng, E.L., Rodriguez, B.L., Blanchette, P.L., Havlik, R.J., Wergowske, G., and Chiu, D. (1996). Prevalence of dementia in older Japanese-American men in Hawaii: The Honolulu-Asia aging study. *JAMA, 276*(12), 955–960.

Page 26, *Other studies have shown that in the United States, children of immigrants*: Grant, W.B. (2014). Trends in diet and Alzheimer's disease during the nutrition transition in Japan and developing countries. *Journal of Alzheimer's Disease, 38*(3), 611–620.

Page 26, *When Jeanne Calment turned ninety*: Robine, J.M., and Allard, M. (1999). Jeanne Calment: Validation of the duration of her life. In B. Jeune and J.W. Vaupel (Eds.), *Validation of Exceptional Longevity* (Vol. 6, pp. 145–172). Odense, Denmark: Odense University Press.

Page 27, *Alzheimer's Disease International estimates that China*: Chan, K.Y., Wang, W., Wu, J.J., Liu, L., Theodoratou, E., Car, J., Middleton, L., Russ, T.C., Deary, I.J., Campbell, H., and Rudan, I. (2013). Epidemiology of Alzheimer's disease and other forms of dementia in China, 1990–2010: A systematic review and analysis. *The Lancet, 381*(9882), 2016–2023.

Page 27, *India is experiencing a similar increase in Alzheimer's cases*: Mathuranath, P.S., George, A., Ranjith, N., Justus, S., Kumar, M.S., Menon, R., Sarma, P.S., and Verghese, J. (2012). Incidence of Alzheimer's disease in India: A 10 years follow-up study. *Neurology India, 60*(6), 625–630.

Page 28, *In early childhood, physical and emotional trauma*: Lupien, S.J., McEwen, B.S., Gunnar, M.R., and Heim, C. (2009). Effects of stress throughout the life span on the brain, behaviour and cognition. *Nature Reviews Neuroscience, 10*(6), 434–445; Tyrka, A.R., Price, L.H., Kao, H.T., Porton, B., Marsella, S.A., and

Carpenter, L.L. (2010). Childhood maltreatment and telomere shortening: Preliminary support for an effect of early stress on cellular aging. *Biological Psychiatry, 67*(6), 531–534.

Page 28, *Atherosclerosis (hardening of the arteries that supply oxygen to the body)*: Beauloye, V., Zech, F., Mong, H.T.T. Clapuyt, P., Maes, M., and Brichard, S.M. (2007). Determinants of early atherosclerosis in obese children and adolescents. *The Journal of Clinical Endocrinology & Metabolism, 92*(8), 3025–3032.

Page 28, *A 2013 study in* Radiology *found that repetitive "heading" in soccer*: Lipton, M.L., Kim, N., Zimmerman, M.E., Kim, M., Stewart, W.F., Branch, C.A., and Lipton, R.B. (2013). Soccer heading is associated with white matter microstructural and cognitive abnormalities. *Radiology, 268*(3), 850–857.

Page 28, *In our twenties and thirties, we continue to accumulate*: Barnes, D.E., Kaup, A., Kirby, K.A., Byers, A.L., Diaz-Arrastia, R., and Yaffe, K. (2014). Traumatic brain injury and risk of dementia in older veterans. *Neurology, 83*(4), 312–319; Gardner, R.C., and Yaffe, K. (2014). Traumatic brain injury may increase risk of young onset dementia. *Annals of Neurology, 75*(3), 339; LoBue, C., Denney, D., Hynan, L.S., Rossetti, H.C., Lacritz, L.H., Hart Jr., J., Womack, K.B., Woon, F.L., and Cullum, C.M. (2016). Self-reported traumatic brain injury and mild cognitive impairment: Increased risk and earlier age of diagnosis. *Journal of Alzheimer's Disease, 51*(3), 727–736.

Page 29, *By the time we reach our sixties and seventies*: Bateman, R.J., Xiong, C., Benzinger, T.L., Fagan, A.M., Goate, A., Fox, N.C., Marcus, D.S., Cairns, N.J., Xie, X., Blazey, T.M., and Holtzman, D.M. (2012). Clinical and biomarker changes in dominantly inherited Alzheimer's disease. *New England Journal of Medicine, 367*(9), 795–804.

Page 29, *A recent study published in* Alzheimer's Research & Therapy: Cummings, J.L., Morstorf, T., and Zhong, K. (2014). Alzheimer's disease drug-development pipeline: few candidates, frequent failures. *Alzheimer's Research & Therapy, 6*(4), 37.

Page 31, *Modern medical research is fundamentally misguided*: Tanzi, R.E., and Bertram, L. (2005). Twenty years of the Alzheimer's disease amyloid hypothesis: A genetic perspective. *Cell, 120*(4), 545–555; Drachman, D.A. (2014). The amyloid hypothesis, time to move on: Amyloid is the downstream result, not cause, of Alzheimer's disease. *Alzheimer's & Dementia, 10*(3), 372–380; de la Torre, J.C. (2012). A turning point for Alzheimer's disease? *Biofactors, 38*(2), 78–83.

Page 32, *Alzheimer's drugs are developed and tested on animal models*: Laurijssens, B., Aujard, F., and Rahman, A. (2013). Animal models of Alzheimer's disease and drug development. *Drug Discovery Today: Technologies, 10*(3), e319–e327.

Page 33, *In recent years, Alzheimer's models have progressed to some extent*: Zhang, S., Lv, Z., Zhang, S., Liu, L., Li, Q., Gong, W., Sha, H., and Wu, H. (2017). Characterization of human induced pluripotent stem cell (iPSC) line from a 72-year-old male patient with later onset Alzheimer's disease. *Stem Cell Research, 19*, 34–36; Zhang, W., Jiao, B., Zhou, M., Zhou, T., and Shen, L. (2016). Modeling Alzheimer's disease with induced pluripotent stem cells: Current challenges and future concerns. *Stem Cells International*. doi:10.1155/2016:7828049.

Page 35, *And this is in spite of many researchers who now acknowledge that lifestyle*: de la Torre, J.C. (2010). Alzheimer's disease is incurable but preventable. *Journal of Alzheimer's Disease, 20*(3), 861–870.

Page 36, *Thanks to Dean Ornish's incredible Lifestyle Heart Trial in 1990*: Ornish, D., Brown, S.E., Billings, J.H., Scherwitz, L.W., Armstrong, W.T., Ports, T.A., McLanahan, S.M., Kirkeeide, R.L., Gould, K.L., and Brand, R.J. (1990). Can lifestyle changes reverse coronary heart disease?: The Lifestyle Heart Trial. *The Lancet, 336*(8708), 129–133; Ornish, D., Scherwitz, L.W., Billings, J.H., Gould, K.L., Merritt, T.A., Sparler, S., Armstrong, W.T., Ports, T.A., Kirkeeide, R.L., Hogeboom, C., and Brand, R.J. (1998). Intensive lifestyle changes for reversal of coronary heart disease. *JAMA, 280*(23), 2001–2007.

Page 37, *A landmark study published in the* New England Journal of Medicine: Diabetes Prevention Program Research Group. (2002). Reduction in the incidence of type 2 diabetes with lifestyle intervention or metformin. *New England Journal of Medicine, 2002*(346), 393–403.

Page 37, *A follow-up study conducted four years later*: Ratner, R.E., and Diabetes Prevention Program Research Group, D. (2006). An update on the diabetes prevention program. *Endocrine Practice, 12*(Suppl. 1), 20–24.

CHAPTER 2. THE POWER OF LIFESTYLE MEDICINE

Page 40, *A third of its roughly twenty-five thousand residents*: Butler, T.L., Fraser, G.E., Beeson, W.L., Knutsen, S.F., Herring, R.P., Chan, J., Sabaté, J., Montgomery, S., Haddad, E., Preston-Martin, S., and Bennett, H. (2008). Cohort profile: The Adventist Health Study-2 (AHS-2). *International Journal of Epidemiology, 37*(2), 260–265.

Page 40, *This unusually healthy lifestyle results*: Fraser, G.E., and Shavlik, D.J. (2001). Ten years of life: Is it a matter of choice? *Archives of Internal Medicine, 161*(13), 1645–1652.

Page 41, *A 2007 study found that Adventists who ate a plant-based diet*: Tonstad, S., Butler, T., Yan, R., and Fraser, G.E. (2009). Type of vegetarian diet, body weight, and prevalence of type 2 diabetes. *Diabetes Care, 32*(5), 791–796.

Page 41, *Another study of the Adventist population found that vegetarians*: Tantamango-Bartley, Y., Jaceldo-Siegl, K., Jing, F.A.N., and Fraser, G. (2012). Vegetarian diets and the incidence of cancer in a low-risk population. *Cancer Epidemiology, Biomarkers and Prevention, 22*(2), 286-294.

Page 41, *In a 2003 study published in the* American Journal of Clinical Nutrition: Singh, P.N., Sabaté, J., and Fraser, G.E. (2003). Does low meat consumption increase life expectancy in humans? *The American Journal of Clinical Nutrition, 78*(3), 526S–532S.

Page 41, *A 1993 study titled "The Incidence of Dementia and Intake of Animal Products,"*: Giem, P., Beeson, W.L., and Fraser, G.E. (1993). The incidence of dementia and intake of animal products: Preliminary findings from the Adventist Health Study. *Neuroepidemiology, 12*(1), 28–36.

Page 41, *Numerous other studies have found*: Fraser, G.E., Sabate, J., Beeson, W.L., and Strahan, T.M. (1992). A possible protective effect of nut consumption on risk of coronary heart disease: The Adventist Health Study. *Archives of Internal Medicine, 152*(7), 1416–1424; Fraser, G.E., Beeson, W.L., and Phillips, R.L. (1991). Diet and lung cancer in California Seventh-day Adventists. *American Journal of Epidemiology, 133*(7), 683–693; Mills, P.K., Beeson, W.L., Abbey, D.E., Fraser, G.E., and Phillips, R.L. (1988). Dietary habits and past medical history as related to fatal pancreas cancer risk among Adventists. *Cancer, 61*(12), 2578–2585.

Page 41, *Loma Linda is also America's only "Blue Zone,"*: Buettner, D. (2012). *The Blue Zones: 9 Lessons for Living Longer from the People Who've Lived the Longest.* National Geographic Books.

Page 44, *They'd found gender differences in elderly populations*: Barrett-Connor, E., and Kritz-Silverstein, D. (1999). Gender differences in cognitive function with age: the Rancho Bernardo study. *Journal of the American Geriatrics Society, 47*(2), 159–164; Edelstein, S. L., Kritz-Silverstein, D., and Barrett-Connor, E. (1998). Prospective association of smoking and alcohol use with cognitive function in an elderly cohort. *Journal of Women's Health, 7*(10), 1271–1281.

Page 44, *The Nurse's Health Study and the Health Professional Follow-Up Study*: Joshipura, K.J., Ascherio, A., Manson, J.E., Stampfer, M.J., Rimm, E.B., Speizer, F.E., Hennekens, C.H., Spiegelman, D., and Willett, W.C. (1999). Fruit and vegetable intake in relation to risk of ischemic stroke. *JAMA, 282*(13), 1233–1239.

Page 44, *A separate analysis of the Nurse's Health Study*: Fung, T.T., Rexrode, K.M., Mantzoros, C.S., Manson, J.E., Willett, W.C., and Hu, F.B. (2009). Mediterranean diet and incidence of and mortality from coronary heart disease and stroke in women. *Circulation, 119*(8), 1093–1100.

Page 44, *The Cardiovascular Health Study revealed that obesity*: Fitzpatrick, A.L., Kuller, L.H., Lopez, O.L., Diehr, P., O'Meara, E.S., Longstreth, W.T., and Luchsinger, J.A. (2009). Midlife and late-life obesity and the risk of dementia: Cardiovascular health study. *Archives of Neurology, 66*(3), 336–342.

Page 44, *Scientists at Columbia University*: Luchsinger, J.A., Tang, M.X., Shea, S., and Mayeux, R. (2004). Hyperinsulinemia and risk of Alzheimer disease. *Neurology, 63*(7), 1187–1192.

Page 46, *As we stated earlier, partners of those who develop*: Alzheimer's Association. (2017). 2017 Alzheimer's disease facts and figures. *Alzheimer's & Dementia, 13*(4), 325–373; Norton, M.C., Smith, K.R., Østbye, T., Tschanz, J.T., Corcoran, C., Schwartz, S., Piercy, K.W., Rabins, P.V., Steffens, D.C., Skoog, I., and Breitner, J. (2010). Greater risk of dementia when spouse has dementia? The Cache County study. *Journal of the American Geriatrics Society, 58*(5), 895–900.

Page 46, *Together we did comprehensive reviews of nutrition*: Sherzai, A., Heim, L.T., Boothby, C., and Sherzai, A.D. (2012). Stroke, food groups, and dietary patterns: A systematic review. *Nutrition Reviews, 70*(8), 423–435; Sherzai, A.Z., Tagliati, M., Park, K., Pezeshkian, S., and Sherzai, D. (2016). Micronutrients and risk of Parkinson's disease: A systematic review. *Gerontology and Geriatric Medicine, 2*, doi:10.1177/2333721416644286.

Page 46, *One study by researchers at Columbia University found*: Scarmeas, N., Stern, Y., Tang, M.X., Mayeux, R., and Luchsinger, J.A. (2006). Mediterranean diet and risk for Alzheimer's disease. *Annals of Neurology, 59*(6), 912–921.

Page 47, *The same researchers looked at eating patterns and the risk*: Scarmeas, N., Stern, Y., Mayeux, R., Manly, J.J., Schupf, N., and Luchsinger, J.A. (2009). Mediterranean diet and mild cognitive impairment. *Archives of Neurology, 66*(2), 216–225.

Page 47, *Another study in our comprehensive review found a similar pattern for Parkinson's disease*: Alcalay, R.N., Gu, Y., Mejia-Santana, H., Cote, L., Marder, K.S., and Scarmeas, N. (2012). The association between Mediterranean diet adherence and Parkinson's disease. *Movement Disorders, 27*(6), 771–774.

Page 49, *The Framingham Longitudinal Study, a famous longitudinal study*: Tan, Z.S., Beiser, A.S., Au, R., Kelly-Hayes, M., Vasan, R.S., Auerbach, S., Murabito, J., Pikula, A., Wolf, P.A., and Seshadri, S.S.

(2010). Physical activity and the risk of dementia: The Framingham Study. *Alzheimer's & Dementia, 6*(4), S68.

Page 49, *Chronic stress was shown to decrease the level of brain-derived neurotrophic factor*: Rothman, S.M., and Mattson, M.P. 2010. Adverse stress, hippocampal networks, and Alzheimer's disease. *Neuromolecular Medicine, 12*(1), 56–70.

Page 49, *Researchers at Washington University in St. Louis*: Kang, J.E., Lim, M.M., Bateman, R.J., Lee, J.J., Smyth, L.P., Cirrito, J.R., Fujiki, N., Nishino, S., and Holtzman, D.M. (2009). Amyloid-β dynamics are regulated by orexin and the sleep-wake cycle. *Science, 326*(5955), 1005–1007.

Page 49, *Several studies from the mid-1990s found an inverse relationship*: Stern, Y., Gurland, B., Tatemichi, T.K., Tang, M.X., Wilder, D., and Mayeux, R. (1994). Influence of education and occupation on the incidence of Alzheimer's disease. *JAMA, 271*(13), 1004–1010; Stern, Y., Alexander, G.E., Prohovnik, I., and Mayeux, R. (1992). Inverse relationship between education and parietotemporal perfusion deficit in Alzheimer's disease. *Annals of Neurology, 32*(3), 371–375; Ott, A., Breteler, M.M., Van Harskamp, F., Claus, J.J., Van Der Cammen, T.J., Grobbee, D.E., and Hofman, A. (1995). Prevalence of Alzheimer's disease and vascular dementia: association with education. The Rotterdam study. *British Medical Journal, 310*(6985), 970–973.

Page 49, *We also read a prominent study conducted at Rush University*: Morris, M.C., Tangney, C.C., Wang, Y., Sacks, F.M., Bennett, D.A., and Aggarwal, N.T. (2015). MIND diet associated with reduced incidence of Alzheimer's disease. *Alzheimer's & Dementia, 11*(9), 1007–1014.

Page 49, *She analyzed the California Teachers Study*: Sherzai, A.Z., Ma, H., Horn-Ross, P., Canchola, A.J., Voutsinas, J., Willey, J.Z., Gu, Y., Scarmeas, N., Sherzai, D., Bernstein, L., and Elkind, M.S. (2015). Abstract MP85: Mediterranean Diet and Incidence of Stroke in the California Teachers Study. *Circulation, 131*(Suppl. 1), AMP85.

Page 58, *When you address vascular risk factors like high blood pressure, high cholesterol*: Norton, S., Matthews, F.E., Barnes, D.E., Yaffe, K., and Brayne, C. (2014). Potential for primary prevention of Alzheimer's disease: An analysis of population-based data. *The Lancet Neurology, 13*(8), 788–794.

CHAPTER 3. NUTRITION

Page 86, *In a new study published in 2017, researchers at Columbia University*: Gardener, H., Dong, C., Rundek, T., McLaughlin, C., Cheung, K., Elkind, M., Sacco, R., and Wright, C. (2017). Diet Clusters in Relation to Cognitive Performance and Decline in the Northern Manhattan Study (S15. 003). *Neurology, 88*(16), S15–003.

Page 86, *Research over the years has shown*: Simons, M., Keller, P., Dichgans, J., and Schulz, J.B. (2001). Cholesterol and Alzheimer's disease Is there a link? *Neurology, 57*(6), 1089–1093.

Page 86, *The Chicago Health and Aging Project*: Morris, M.C., Evans, D.A., Bienias, J.L., Tangney, C.C., Bennett, D.A., Aggarwal, N., Schneider, J., and Wilson, R.S. (2003). Dietary fats and the risk of incident Alzheimer's disease. *Archives of Neurology, 60*(2), 194–200.

Page 86, *Scientists looked at nearly 9,900 patients*: Solomon, A., Kivipelto, M., Wolozin, B., Zhou, J., and Whitmer, R.A. (2009). Midlife serum cholesterol and increased risk of Alzheimer's and vascular dementia three decades later. *Dementia and Geriatric Cognitive Disorders, 28*(1), 75–80.

Page 87, *Researchers for the Women's Health Study at Harvard*: Okereke, O.I., Rosner, B.A., Kim, D.H., Kang, J.H., Cook, N.R., Manson, J.E., Buring, J.E., Willett, W.C., and Grodstein, F. (2012). Dietary fat types and 4-year cognitive change in community-dwelling older women. *Annals of Neurology, 72*(1), 124–134.

Page 87, *In one such landmark study published in the* Journal of the American Medical Association *in 2016*: Song, M., Fung, T.T., Hu, F.B., Willett, W.C., Longo, V.D., Chan, A.T., and Giovannucci, E.L. (2016). Association of animal and plant protein intake with all-cause and cause-specific mortality. *JAMA Internal Medicine, 176*(10), 1453–1463.

Page 87, *The Iowa Women's Health Study*: Kelemen, L.E., Kushi, L.H., Jacobs, D.R., and Cerhan, J.R. (2005). Associations of dietary protein with disease and mortality in a prospective study of postmenopausal women. *American Journal of Epidemiology, 161*(3), 239–249.

Page 87, *Additionally, a 2003 study published in* Metabolism: Jenkins, D.J., Kendall, C.W., Marchie, A., Faulkner, D., Vidgen, E., Lapsley, K.G., Trautwein, E.A., Parker, T.L., Josse, R.G., Leiter, L.A., and Connelly, P.W. (2003). The effect of combining plant sterols, soy protein, viscous fibers, and almonds in treating hypercholesterolemia. *Metabolism, 52*(11), 1478–1483.

Page 88, *But plant-based fats, like the mono- and polyunsaturated fats*: Bazinet, R.P., and Layé, S. (2014). Polyunsaturated fatty acids and their metabolites in brain function and disease. *Nature Reviews Neuroscience, 15*(12), 771–785.

Page 88, *Omega-3 fatty acids (found in nuts, seeds, marine algae, and fish)*: Dyall, S.C. (2015). Long-chain omega-3 fatty acids and the brain: A review of the independent and shared effects of EPA, DPA and DHA. *Frontiers in Aging Neuroscience, 7,* 52.

Page 88, *A 2014 study conducted by researchers at UCSF*: Pottala, J.V., Yaffe, K., Robinson, J.G., Espeland, M.A., Wallace, R., and Harris, W.S. (2014). Higher RBC EPA+ DHA corresponds with larger total brain and hippocampal volumes WHIMS-MRI Study. *Neurology, 82*(5), 435–442.

Page 88, *The Framingham Longitudinal Study, the highly regarded longitudinal study*: Tan, Z.S., Harris, W.S., Beiser, A.S., Au, R., Himali, J.J., Debette, S., Pikula, A., DeCarli, C., Wolf, P.A., Vasan, R.S., and Robins, S.J. (2012). Red blood cell omega-3 fatty acid levels and markers of accelerated brain aging. *Neurology, 78*(9), 658–664.

Page 88, *Another randomized controlled trial showed that omega-3s*: Witte, A.V., Kerti, L., Hermannstädter, H.M., Fiebach, J.B., Schreiber, S.J., Schuchardt, J.P., Hahn, A., and Flöel, A. (2013). Long-chain omega-3 fatty acids improve brain function and structure in older adults. *Cerebral Cortex.* doi:10.1093/cercor/bht163.

Page 89, *While it's true that fish are rich in omega-3s, farmed fish and large predatory fish*: Hong, M.Y., Lumibao, J., Mistry, P., Saleh, R., and Hoh, E. (2015). Fish oil contaminated with persistent organic pollutants reduces antioxidant capacity and induces oxidative stress without affecting its capacity to lower lipid concentrations and systemic inflammation in rats. *The Journal of Nutrition, 145*(5), 939–944; Shaw, S.D., Brenner, D., Berger, M.L., Carpenter, D.O., and Kannan, K. (2007). PCBs, PCDD/Fs, and organochlorine pesticides in farmed Atlantic salmon from Maine, Eastern Canada, and Norway, and wild salmon from Alaska. *Environmental Science & Technology, 41*(11), 4180; Wenstrom, K.D. (2014). The FDA's new advice on fish: It's complicated. *American Journal of Obstetrics and Gynecology, 211*(5), 475–478; Gribble, M.O., Karimi, R., Feingold, B.J., Nyland, J.F., O'Hara, T.M., Gladyshev, M.I., and Chen, C.Y. (2016). Mercury, selenium and fish oils in marine food webs and implications for human health. *Journal of the Marine Biological Association of the United Kingdom, 96*(01), 43–59.

Page 90, *Historically, the Paleo diet was consumed*: Turner, B.L., and Thompson, A.L. (2013). Beyond the Paleolithic prescription: Incorporating diversity and flexibility in the study of human diet evolution. *Nutrition Reviews, 71*(8), 501–510; Milton, K. (2000). Back to basics: Why foods of wild primates have relevance for modern human health. *Nutrition, 16*(7), 480–483; Konner, M., and Eaton, S.B. (2010). Paleolithic nutrition twenty-five years later. *Nutrition in Clinical Practice, 25*(6), 594–602.

Page 91, *Several years ago there emerged*: Newport, M.T., VanItallie, T.B., Kashiwaya, Y., King, M.T., and Veech, R.L. (2015). A new way to produce hyperketonemia: Use of ketone ester in a case of Alzheimer's disease. *Alzheimer's & Dementia, 11*(1), 99–103.

Page 91, *Researchers are currently studying the effects of medium-chain fatty acids*: Willett, W.C. (2011). Ask the Doctor. I have started noticing more coconut oil at the grocery store and have heard it is better for you that a lot of other oils. Is that true? *Harvard Health Letter, 36*(7), 7.

Page 92, *The popular misconception is that Eskimos live longer*: Dyerberg, J., Bang, H.O. and Hjorne, N. (1975). Fatty acid composition of the plasma lipids in Greenland Eskimos. *The American Journal of Clinical Nutrition, 28*(9), 958–966.

Page 92, *In the groundbreaking paper published in the* Canadian Journal of Cardiology: Fodor, J.G., Helis, E., Yazdekhasti, N., and Vohnout, B. (2014). "Fishing" for the origins of the "Eskimos and heart disease" story: facts or wishful thinking? *Canadian Journal of Cardiology, 30*(8), 864–868.

Page 92, *Plant-centered diets first captured the attention of the scientific community*: Keys, A., Menotti, A., Aravanis, C., Blackburn, H., Djordević, B.S., Buzina, R., Dontas, A.S., Fidanza, F., Karvonen, M.J., Kimura, N., and Mohaček, I. (1984). The seven countries study: 2,289 deaths in 15 years. *Preventive Medicine, 13*(2), 141–154.

Page 93, *In one study, Columbia University researchers examined*: Scarmeas, N., Luchsinger, J.A., Mayeux, R., and Stern, Y. (2007). Mediterranean diet and Alzheimer disease mortality. *Neurology, 69*(11), 1084–1093; Gu, Y., Luchsinger, J.A., Stern, Y., and Scarmeas, N. (2010). Mediterranean diet, inflammatory and metabolic biomarkers, and risk of Alzheimer's disease. *Journal of Alzheimer's Disease, 22*(2), 483–492.

Page 93, *When the DASH diet was evaluated in a clinical trial*: Wengreen, H., Munger, R.G., Cutler, A., Quach, A., Bowles, A., Corcoran, C., Tschanz, J.T., Norton, M.C., and Welsh-Bohmer, K.A. (2013). Prospective study of dietary approaches to stop hypertension—and Mediterranean-style dietary patterns and age-related cognitive change: The Cache County Study on Memory, Health and Aging. *The American Journal of Clinical Nutrition, 98*(5), 1263–1271.

Page 93, *The MIND diet is a hybrid of the Mediterranean and DASH diets*: Morris, M.C., Tangney, C.C., Wang, Y., Sacks, F.M., Bennett, D.A., and Aggarwal, N.T. (2015). MIND diet associated with reduced incidence of Alzheimer's disease. *Alzheimer's & Dementia, 11*(9), 1007–1014; Morris, M.C.,

Tangney, C.C., Wang, Y., Sacks, F.M., Barnes, L.L., Bennett, D.A., and Aggarwal, N.T. (2015). MIND diet slows cognitive decline with aging. *Alzheimer's & Dementia, 11*(9), 1015–1022; Morris, M.C., Tangney, C.C., Wang, Y., Barnes, L.L., Bennett, D.A., and Aggarwal, N. (2014). MIND diet score more predictive than DASH or Mediterranean diet scores. *Alzheimer's & Dementia: The Journal of the Alzheimer's Association, 10*(4), P166.

Page 94, *One study showed that when people switch from red meat to white meat*: Vergnaud, A.C., Norat, T., Romaguera, D., Mouw, T., May, A.M., Travier, N., Luan, J.A., Wareham, N., Slimani, N., Rinaldi, S., and Couto, E. (2010). Meat consumption and prospective weight change in participants of the EPIC-PANACEA study. *The American Journal of Clinical Nutrition, 92*(2), 398–407.

Page 94, *Poultry, just like red meat, increases your risk for both vascular disease and dementia*: Maki, K.C., Van Elswyk, M.E., Alexander, D.D., Rains, T.M., Sohn, E.L., and McNeill, S. (2012). A meta-analysis of randomized controlled trials that compare the lipid effects of beef versus poultry and/or fish consumption. *Journal of Clinical Lipidology, 6*(4), 352–361.

Page 95, *Beans are high in antioxidants, phytonutrients, plant protein*: Kokubo, Y., Iso, H., Ishihara, J., Okada, K., Inoue, M., and Tsugane, S. (2007). Association of dietary intake of soy, beans, and isoflavones with risk of cerebral and myocardial infarctions in Japanese populations. *Circulation, 116*(22), 2553–2562.

Page 96, *Harvard longitudinal study conducted on 16,000 nurses*: Devore, E.E., Kang, J.H., Breteler, M., and Grodstein, F. (2012). Dietary intakes of berries and flavonoids in relation to cognitive decline. *Annals of Neurology, 72*(1), 135–143.

Page 96, *Rich in lutein and zeaxanthin, carotenoid antioxidants*: Kang, J.H., Ascherio, A., and Grodstein, F. (2005). Fruit and vegetable consumption and cognitive decline in aging women. *Annals of Neurology, 57*(5), 713–720.

Page 96, *The caffeine in coffee is an adenosine receptor antagonist*: Arendash, G.W., and Cao, C. (2010). Caffeine and coffee as therapeutics against Alzheimer's disease. *Journal of Alzheimer's Disease, 20*(S1), 117–126; Liu, Q.P., Wu, Y.F., Cheng, H.Y., Xia, T., Ding, H., Wang, H., Wang, Z.M., and Xu, Y. (2016). Habitual coffee consumption and risk of cognitive decline/dementia: A systematic review and meta-analysis of prospective cohort studies. *Nutrition, 32*(6), 628–636; Sugiyama, K., Tomata, Y., Kaiho, Y., Honkura, K., Sugawara, Y., and Tsuji, I. (2016). Association between coffee consumption and incident risk of disabling dementia in elderly Japanese: The Ohsaki Cohort 2006 Study. *Journal of Alzheimer's Disease, 50*(2), 491–500.

Page 96, *Excellent source of monounsaturated fatty acids*: Berr, C., Portet, F., Carriere, I., Akbaraly, T.N., Feart, C., Gourlet, V., Combe, N., Barberger-Gateau, P. and Ritchie, K. (2009). Olive oil and cognition: results from the three-city study. *Dementia and Geriatric Cognitive Disorders, 28*(4), 357–364.

Page 97, *Nuts provide the highest source of healthy unsaturated fats*: Muthaiyah, B., Essa, M.M., Chauhan, V., and Chauhan, A. (2011). Protective effects of walnut extract against amyloid beta peptide-induced cell death and oxidative stress in PC12 cells. *Neurochemical research, 36*(11), 2096–2103; Poulose, S.M., Miller, M.G., and Shukitt-Hale, B. (2014). Role of walnuts in maintaining brain health with age. *The Journal of Nutrition, 144*(4), 561S–566S. Shytle, R.D., Tan, J., Bickford, P.C., Rezai-Zadeh, K., Hou, L., Zeng, J., Sanberg, P.R., Sanberg, C.D., Alberte, R.S., Fink, R.C., and Roschek, B. Jr. (2012). Optimized turmeric extract reduces β-amyloid and phosphorylated tau protein burden in Alzheimer's transgenic mice. *Current Alzheimer Research, 9*(4), 500–506; Ringman, J.M., Frautschy, S.A., Cole, G.M., Masterman, D.L., and Cummings, J.L. (2005). A potential role of the curry spice curcumin in Alzheimer's disease. *Current Alzheimer Research, 2*(2), 131–136; Shytle, R.D., Bickford, P.C., Rezai-zadeh, K., Hou, L., Zeng, J., Tan, J., Sanberg, P.R., Sanberg, C.D., Roschek, J., Fink, R.C., and Alberte, R.S. (2009). Optimized turmeric extracts have potent anti-amyloidogenic effects. *Current Alzheimer Research, 6*(6), 564–571.

Page 97, *High-powered, plant-based omega-3s*: Eckert, G.P., Franke, C., Nöldner, M., Rau, O., Wurglics, M., Schubert-Zsilavecz, M., and Müller, W.E. (2010). Plant derived omega-3-fatty acids protect mitochondrial function in the brain. *Pharmacological Research, 61*(3), 234–241; Bradbury, J. (2011). Docosahexaenoic acid (DHA): An ancient nutrient for the modern human brain. *Nutrients, 3*(5), 529–554; Valenzuela, R.W., Sanhueza, J., and Valenzuela, A. (2012). Docosahexaenoic acid (DHA), an important fatty acid in aging and the protection of neurodegenerative diseases. *Journal of Nutritional Therapeutics, 1*(1), 63–72; Witte, A.V., Kerti, L., Hermannstädter, H.M., Fiebach, J.B., Schreiber, S.J., Schuchardt, J.P., Hahn, A., and Flöel, A. (2013). Long-chain omega-3 fatty acids improve brain function and structure in older adults. *Cerebral Cortex, 24*(11), 3059–3068.

Page 98, *Green tea contains green tea catechin*: Tomata, Y., Sugiyama, K., Kaiho, Y., Honkura, K., Watanabe, T., Zhang, S., Sugawara, Y., and Tsuji, I., 2016. Green tea consumption and the risk of incident dementia in elderly Japanese: The Ohsaki Cohort 2006 Study. *The American Journal of Geriatric Psychiatry, 24*(10), 881–889.

Page 98, *Packed with cholesterol-lowering fiber, complex carbohydrates, protein*: Flight, I., and Clifton, P. (2006). Cereal grains and legumes in the prevention of coronary heart disease and stroke: A review of the literature. *European Journal of Clinical Nutrition, 60*(10), 1145–1159; McKeown, N.M., Meigs, J.B., Liu, S., Wilson, P.W., and Jacques, P.F. (2002). Whole-grain intake is favorably associated with metabolic risk factors for type 2 diabetes and cardiovascular disease in the Framingham Offspring Study. *The American Journal of Clinical Nutrition, 76*(2), 390–398; Mellen, P.B., Walsh, T.F., and Herrington, D.M. (2008). Whole grain intake and cardiovascular disease: A meta-analysis. *Nutrition, Metabolism and Cardiovascular Diseases, 18*(4), 283–290; Ross, A.B., Bruce, S.J., Blondel-Lubrano, A., Oguey-Araymon, S., Beaumont, M., Bourgeois, A., Nielsen-Moennoz, C., Vigo, M., Fay, L.B., Kochhar, S., and Bibiloni, R. (2011). A whole-grain cereal-rich diet increases plasma betaine, and tends to decrease total and LDL-cholesterol compared with a refined-grain diet in healthy subjects. *British Journal of Nutrition, 105*(10), 1492–1502; Ye, E.Q., Chacko, S.A., Chou, E.L., Kugizaki, M., and Liu, S. (2012). Greater whole-grain intake is associated with lower risk of type 2 diabetes, cardiovascular disease, and weight gain. *The Journal of Nutrition, 142*(7), 1304–1313; Montonen, J., Knekt, P., Järvinen, R., Aromaa, A., and Reunanen, A. (2003). Whole-grain and fiber intake and the incidence of type 2 diabetes. *The American Journal of Clinical Nutrition, 77*(3), 622–629.

Page 103, *The American Heart Association has set the limits for daily added sugar*: Johnson, R.K., Appel, L.J., Brands, M., Howard, B.V., Lefevre, M., Lustig, R.H., Sacks, F., Steffen, L.M., and Wylie-Rosett, J. (2009). Dietary sugars intake and cardiovascular health. *Circulation, 120*(11), 1011–1020; Francis, H.M., and Stevenson, R.J. (2011). Higher reported saturated fat and refined sugar intake is associated with reduced hippocampal-dependent memory and sensitivity to interoceptive signals. *Behavioral Neuroscience, 125*(6), 943; Kanoski, S.E., and Davidson, T.L. (2011). Western diet consumption and cognitive impairment: Links to hippocampal dysfunction and obesity. *Physiology & Behavior, 103*(1), 59–68; Moreira, P.I. (2013). High-sugar diets, type 2 diabetes and Alzheimer's disease. *Current Opinion in Clinical Nutrition & Metabolic Care, 16*(4), 440–445.

Page 108, *A 2017 report on The Framingham Longitudinal Study*: Pase, M.P., Himali, J.J., Jacques, P.F., DeCarli, C., Satizabal, C.L., Aparicio, H., Vasan, R.S., Beiser, A.S., and Seshadri, S. (2017). Sugary beverage intake and preclinical Alzheimer's disease in the community. *Alzheimer's & Dementia.* doi:10.1016/j.jalz.2017.01.024.

Page 108, *Another study published in 2015*: Willette, A.A., Bendlin, B.B., Starks, E.J., Birdsill, A.C., Johnson, S.C., Christian, B.T., Okonkwo, O.C., La Rue, A., Hermann, B.P., Koscik, R.L., and Jonaitis, E.M. (2015). Association of insulin resistance with cerebral glucose uptake in late middle–aged adults at risk for Alzheimer disease. *JAMA Neurology, 72*(9), 1013–1020.

Page 108, *In our own analysis of a large national sample*: Sherzai, A., Yu, J., Talbot, K., Shaheen, M., and Sherzai, D. (2016). Abstract P167: Insulin Resistance and Cognitive Status Among Adults 50 Years and Older: Data from National Health and Nutrition Examination Survey (NHANES). *Circulation, 133*, AP167.

Page 113, *A 2016 study published in the* Neurobiology of Aging: Ronan, L., Alexander-Bloch, A.F., Wagstyl, K., Farooqi, S., Brayne, C., Tyler, L.K., and Fletcher, P.C. (2016). Obesity associated with increased brain age from midlife. *Neurobiology of Aging, 47*, 63–70; Luchsinger, J.A., Tang, M.X., Shea, S., and Mayeux, R. (2002). Caloric intake and the risk of Alzheimer disease. *Archives of Neurology, 59*(8), 1258–1263.

Page 118, *Though proton pump inhibitors improve the gastric function*: Gomm, W., von Holt, K., Thomé, F., Broich, K., Maier, W., Fink, A., Doblhammer, G., and Haenisch, B. (2016). Association of proton pump inhibitors with risk of dementia: a pharmacoepidemiological claims data analysis. *JAMA Neurology, 73*(4), 410–416.

Page 118, *Statins, which lower LDL ("bad") cholesterol*: Daneschvar, H.L., Aronson, M.D., and Smetana, G.W. (2015). Do statins prevent Alzheimer's disease? A narrative review. *European Journal of Internal Medicine, 26*(9), 666–669; Rockwood, K., Kirkland, S., Hogan, D.B., MacKnight, C., Merry, H., Verreault, R., Wolfson, C., and McDowell, I. (2002). Use of lipid-lowering agents, indication bias, and the risk of dementia in community-dwelling elderly people. *Archives of Neurology, 59*(2), 223–227; Liang, T., Li, R., and Cheng, O. (2015). Statins for treating Alzheimer's disease: truly ineffective? *European Neurology, 73*(5-6), 360–366; Zissimopoulos, J.M., Barthold, D., Brinton, R.D., and Joyce, G. (2017). Sex and race differences in the association between statin use and the incidence of Alzheimer disease. *JAMA Neurology, 74*(2), 225–232.

Page 119, *A new study from Iran looked at the effects of drinking fermented yogurt*: Akbari, E., Asemi, Z., Kakhaki, R.D., Bahmani, F., Kouchaki, E., Tamtaji, O.R., Hamidi, G.A., and Salami, M. (2016). Effect of probiotic supplementation on cognitive function and metabolic status in Alzheimer's disease: a randomized, double-blind and controlled trial. *Frontiers in Aging Neuroscience, 10*(8), 256.

Page 119, *Given what we know now, our recommendation is again to focus on whole foods*: Cepeda, M.S., Katz, E.G., and Blacketer, C. (2016). Microbiome-gut-brain axis: Probiotics and their association with depression. *The Journal of Neuropsychiatry and Clinical Neurosciences, 29*(1), 39–44.

Page 120, *Recent studies have found that androgen deprivation therapy*: Khosrow-Khavar, F., Rej, S., Yin, H., Aprikian, A., and Azoulay, L. (2016). Androgen deprivation therapy and the risk of dementia in patients with prostate cancer. *Journal of Clinical Oncology, 35*(2), 201–207.

Page 120, *A 2016 study in* Neuroepidemiology *concluded*: Islam, M.M., Iqbal, U., Walther, B., Atique, S., Dubey, N.K., Nguyen, P.A., Poly, T.N., Masud, J.H.B., Li, Y.C. and Shabbir, S.A. (2016). Benzodiazepine Use and Risk of Dementia in the Elderly Population: A Systematic Review and Meta-Analysis. *Neuroepidemiology, 47*(3–4), 181–191.

CHAPTER 4. EXERCISE

Page 147, *Anything that reduces blood flow*: Querido, J.S., and Sheel, A.W. (2007). Regulation of cerebral blood flow during exercise. *Sports Medicine, 37*(9), 765–782.

Page 147, *Many studies have shown that regular aerobic activity*: Thompson, P.D., Buchner, D., Piña, I.L., Balady, G.J., Williams, M.A., Marcus, B.H., Berra, K., Blair, S.N., Costa, F., Franklin, B., and Fletcher, G.F. (2003). Exercise and physical activity in the prevention and treatment of atherosclerotic cardiovascular disease. *Arteriosclerosis, Thrombosis, and Vascular Biology, 23*(8), e42–e49; Palmefors, H., DuttaRoy, S., Rundqvist, B., and Börjesson, M. (2014). The effect of physical activity or exercise on key biomarkers in atherosclerosis—a systematic review. *Atherosclerosis, 235*(1), 150–161; Chomistek, A.K., Manson, J.E., Stefanick, M.L., Lu, B., Sands-Lincoln, M., Going, S.B., Garcia, L., Allison, M.A., Sims, S.T., LaMonte, M.J., and Johnson, K.C. (2013). Relationship of sedentary behavior and physical activity to incident cardiovascular disease: Results from the Women's Health Initiative. *Journal of the American College of Cardiology, 61*(23), 2346–2354.

Page 147, *A 2010 meta-analysis of fifteen studies*: Sofi, F., Valecchi, D., Bacci, D., Abbate, R., Gensini, G.F., Casini, A., and Macchi, C. (2011). Physical activity and risk of cognitive decline: A meta-analysis of prospective studies. *Journal of Internal Medicine, 269*(1), 107–117.

Page 147, *Researchers at the University of Lisbon*: Frederiksen, K.S., Verdelho, A., Madureira, S., Bäzner, H., O'Brien, J.T., Fazekas, F., Scheltens, P., Schmidt, R., Wallin, A., Wahlund, L.O., and Erkinjunttii, T. (2015). Physical activity in the elderly is associated with improved executive function and processing speed: the LADIS Study. *International Journal of Geriatric Psychiatry, 30*(7), 744–750.

Page 147, *The 2010 Framingham Longitudinal Study*: Tan, Z.S., Beiser, A.S., Au, R., Kelly-Hayes, M., Vasan, R.S., Auerbach, S., Murabito, J., Pikula, A., Wolf, P.A., and Seshadri, S.S. (2010). Physical activity and the risk of dementia: The Framingham Study. *Alzheimer's & Dementia, 6*(4), S68.

Page 147, *In another study at Harvard of more than 18,000 women*: Weuve, J., Kang, J.H., Manson, J.E., Breteler, M.M., Ware, J.H. and Grodstein, F., 2004. Physical activity, including walking, and cognitive function in older women. *JAMA, 292*(12), 1454–1461.

Page 147, *Researchers at the University of Pittsburgh found*: Erickson, K.I., Voss, M.W., Prakash, R.S., Basak, C., Szabo, A., Chaddock, L., Kim, J.S., Heo, S., Alves, H., White, S.M., and Wojcicki, T.R. (2011). Exercise training increases size of hippocampus and improves memory. *Proceedings of the National Academy of Sciences, 108*(7), 3017–3022.

Page 147, *Scientists at Wake Forest University compared*: Baker, L.D. (2016). Exercise and memory decline. *Alzheimer's & Dementia, 12*(7), P220–P221.

Page 148, *High blood pressure in midlife is clearly*: Gottesman, R.F., Schneider, A.L., Albert, M., Alonso, A., Bandeen-Roche, K., Coker, L., Coresh, J., Knopman, D., Power, M.C., Rawlings, A. and Sharrett, A.R. (2014). Midlife hypertension and 20-year cognitive change: the atherosclerosis risk in communities neurocognitive study. *JAMA Neurology, 71*(10), 1218–1227; Kivipelto, M., Helkala, E.L., Laakso, M.P., Hanninen, T., Hallikainen, M., Alhainen, K., Iivonen, S., Mannermaa, A., Tuomilehto, J., Nissinen, A., and Soininen, H. (2002). Apolipoprotein E ε4 allele, elevated midlife total cholesterol level, and high midlife systolic blood pressure are independent risk factors for late-life Alzheimer disease. *Annals of Internal Medicine, 137*(3), 149–155.

Page 149, *This study looked at lifetime recreational activity*: Torres, E.R., Merluzzi, A.P., Zetterberg, H., Blennow, K., Carlsson, C.M., Okonkwo, O.C., Asthana, S., Johnson, S.C., and Bendlin, B.B. (2016). Lifetime recreational physical activity is associated with CSF amyloid in cognitively asymptomatic adults. *Alzheimer's & Dementia, 12*(7), P591–P592.

Page 149, *There is evidence, however, that aerobic exercise can enhance connectivity*: Rajab, A.S., Crane, D.E., Middleton, L.E., Robertson, A.D., Hampson, M., and MacIntosh, B.J. (2014). A single session of exercise increases connectivity in sensorimotor-related brain networks: a resting-state fMRI study in young healthy adults. *Frontiers in Human Neuroscience, 8*, 625.

Page 151, *Aerobic activity has been shown to increase the synthesis of BDNF*: Gómez-Pinilla, F., Ying, Z., Roy, R.R., Molteni, R., and Edgerton, V.R. (2002). Voluntary exercise induces a BDNF-mediated mechanism that promotes neuroplasticity. *Journal of Neurophysiology, 88*(5), 2187–2195; Cotman, C.W., Berchtold, N.C., and Christie, L.A. (2007). Exercise builds brain health: Key roles of growth factor cascades and inflammation. *Trends in Neurosciences, 30*(9), 464–472; Huang, T., Larsen, K.T., Ried-Larsen, M., Møller, N.C., and Andersen, L.B. (2014). The effects of physical activity and exercise on brain-derived neurotrophic factor in healthy humans: A review. *Scandinavian Journal of Medicine & Science in Sports, 24*(1), 1–10; de Melo Coelho, F.G., Gobbi, S., Andreatto, C.A.A., Corazza, D.I., Pedroso, R.V., and Santos-Galduróz, R.F. (2013). Physical exercise modulates peripheral levels of brain-derived neurotrophic factor (BDNF): A systematic review of experimental studies in the elderly. *Archives of Gerontology and Geriatrics, 56*(1), 10–15.

Page 151, *Other important factors that promote neuroplasticity*: Maass, A., Düzel, S., Brigadski, T., Goerke, M., Becke, A., Sobieray, U., Neumann, K., Lövdén, M., Lindenberger, U., Bäckman, L., and Braun-Dullaeus, R. (2016). Relationships of peripheral IGF-1, VEGF and BDNF levels to exercise-related changes in memory, hippocampal perfusion and volumes in older adults. *Neuroimage, 131*, 142–154.

Page 151, *In a systematic review and meta-analysis of forty-three studies*: Hammonds, T.L., Gathright, E.C., Goldstein, C.M., Penn, M.S., and Hughes, J.W. (2016). Effects of exercise on c-reactive protein in healthy patients and in patients with heart disease: A meta-analysis. *Heart & Lung: The Journal of Acute and Critical Care, 45*(3), 273–282.

Page 151, *Researchers at UCSF found that people who carry the klotho gene*: Yokoyama, J., Sturm, V., Bonham, L., Klein, E., Arfanakis, K., Yu, L., Coppola, G., Kramer, J., Bennett, D., Miller, B., and Dubal, D.B. (2015). Variation in longevity gene KLOTHO is associated with greater cortical volumes in aging. *Annals of Clinical and Translational Neurology, 2*(3), 215–230.

Page 151, *Other studies show that klotho levels can increase after only twenty minutes*: Matsubara, T., Miyaki, A., Akazawa, N., Choi, Y., Ra, S.G., Tanahashi, K., Kumagai, H., Oikawa, S., and Maeda, S. (2013). Aerobic exercise training increases plasma Klotho levels and reduces arterial stiffness in postmenopausal women. *American Journal of Physiology-Heart and Circulatory Physiology, 306*(3), H348–H355.

Page 152, *Researchers from the University of British Columbia found that twice-weekly*: Bolandzadeh, N., Tam, R., Handy, T.C., Nagamatsu, L.S., Hsu, C.L., Davis, J.C., Dao, E., Beattie, B.L., and Liu-Ambrose, T. (2015). Resistance Training and White Matter Lesion Progression in Older Women: Exploratory Analysis of a 12-Month Randomized Controlled Trial. *Journal of the American Geriatrics Society, 63*(10), 2052–2060; Nagamatsu, L.S., Handy, T.C., Hsu, C.L., Voss, M., and Liu-Ambrose, T. (2012). Resistance training promotes cognitive and functional brain plasticity in seniors with probable mild cognitive impairment. *Archives of Internal Medicine, 172*(8), 666–668.

Page 152, *Researchers at the University of Florida found that adults*: Yarrow, J.F., White, L.J., McCoy, S.C., and Borst, S.E. (2010). Training augments resistance exercise induced elevation of circulating brain derived neurotrophic factor (BDNF). *Neuroscience Letters, 479*(2), 161–165.

Page 152, *In a study at the University of British Columbia*: Liu-Ambrose, T., Nagamatsu, L.S., Voss, M.W., Khan, K.M., and Handy, T.C. (2012). Resistance training and functional plasticity of the aging brain: A 12-month randomized controlled trial. *Neurobiology of Aging, 33*(8), 1690–1698.

Page 153, *Serum homocysteine, which leads to inflammation*: Vincent, K.R., Braith, R.W., Bottiglieri, T., Vincent, H.K., and Lowenthal, D.T. (2003). Homocysteine and lipoprotein levels following resistance training in older adults. *Preventive Cardiology, 6*(4), 197–203.

Page 153, *A study published in the* Journal of the American Geriatric Society: Mavros, Y., Gates, N., Wilson, G.C., Jain, N., Meiklejohn, J., Brodaty, H., Wen, W., Singh, N., Baune, B.T., Suo, C., and Baker, M.K. (2016). Mediation of Cognitive Function Improvements by Strength Gains After Resistance Training in Older Adults with Mild Cognitive Impairment: Outcomes of the Study of Mental and Resistance Training. *Journal of the American Geriatrics Society, 65*(3), 550–559.

Page 153, *Another new study in the* American Journal of Geriatric Psychiatry: Bossers, W.J., van der Woude, L.H., Boersma, F., Hortobágyi, T., Scherder, E.J., and van Heuvelen, M.J. (2015). A 9-week aerobic and strength training program improves cognitive and motor function in patients with dementia: a randomized, controlled trial. *The American Journal of Geriatric Psychiatry, 23*(11), 1106–1116.

Page 155, *A 2016 study from Thailand found*: Sungkarat, S., Boripuntakul, S., Chattipakorn, N., Watcharasaksilp, K., and Lord, S.R. (2016). Effects of tai chi on cognition and fall risk in older adults with mild cognitive impairment: a randomized controlled trial. *Journal of the American Geriatrics Society, 65*(4), 721–727.

Page 155, *Another study from 2012 found that a forty-week tai chi program*: Mortimer, J.A., Ding, D., Borenstein, A.R., DeCarli, C., Guo, Q., Wu, Y., Zhao, Q., and Chu, S. (2012). Changes in brain volume and cognition in a randomized trial of exercise and social interaction in a community-based sample of non-demented Chinese elders. *Journal of Alzheimer's Disease, 30*(4), 757–766.

Page 155, *Additionally, a 2016 study at St. Luke's Hospital*: Del Moral, M.C.O., Dominguez, J.C., and Natividad, B.P. (2016). An observational study on the cognitive effects of ballroom dancing among Filipino elderly with MCI. *Alzheimer's & Dementia, 12*(7), P791.

Page 159, *Not surprisingly, they found that those individuals who spent the most time watching television*: Hoang, T.D., Reis, J., Zhu, N., Jacobs, D.R., Launer, L.J., Whitmer, R.A., Sidney, S. and Yaffe, K. (2016). Effect of early adult patterns of physical activity and television viewing on midlife cognitive function. *JAMA Psychiatry, 73*(1), 73–79.

Page 159, *Another study showed that sedentary behavior*: Klaren, R.E., Hubbard, E.A., Wetter, N.C., Sutton, B.P., and Motl, R.W. (2017). Objectively measured sedentary behavior and brain volumetric measurements in multiple sclerosis. *Neurodegenerative Disease Management, 7*(1), 31–37.

CHAPTER 5. UNWIND

Page 181, *Cortisol has also been linked to shrinkage of the hippocampus*: McLaughlin, K.J., Gomez, J.L., Baran, S.E., and Conrad, C.D. (2007). The effects of chronic stress on hippocampal morphology and function: an evaluation of chronic restraint paradigms. *Brain Research, 1161,* 56–64; Tynan, R.J., Naicker, S., Hinwood, M., Nalivaiko, E., Buller, K.M., Pow, D.V., Day, T.A., and Walker, F.R. (2010). Chronic stress alters the density and morphology of microglia in a subset of stress-responsive brain regions. *Brain, Behavior, and Immunity, 24*(7), 1058–1068.

Page 181, *New evidence indicates that uncontrolled stress and high cortisol levels*: Heim, C., and Binder, E.B. (2012). Current research trends in early life stress and depression: Review of human studies on sensitive periods, gene–environment interactions, and epigenetics. *Experimental Neurology, 233*(1), 102–111.

Page 181, *Uncontrolled stress appears to inhibit the production*: Slavich, G.M., and Irwin, M.R. (2014). From stress to inflammation and major depressive disorder: A social signal transduction theory of depression. *Psychological Bulletin, 140*(3), 774–815.

Page 182, *A study conducted by researchers at McGill University*: Lupien, S.J., de Leon, M., De Santi, S., Convit, A., Tarshish, C., Nair, N.P.V., Thakur, M., McEwen, B.S., Hauger, R.L., and Meaney, M.J. (1998). Cortisol levels during human aging predict hippocampal atrophy and memory deficits. *Nature Neuroscience, 1*(1), 69–73.

Page 183, *Uncontrolled stress has consistently been associated with weight gain*: Torres, S.J., and Nowson, C.A. (2007). Relationship between stress, eating behavior, and obesity. *Nutrition, 23*(11), 887–894.

Page 186, *A 2011 study in the* Proceedings of the National Academy of Sciences: Clapp, W.C., Rubens, M.T., Sabharwal, J., and Gazzaley, A. (2011). Deficit in switching between functional brain networks underlies the impact of multitasking on working memory in older adults. *Proceedings of the National Academy of Sciences, 108*(17), 7212–7217.

Page 186, *A 2014 comprehensive review and meta-analysis*: Goyal, M., Singh, S., Sibinga, E.M., Gould, N.F., Rowland-Seymour, A., Sharma, R., Berger, Z., Sleicher, D., Maron, D.D., Shihab, H.M. and Ranasinghe, P.D. (2014). Meditation programs for psychological stress and well-being: a systematic review and meta-analysis. *JAMA Internal Medicine, 174*(3), 357–368.

Page 186, *In a study conducted at Harvard Massachusetts General Hospital*: Lazar, S.W., Kerr, C.E., Wasserman, R.H., Gray, J.R., Greve, D.N., Treadway, M.T., McGarvey, M., Quinn, B.T., Dusek, J.A., Benson, H., and Rauch, S.L. (2005). Meditation experience is associated with increased cortical thickness. *Neuroreport, 16*(17), 1893–1897.

Page 187, *Another study matched Zen practitioners*: Pagnoni, G., and Cekic, M. (2007). Age effects on gray matter volume and attentional performance in Zen meditation. *Neurobiology of Aging, 28*(10), 1623–1627.

Page 187, *A 2015 study at UCLA showed that meditation*: Kurth, F., Cherbuin, N., and Luders, E. (2015). Reduced age-related degeneration of the hippocampal subiculum in long-term meditators. *Psychiatry Research: Neuroimaging, 232*(3), 214–218.

Page 187, *Researchers at the University of Pittsburgh showed*: Taren, A.A., Creswell, J.D., and Gianaros, P.J. (2013). Dispositional mindfulness co-varies with smaller amygdala and caudate volumes in community adults. *PLoS One, 8*(5), e64574; Taren, A.A., Gianaros, P.J., Greco, C.M., Lindsay, E.K., Fairgrieve, A.,

Brown, K.W., Rosen, R.K., Ferris, J.L., Julson, E., Marsland, A.L., and Bursley, J.K. (2015). Mindfulness meditation training alters stress-related amygdala resting state functional connectivity: A randomized controlled trial. *Social Cognitive and Affective Neuroscience, 10*(12), 1758–1768.

Page 190, *A 2016 review also found that yoga*: Mathersul, D.C., and Rosenbaum, S. (2016). The Roles of Exercise and Yoga in Ameliorating Depression as a Risk Factor for Cognitive Decline. *Evidence-Based Complementary and Alternative Medicine, 2016*, 4612953; Oken, B.S., Zajdel, D., Kishiyama, S., Flegal, K., Dehen, C., Haas, M., Kraemer, D.F., Lawrence, J., and Leyva, J. (2006). Randomized, controlled, six-month trial of yoga in healthy seniors: Effects on cognition and quality of life. *Alternative Therapies in Health and Medicine, 12*(1), 40–47.

Page 191, *A study published in* Frontiers of Psychology *in 2011*: Koelsch, S., Fuermetz, J., Sack, U., Bauer, K., Hohenadel, M., Wiegel, M., Kaisers, U., and Heinke, W. (2011). Effects of music listening on cortisol levels and propofol consumption during spinal anesthesia. *Frontiers in Psychology, 2*, 58.

Page 191, *The Harvard Grant Study has shown over the course of seventy-five years*: Waldinger, R.J., and Schulz, M.S. (2010). What's love got to do with it? Social functioning, perceived health, and daily happiness in married octogenarians. *Psychology and Aging, 25*(2), 422–431.

Page 192, *A 2010 study at Rush University looked at American and Japanese elderly*: Boyle, P.A., Buchman, A.S., Barnes, L.L., and Bennett, D.A. (2010). Effect of a purpose in life on risk of incident Alzheimer disease and mild cognitive impairment in community-dwelling older persons. *Archives of General Psychiatry, 67*(3), 304–310; Kaplin, A., and Anzaldi, L. (2015, May). New movement in neuroscience: A purpose-driven life. *Cerebrum, 7*.

CHAPTER 6. RESTORE

Page 202, *A follow-up study at Harvard showed that residents*: Landrigan, C.P., Rothschild, J.M., Cronin, J.W., Kaushal, R., Burdick, E., Katz, J.T., Lilly, C.M., Stone, P.H., Lockley, S.W., Bates, D.W., and Czeisler, C.A. (2004). Effect of reducing interns' work hours on serious medical errors in intensive care units. *New England Journal of Medicine, 351*(18), 1838–1848.

Page 202, *Sleep was designed especially for the brain*: Diekelmann, S., and Born, J. (2010). The memory function of sleep. *Nature Reviews Neuroscience, 11*(2), 114–126; Smith, C. (1995). Sleep states and memory processes. *Behavioural Brain Research, 69*(1), 137–145.

Page 205, *Studies have shown that long-term night-shift workers*: Rouch, I., Wild, P., Ansiau, D., and Marquié, J.C. (2005). Shiftwork experience, age and cognitive performance. *Ergonomics, 48*(10), 1282–1293.

Page 205, *A 2001 study in* Nature Neuroscience *examined the cognitive performance*: Cho, K. (2001). Chronic "jet lag" produces temporal lobe atrophy and spatial cognitive deficits. *Nature Neuroscience, 4*(6), 567–568; Drummond, S.P., Brown, G.G., Gillin, J.C., Stricker, J.L., Wong, E.C., and Buxton, R.B. (2000). Altered brain response to verbal learning following sleep deprivation. *Nature, 403*(6770), 655–657.

Page 205, *Other studies have found that TNF*: Mullington, J.M., Haack, M., Toth, M., Serrador, J.M., and Meier-Ewert, H.K. (2009). Cardiovascular, inflammatory, and metabolic consequences of sleep deprivation. *Progress in Cardiovascular Diseases, 51*(4), 294–302; Haack, M., Sanchez, E., and Mullington, J.M. (2007). Elevated inflammatory markers in response to prolonged sleep restriction are associated with increased pain experience in healthy volunteers. *Sleep, 30*(9), 1145–1152; Clark, I.A., and Vissel, B. (2014). Inflammation-sleep interface in brain disease: TNF, insulin, orexin. *Journal of Neuroinflammation, 11*(1), 51.

Page 206, *People who sleep nine hours per night usually perform worse*: Ferrie, J.E., Shipley, M.J., Akbaraly, T.N., Marmot, M.G., Kivimaki, M., and Singh-Manoux, A. (2011). Change in sleep duration and cognitive function: findings from the Whitehall II Study. *Sleep, 34*(5), 565–573.

Page 207, *In 2009, researchers at Washington University in St. Louis*: Kang, J.E., Lim, M.M., Bateman, R.J., Lee, J.J., Smyth, L.P., Cirrito, J.R., Fujiki, N., Nishino, S., and Holtzman, D.M. (2009). Amyloid-β dynamics are regulated by orexin and the sleep-wake cycle. *Science, 326*(5955), 1005–1007.

Page 207, *Just four years later, researchers at Oregon Health & Science University*: Xie, L., Kang, H., Xu, Q., Chen, M. J., Liao, Y., Thiyagarajan, M., O'Donnell, J., Christensen, D.J., Nicholson, C., Iliff, J.J., and Takano, T. (2013). Sleep drives metabolite clearance from the adult brain. *Science, 342*(6156), 373–377; Ooms, S., Overeem, S., Besse, K., Rikkert, M.O., Verbeek, M., and Claassen, J.A. (2014). Effect of 1 night of total sleep deprivation on cerebrospinal fluid β-amyloid 42 in healthy middle-aged men: A randomized clinical trial. *JAMA Neurology, 71*(8), 971–977.

Page 208, *One study found that individuals who sleep appropriately spend 11 percent less*: Kapur, V.K., Redline, S., Nieto, F.J., Young, T.B., Newman, A.B., and Henderson, J.A. (2002). The relationship between chronically disrupted sleep and healthcare use. *Sleep, 25*(3), 289–296.

Page 208, *Better sleep leads to fewer colds and immune-related disorders*: Gamaldo, C.E., Shaikh, A.K., and McArthur, J.C. (2012). The sleep-immunity relationship. *Neurologic Clinics, 30*(4), 1313–1343; Bollinger, T., Bollinger, A., Oster, H., and Solbach, W. (2010). Sleep, immunity, and circadian clocks: A mechanistic model. *Gerontology, 56*(6), 574–580.

Page 208, *There is a direct correlation between restorative sleep*: Ford, D.E., and Cooper-Patrick, L. (2001). Sleep disturbances and mood disorders: An epidemiologic perspective. *Depression and Anxiety, 14*(1), 3–6.

Page 208, *One study found that college students*: Brown, F.C., Buboltz Jr., W.C., and Soper, B. (2002). Relationship of sleep hygiene awareness, sleep hygiene practices, and sleep quality in university students. *Behavioral Medicine, 28*(1), 33–38.

Page 208, *A good night's sleep can also help us process emotions*: Mauss, I.B., Troy, A.S., and LeBourgeois, M.K. (2013). Poorer sleep quality is associated with lower emotion-regulation ability in a laboratory paradigm. *Cognition & Emotion, 27*(3), 567–576.

Page 209, *A 2005 review in* Neurology *found*: Durmer, J.S., and Dinges, D.F. (2005, March). Neurocognitive consequences of sleep deprivation. *Seminars in Neurology, 25* (1), 117–129. Copyright © 2005 by Thieme Medical Publishers, Inc., 333 Seventh Avenue, New York, NY 10001, USA.

Page 209, *People who sleep well have better short-term*: Maquet, P. (2001). The role of sleep in learning and memory. *Science, 294*(5544), 1048–1052; Curcio, G., Ferrara, M., and De Gennaro, L. (2006). Sleep loss, learning capacity and academic performance. *Sleep Medicine Reviews, 10*(5), 323–337; Yang, G., Lai, C.S.W., Cichon, J., Ma, L., Li, W., and Gan, W.B. (2014). Sleep promotes branch-specific formation of dendritic spines after learning. *Science, 344*(6188), 1173–1178.

Page 209, *Lack of sleep can blunt our responses to the environment*: Ayalon, R.D., and Friedman, F. (2008). The effect of sleep deprivation on fine motor coordination in obstetrics and gynecology residents. *American Journal of Obstetrics and Gynecology, 199*(5), 576, e1–5.

Page 209, *Better sleepers are less likely to abuse alcohol*: Wallen, G.R., Brooks, M.A.T., Whiting, M.B., Clark, R., Krumlauf, M.M.C., Yang, L., Schwandt, M.L., George, D.T., and Ramchandani, V.A. (2014). The prevalence of sleep disturbance in alcoholics admitted for treatment: A target for chronic disease management. *Family & Community Health, 37*(4), 288–297.

Page 209, *Adults who slept seven to eight hours per night*: Green, M.J., Espie, C.A., Popham, F., Robertson, T., and Benzeval, M. (2017). Insomnia symptoms as a cause of type 2 diabetes Incidence: A 20 year cohort study. *BMC Psychiatry, 17*(1), 94; Bonnet, M.H., Burton, G.G., and Arand, D.L. (2014). Physiological and medical findings in insomnia: Implications for diagnosis and care. *Sleep Medicine Reviews, 18*(2), 111–122.

Page 210, *Lack of quality sleep increases the risk of stroke*: Wu, M.P., Lin, H.J., Weng, S.F., Ho, C.H., Wang, J.J., and Hsu, Y.W. (2014). Insomnia subtypes and the subsequent risks of stroke. *Stroke, 45*(5), 1349–1354.

Page 210, *This benefit was illustrated in a study where forty-three women*: Calhoun, A.H., and Ford, S. (2007). Behavioral sleep modification may revert transformed migraine to episodic migraine. *Headache: The Journal of Head and Face Pain, 47*(8), 1178–1183.

Page 210, *In a thirteen-year study of 500 individuals*: Hasler, G., Buysse, D.J., Klaghofer, R., Gamma, A., Ajdacic, V., Eich, D., Rössler, W., and Angst, J. (2004). The association between short sleep duration and obesity in young adults: a 13-year prospective study. *Sleep, 27*(4), 661–666.

Page 210, *A new study from 2017 revealed that sleep deprivation*: Bellesi, M., de Vivo, L., Chini, M., Gilli, F., Tononi, G., and Cirelli, C. (2017). Sleep Loss Promotes Astrocytic Phagocytosis and Microglial Activation in Mouse Cerebral Cortex. *Journal of Neuroscience, 37*(21), 5263–5273.

Page 213, *Many people taking sleep medication assume*: de Gage, S.B., Bégaud, B., Bazin, F., Verdoux, H., Dartigues, J.F., Pérès, K., Kurth, T., and Pariente, A. (2012). Benzodiazepine use and risk of dementia: Prospective population based study. *British Medical Journal, 345*, e6231.

Page 217, *Research suggests that the lack of oxygen and blood flow to the brain*: Osorio, R.S., Gumb, T., Pirraglia, E., Varga, A.W., Lu, S.E., Lim, J., Wohlleber, M.E., Ducca, E.L., Koushyk, V., Glodzik, L., and Mosconi, L. (2015). Sleep-disordered breathing advances cognitive decline in the elderly. *Neurology, 84*(19), 1964–1971; Lutsey, P.L., Bengtson, L.G., Punjabi, N.M., Shahar, E., Mosley, T.H., Gottesman, R.F., Wruck, L.M., MacLehose, R.F., and Alonso, A. (2016). Obstructive sleep apnea and 15-year cognitive decline: The Atherosclerosis Risk in Communities (ARIC) study. *Sleep, 39*(2), 309–316; Gagnon, K., Baril, A.A., Gagnon, J.F., Fortin, M., Decary, A., Lafond, C., Desautels, A., Montplaisir, J., and Gosselin, N. (2014). Cognitive impairment in obstructive sleep apnea. *Pathologie Biologie, 62*(5), 233–240.

Page 217, *In our own research, published in* Circulation *in 2015*: Sherzai, A.Z., Willey, J.Z., Vega, S., and Sherzai, D. (2015). The Association Between Chronic Obstructive Pulmonary Disease and Cognitive

Status in an Elderly Sample Using the Third National Health and Nutrition Examination Survey. *Circulation, 131*(Suppl. 1), AP125.

Page 217, *In a review and meta-analysis of seven studies published in 2015*: Bubu, O.M., Utuama, O., Umasabor-Bubu, O.Q., and Schwartz, S. (2015). Obstructive sleep apnea and Alzheimer's disease: A systematic review and meta-analytic approach. *Alzheimer's & Dementia, 11*(7), P452.

CHAPTER 7. OPTIMIZE

Page 235, *Cognitive reserve, on the other hand*: Stern, Y. (2002). What is cognitive reserve? Theory and research application of the reserve concept. *Journal of the International Neuropsychological Society, 8*(03), 448–460; Alexander, G.E., Furey, M.L., Grady, C.L., Pietrini, P., Brady, D.R., Mentis, M.J., and Schapiro, M.B. (1997). Association of premorbid intellectual function with cerebral metabolism in Alzheimer's disease: Implications for the cognitive reserve hypothesis. *American Journal of Psychiatry, 154*(2), 165–172; Meng, X., and D'Arcy, C. (2012). Education and dementia in the context of the cognitive reserve hypothesis: A systematic review with meta-analyses and qualitative analyses. *PloS One, 7*(6), e38268; Scarmeas, N., and Stern, Y. (2003). Cognitive reserve and lifestyle. *Journal of Clinical and Experimental Neuropsychology, 25*(5), 625–633; Stern, Y., Albert, S., Tang, M.X., and Tsai, W.Y. (1999). Rate of memory decline in AD is related to education and occupation cognitive reserve? *Neurology, 53*(9), 1942–1942.

Page 236, *In a randomized longitudinal study conducted by the University of Florida*: Edwards, J.D., Xu, H., Clark, D., Ross, L.A., and Unverzagt, F.W. (2016). The ACTIVE study: what we have learned and what is next? Cognitive training reduces incident dementia across ten years. *Alzheimer's & Dementia, 12*(7), 212.

Page 237, *One such study, published in* Neuron *in 2017*: Dresler, M., Shirer, W.R., Konrad, B.N., Müller, N.C., Wagner, I.C., Fernández, G., Czisch, M., and Greicius, M.D. (2017). Mnemonic training reshapes brain networks to support superior memory. *Neuron, 93*(5), 1227–1235.

Page 239, *A 2006 study at University College London identified*: Maguire, E.A., Woollett, K., and Spiers, H.J. (2006). London taxi drivers and bus drivers: A structural MRI and neuropsychological analysis. *Hippocampus, 16*(12), 1091–1101; Woollett, K., Spiers, H.J., and Maguire, E.A. (2009). Talent in the taxi: A model system for exploring expertise. *Philosophical Transactions of the Royal Society B: Biological Sciences, 364*(1522), 1407–1416.

Page 239, *There is evidence that second languages (or early bilingualism)*: Craik, F.I., Bialystok, E., and Freedman, M. (2010). Delaying the onset of Alzheimer disease: Bilingualism as a form of cognitive reserve. *Neurology, 75*(19), 1726–1729.

Page 239, *In 2014, researchers at Ghent University*: Woumans, E., Santens, P., Sieben, A., Versijpt, J., Stevens, M., and Duyck, W. (2015). Bilingualism delays clinical manifestation of Alzheimer's disease. *Bilingualism: Language and Cognition, 18*(03), 568–574.

Page 239, *A 2016 study conducted by the NIH found*: Perani, D., Farsad, M., Ballarini, T., Lubian, F., Malpetti, M., Fracchetti, A., Magnani, G., March, A., and Abutalebi, J. (2017). The impact of bilingualism on brain reserve and metabolic connectivity in Alzheimer's dementia. *Proceedings of the National Academy of Sciences, 114*(7), 1690–1695.

Page 239, *Another study conducted in Spain in 2016*: Estanga, A., Ecay-Torres, M., Ibañez, A., Izagirre, A., Villanua, J., Garcia-Sebastian, M., Gaspar, M.T.I., Otaegui-Arrazola, A., Iriondo, A., Clerigue, M., and Martinez-Lage, P. (2017). Beneficial effect of bilingualism on Alzheimer's disease CSF biomarkers and cognition. *Neurobiology of Aging, 50*, 144–151.

Page 239, *Researchers have found a similar phenomenon in musicians*: Sluming, V., Barrick, T., Howard, M., Cezayirli, E., Mayes, A., and Roberts, N. (2002). Voxel-based morphometry reveals increased gray matter density in Broca's area in male symphony orchestra musicians. *Neuroimage, 17*(3), 1613–1622; Gaser, C., and Schlaug, G. (2003). Gray matter differences between musicians and nonmusicians. *Annals of the New York Academy of Sciences, 999*(1), 514–517.

Page 239, *A study published in the* New England Journal of Medicine *in 2003*: Verghese, J., Lipton, R.B., Katz, M.J., Hall, C.B., Derby, C.A., Kuslansky, G., Ambrose, A.F., Sliwinski, M., and Buschke, H. (2003). Leisure activities and the risk of dementia in the elderly. *New England Journal of Medicine, 2003*(348), 2508–2516.

Page 240, *A study published in 2007 looked at a group of British individuals*: Roe, C.M., Xiong, C., Miller, J.P., and Morris, J.C. (2007). Education and Alzheimer disease without dementia support for the cognitive reserve hypothesis. *Neurology, 68*(3), 223–228; Cobb, J.L., Wolf, P.A., Au, R., White, R., and D'Agostino, R.B. (1995). The effect of education on the incidence of dementia and Alzheimer's disease in the Framingham Study. *Neurology, 45*(9), 1707–1712; Amieva, H., Mokri, H., Le Goff, M., Meillon, C.,

Jacqmin-Gadda, H., Foubert-Samier, A., Orgogozo, J.M., Stern, Y., and Dartigues, J.F. (2014). Compensatory mechanisms in higher-educated subjects with Alzheimer's disease: A study of 20 years of cognitive decline. *Brain, 137*(4), 1167–1175.

Page 240, *And education doesn't have to take place early in life to be protective*: in a 2011 study conducted in Brazil: da Silva, E.M., Farfel, J., Apolinario, D., Magaldi, R., Nitrini, R., and Jacob-Filho, W. (2011). Formal education after 60 years improves cognitive performance. *Alzheimer's & Dementia, 7*(4), S503.

Page 240, *New research from 2016 by scientists at the Wisconsin Alzheimer's Disease Research Center*: Boots, E.A., Schultz, S.A., Oh, J.M., Racine, A.M., Koscik, R.L., Gallagher, C.L., Carlsson, C.M., Rowley, H.A., Bendlin, B.B., Asthana, S., and Sager, M.A. (2016). Occupational complexity, cognitive reserve, and white matter hyperintensities: Findings from the Wisconsin Registry for Alzheimer's Prevention. *Alzheimer's & Dementia, 12*(7), P130.

Page 241, *Another new study at Massachusetts General Hospital*: Sun, F.W., Stepanovic, M.R., Andreano, J., Barrett, L.F., Touroutoglou, A., and Dickerson, B.C. (2016). Youthful brains in older adults: Preserved neuroanatomy in the default mode and salience networks contributes to youthful memory in superaging. *Journal of Neuroscience, 36*(37), 9659–9668.

Page 241, *In a systematic review of virtual reality cognitive training*: Coyle, H., Traynor, V., and Solowij, N. (2015). Computerized and virtual reality cognitive training for individuals at high risk of cognitive decline: systematic review of the literature. *The American Journal of Geriatric Psychiatry, 23*(4), 335–359.

Page 245, *A 2013 study published in the* Journal of the American Medical Association Internal Medicine: Lin, F.R., Metter, E.J., O'Brien, R.J., Resnick, S.M., Zonderman, A.B., and Ferrucci, L. (2011). Hearing loss and incident dementia. *Archives of Neurology, 68*(2), 214–220.

Page 245, *Other studies have found that visual impairment*: Valentijn, S.A., Van Boxtel, M.P., Van Hooren, S.A., Bosma, H., Beckers, H.J., Ponds, R.W., and Jolles, J. (2005). Change in sensory functioning predicts change in cognitive functioning: Results from a 6-year follow-up in the Maastricht Aging Study. *Journal of the American Geriatrics Society, 53*(3), 374–380.

Page 246, *A study conducted in the Netherlands in 2013 found that engaging in music*: Burggraaf, J.L.I., Elffers, T.W., Segeth, F.M., Austie, F.M.C., Plug, M.B., Gademan, M.G.J., Maan, A.C., Man, S., de Muynck, M., Soekkha, T., and Simonsz, A. (2013). Neurocardiological differences between musicians and control subjects. *Netherlands Heart Journal, 21*(4), 183–188; Kunikullaya, K.U., Goturu, J., Muradi, V., Hukkeri, P.A., Kunnavil, R., Doreswamy, V., Prakash, V.S., and Murthy, N.S. (2016). Combination of music with lifestyle modification versus lifestyle modification alone on blood pressure reduction—A randomized controlled trial. *Complementary Therapies in Clinical Practice, 23*, 102–109.

Page 248, *One study found that people who don't engage in social activity*: Holwerda, T.J., van Tilburg, T.G., Deeg, D.J., Schutter, N., Van, R., Dekker, J., Stek, M.L., Beekman, A.T., and Schoevers, R.A. (2016). Impact of loneliness and depression on mortality: results from the Longitudinal Aging Study Amsterdam. *The British Journal of Psychiatry, 209*(2), 127–34.

Page 249, *The Blue Zones all have a strong social dimension*: Poulain, M., Herm, A., and Pes, G. (2013). The Blue Zones: Areas of exceptional longevity around the world. *Vienna Yearbook of Population Research, 11*, 87–108.

Page 249, *The renowned Grant Study at Harvard followed 286 men*: Waldinger, R.J., and Schulz, M.S. (2010). What's love got to do with it? Social functioning, perceived health, and daily happiness in married octogenarians. *Psychology and Aging, 25*(2), 422–431.

Page 249, *The immunologist Esther Sternberg*: Sternberg, E.M. (2001). *The Balance Within: The Science Connecting Health and Emotions.* New York: Macmillan.

Page 249, *One study published in* JAMA Psychiatry: Wilson, R.S., Krueger, K.R., Arnold, S.E., Schneider, J.A., Kelly, J.F., Barnes, L.L., Tang, Y., and Bennett, D.A. (2007). Loneliness and risk of Alzheimer disease. *Archives of General Psychiatry, 64*(2), 234–240.

Page 249, *A 2013 study from the University of New South Wales in Australia*: Lipnicki, D.M., Sachdev, P.S., Crawford, J., Reppermund, S., Kochan, N.A., Trollor, J.N., Draper, B., Slavin, M.J., Kang, K., Lux, O., and Mather, K.A. (2013). Risk factors for late-life cognitive decline and variation with age and sex in the Sydney Memory and Ageing Study. *PloS One, 8*(6), e65841.

Index

Page numbers of illustrations and charts appear in italics.

About the Authors

Drs. Dean and Ayesha Sherzai are highly accomplished neurologists with a longstanding interest in how healthy lifestyles can protect against cognitive decline. Throughout their careers, both physicians have selected universities, fellowships, and research projects that allowed them to study lifestyle factors with some of the field's most accomplished researchers. Additionally, they have many years of experience working directly with patients on how to implement healthy behaviors and make lasting behavioral change. They believe we all have the power to stop many of the most feared neurodegenerative diseases, including Alzheimer's. Their mission is to present the newest scientific data in an accessible way, encouraging healthy habits in families, communities, and organizations worldwide.

Dean Sherzai, M.D., Ph.D., is codirector of the Brain Health and Alzheimer's Prevention Program at Loma Linda University, where he was previously the director of the Memory and Aging Center as well as director of research. During his years at Loma Linda, a Blue Zone community where residents live measurably longer and healthier lives, he was the lead scientist studying the effects of healthy living on cognitive aging. Dean trained in neurology at Georgetown University School of Medicine and completed fellowships in neurodegenerative disease and dementia at the National Institutes of Health and UC–San Diego, where he studied under Dr. Leon Thal, one of the world's most renowned dementia researchers, and Dr. Dilip Jeste, the world's foremost specialist in cognitive aging. He also holds a Ph.D. in health-care leadership with a focus on community health, and a master's in public health from Loma Linda University, where his research focused on the prevention of cognitive decline through lifestyle changes. Dean has won several awards and published numerous scientific papers, including comprehensive reviews on nutrition and neurodegenerative disease and a recent meta-analysis of cognitive training and memory improvement.

Ayesha Sherzai, M.D., is codirector of the Brain Health and Alzheimer's Prevention Program at Loma Linda University, where she leads the

Lifestyle Program for the Prevention of Neurological Diseases. She completed a dual training in preventative medicine and neurology at Loma Linda University, received a master's degree in advanced research methodology from UC–San Diego, and completed a fellowship in lifestyle and vascular brain diseases at Columbia University. She will soon complete a Ph.D. in epidemiology from Loma Linda University, where her dissertation focuses on nutrition and its role in cognitive aging and neurological disease. Ayesha has published more than a dozen scientific papers, and in 2015, she won the American Heart Association's Trudy Bush Fellowship Award for Cardiovascular Disease Research in Women's Health. She is the lead researcher in the landmark study at Loma Linda that investigates the effects of comprehensive lifestyle intervention on individuals at risk for Alzheimer's.

Both of us have dedicated our lives to community, service, and science. It was on an early mission to serve, this one in Afghanistan, that we first met. Our conversation that night in the corner of a crowded room was the beginning of the philosophy we share in this book. Thirteen years, and many fellowships and degrees later, it is our love for each other and our passion for making a difference that motivates us to work day and night, bringing what we learn in the clinic to the greater community. During those thirteen years we also brought two amazing children into the world. Our son, Alex, is a brilliant mathematician and pianist who often helps us frame our questions, and our daughter, Sophia, is a thinker, comedian, and opera singer who adds light and wisdom to every conversation. And we can't forget our beloved dog, Obi Wan Kenobi ("Obi" for short), who recently joined our family and made it complete.

Our mission statement as a family is to help diminish suffering. We hope this book will do just that.